BABIES FOR SALE?

TRANSNATIONAL SURROGACY, HUMAN RIGHTS
AND THE POLITICS OF REPRODUCTION

Edited by Miranda Davies

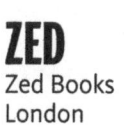

ZED
Zed Books
London

Babies for Sale? Transnational Surrogacy, Human Rights and the Politics of Reproduction
was first published in 2017 by Zed Books Ltd, The Foundry,
17 Oval Way, London SE11 5RR, UK.

www.zedbooks.net

Editorial copyright © Miranda Davies 2017
Copyright in this collection © Zed Books 2017

The right of Miranda Davies to be identified as the editor of this work has been asserted by her in accordance with the Copyright, Designs and Patents Act, 1988.

Typeset in Plantin and Kievit by Swales & Willis Ltd, Exeter, Devon
Index by ed.emery@thefreeuniversity.net
Cover design by www.alice-marwick.co.uk

All rights reserved. No part of this publication may be reproduced, stored in a retrieval system or transmitted in any form or by any means, electronic, mechanical, photocopying or otherwise, without the prior permission of Zed Books Ltd.

A catalogue record for this book is available from the British Library.

ISBN 978-1-78360-702-0 hb
ISBN 978-1-78360-701-3 pb
ISBN 978-1-78360-703-7 pdf
ISBN 978-1-78360-704-4 epub
ISBN 978-1-78360-705-1 mobi

*To dear Sonia
an inspiration!
love Amanda xx*

BABIES FOR SALE?

and from me to Zoë

ABOUT THE EDITOR

Miranda Davies is a writer and editor with a longstanding interest in gender, development and human rights. She has worked for numerous organizations, including Isis International Women's Network, the Central America Committee for Human Rights, Virago, Channel Four, the Rough Guides, Sort Of Books and CoramBAAF Adoption and Fostering Academy, where she is managing editor of *Adoption & Fostering* journal. This is her fourth international anthology for Zed.

CONTENTS

Acknowledgements | viii
Glossary | x
Preface | xiii

Introduction 1
Miranda Davies

PART ONE   RECONSTRUCTING PARENTHOOD

1 Motherhood in fragments: the disaggregation of biology
  and care 19
  Laurel Swerdlow and Wendy Chavkin

2 Constructions of gay men's reproductive desires on commercial
  surrogacy clinic websites 33
  Damien W Riggs and Clemence Due

PART TWO   GLOBAL BABIES: WHO BENEFITS?

3 Transnational surrogacy and the earthquake in Nepal: a
  case study from Israel 49
  Carmel Shalev, Hedva Eyal and Etti Samama

4 Recruiting to give birth: agent-facilitators and the commercial
  surrogacy arrangement in India 65
  Sarojini Nadimpally and Anindita Majumdar

5 Gestational surrogacy: how safe? 82
  Diane Beeson and Abby Lippman

6 The fertility continuum: racism, bio-capitalism and
  post-colonialism in the transnational surrogacy industry 105
  France Winddance Twine

7 Networks of reproduction: politics and practices surrounding
  surrogacy in Romania 123
  Enikő Demény

8 Surrogacy arrangements in austerity Greece: policy considerations in a permissive regime 142
Konstantina Davaki

PART THREE   WHAT ABOUT THE CHILDREN?

9 What are children's 'best interests' in international surrogacy? A social work perspective from the UK 163
Marilyn Crawshaw, Patricia Fronek, Eric Blyth and Andy Elvin

10 What about the children? Citizenship, nationality and the perils of statelessness 185
Marsha Tyson Darling

11 Transnational third-party assisted conception: pursuing the desire for 'origins' information in the internet era 204
Deborah Dempsey and Fiona Kelly

PART FOUR   FEMINIST RESPONSES AROUND THE WORLD

12 Frequently *un*asked questions: understanding and responding to gaps in public knowledge of international surrogacy practices worldwide 221
Ayesha Chatterjee and Sally Whelan (Our Bodies Ourselves)

13 Surrogate motherhood: ethical or commercial? 245
The Centre for Social Research

14 Surrogacy in Mexico 262
Isabel Fulda and Regina Tamés (GIRE)

15 A reproductive justice analysis of genetic technologies: report of a national convening of women of colour and Indigenous women 276
Generations Ahead

16 I donated my eggs and I wouldn't do it again 292
Ari Laurel

17 Swedish feminists against surrogacy 298
Kajsa Ekis Ekman, Linn Hellerström and the Swedish Women's Lobby

PART FIVE   LOOKING AHEAD

18 Mapping feminist views on commercial surrogacy 313
Emma Maniere

19 Transnational commercial surrogacy in India: to ban or
not to ban 328
Amrita Pande

20 Governing transnational surrogacy practices: what role can
national and international regulation play? 344
Sonia Allan

About the authors | 376
Index | 383

ACKNOWLEDGEMENTS

Before I attended the International Forum on Intercountry Adoption and Global Surrogacy in The Hague this book was merely an idea. I am therefore greatly indebted to Kristen Cheney and Karen Smith Rotabi for their vision, energy and superb organizational skills in making it happen.

Among the many experts who also worked so hard to make the Forum such a groundbreaking and inspirational event, I owe a lot to Marcy Darnovsky, for finding space for me in the Global Surrogacy Practices thematic area despite those sessions being so often oversubscribed, and to Marsha Tyson Darling, for giving me the initial confidence to proceed with this project. Marsha not only agreed to contribute early on but introduced me to many of the other Forum participants who came on board. I am also grateful to Deepa Venkatachalam, director of Sama Resource Group for Women and Health, who gave the keynote address on global surrogacy and agreed to commission the chapter on 'agent-facilitators' and recruitment of surrogates in India. Thanks to you all. This book could not have been produced without you.

Closer to home, I'd like to acknowledge the support of Julia Feast and Shaila Shah of CoramBAAF Adoption & Fostering Academy for alerting me to the Forum in the first place. From the early days of *Third World – Second Sex* (Zed Books, 1983), Shaila has witnessed my development as an editor committed to giving voice to women's perspectives around the world. I value her friendship as well as her willingness to offer advice and to share her own considerable editorial skills. For inspiration and encouragement I also owe a huge thank you to another friend and colleague at CoramBAAF, Michelle Bell, who supported this project from the very beginning.

Central to the book's progress has been the input of my dear friend and critical reader, Annabel Hendry. In addition to being an excellent writer and editor, despite being new to the world of transnational commercial surrogacy, she contributed her considerable insights as an anthropologist, trained in the art and science of cross-cultural comparisons, not to mention the importance of empirical research. Without her my task would have been much harder and far less enjoyable.

I'd also like to thank Sonia Allan, who needed to read every chapter in preparation for writing her own, and assured me that I'd got 'a winner'; Jane Cottingham, loyal friend and co-founder of Isis International Women's Network; Hilary Arnold and Natania Jansz, for longstanding friendship and support; and Roger Bullock, commissioning editor of *Adoption & Fostering*, whose encouragement and astonishment that such practices exist helped to reinforce my belief in the importance of the topic.

And last but clearly not least, it would be hard to match the enthusiasm of my daughters, Ella and Lucia Reed, whose strength, humour and faith in my abilities have helped to sustain me along the way.

GLOSSARY

Most of these definitions are taken from the website of the Human Fertilisation and Embryology Authority (HFEA) based in the UK (www.hfea.gov.uk/glossary_c.html).

Amnion   The inner membrane forming the sac in which the embryo develops.

Artificial insemination (AI)   Involves directly inserting sperm into a woman's womb.

Assisted reproductive technologies (ARTs)   The collective term for all techniques used artificially to assist women to carry children, including IVF and ICSI.

Blastocyst   An embryo that has developed for five to six days after fertilization.

Blastocyst transfer   Transfer of an embryo that has developed for five to six days after fertilization.

Cryopreservation   A process where cells, whole tissues or any other substances susceptible to damage caused by chemical reactivity or time are preserved by cooling to sub-zero temperatures.

C-section   An abbreviation of the term 'caesarean section' referring to the delivery of a baby through a surgical incision in the mother's abdomen and uterus.

Donor insemination   The introduction of donor sperm into the vagina, the cervix or the womb itself.

Epigenetic   Heritable changes in gene expression that do not involve changes in the underlying DNA sequence.

Essential thrombocythemia (ET)   A relatively rare disorder in which the body produces too many blood platelets. Since it can cause complications in pregnancy, this is one of the main conditions that potential surrogate mothers are tested for.

Exogenous hormones   Hormones developed or originating outside the organism or body; in other words, artificially induced.

Gamete   The male sperm or female egg which fuse together to form a zygote.

Gestational surrogacy   The most common form of commercial surrogacy, whereby a woman is hired to gestate a fetus grown via embryo transfer and to which she has no genetic tie.

Gonadotropin   Hormones containing follicle-stimulating hormone (FSH), luteinizing hormone (LH) or a combination used to stimulate the ovaries to produce eggs before cycles of IVF treatment. They are delivered through daily injections and can be followed by an injection of human chorionic gonadotrophin (hCG) to trigger the final stage of egg maturation.

Intra-cytoplasmic sperm injection (ICSI)   A technique in which a single sperm is injected into the centre of an egg. The rate of fertilization is usually around 90 per cent.

Intrauterine insemination (IUI)   Process whereby the sperm are placed into the uterus via a plastic tube that is passed through the cervix. More than one treatment is usually needed to achieve pregnancy, sometimes stimulated by progesterone pessaries (or suppositories).

In vitro fertilization (IVF)   IVF treatment involves the fertilization of an egg (or eggs) outside the body. The treatment can be performed using the intended parents' own eggs and sperm or using either donated sperm, donated eggs or both.

Ob-gyn   Physician specializing in medical and surgical care to women who has particular expertise in pregnancy, childbirth and disorders of the reproductive system.

Oocyte   Female gamete (egg).

Ovarian hyperstimulation syndrome (OHSS) The most serious consequence of induction of ovulation as part of assisted conception techniques. It may occur after stimulation of the ovaries into superovulation with drugs such as human chorionic gonadotropin (hCG) and human menopausal gonadotropin.

Paracentesis Procedure whereby fluid from the abdomen is removed through a needle.

Parental Order An order issued by the court to the intended parents of a surrogate child that extinguishes the legal parenthood of the surrogate mother and her partner (if she has one), and reassigns legal parenthood and parental responsibility to the intended parents.

Pre-implantation genetic diagnosis (PGD) Sex selection for non-medical purposes is illegal in the UK but legal in many overseas countries.

Traditional surrogacy Unlike a gestational surrogate, the woman who gives birth has a genetic link to the child she has carried, i.e. using her own eggs.

Zygote The cell formed as a result of fertilization.

PREFACE

Luke and Tony are professionals in their late 30s. After several years together they affirmed their relationship in two civil partnership ceremonies, first in the UK, where Tony was born, and later in Luke's home town of Sydney, where the couple have lived and worked for the past decade.

Not long after celebrating their commitment to one another, the pair began to look into possibilities for starting a family. They had been talking about their shared desire for parenthood for some months and now seemed the right time.

Like most people researching a new venture, especially tech-savvy professionals, their starting point was the internet. With money unlikely to be an obstacle (both are high-earning lawyers), they purchased an online 'egg catalogue' listing the origins, age and mental and physical characteristics of potential 'donors'. Sifting through the range of entries, they decided they would like a baby with what they considered to be 'Swedish' characteristics: 'blonde, blue-eyed, strong and sporty'.

The couple signed up with a surrogacy agency that recommended they opt for an Indian surrogate to carry the baby. Three months down the line and having spent around $3000, for personal reasons they shelved the idea and bought a puppy.

Then came Tony's 40th birthday and the desire for a family resurfaced. Not wishing to delay any further, the couple got in touch with a new agency and had soon committed themselves to using the services of an egg donor in New Zealand and a surrogate in Thailand. The eggs arrived, were fertilized by both men and the resulting embryos swiftly frozen and flown to a small town south of Bangkok. Here, at a designated clinic, the embryos were thawed and implanted into the uterus of the surrogate.

Luke and Tony chatted several times to the donor on Skype and were also in regular contact with the surrogate before and after the pregnancy was confirmed. Two weeks before she was due to give birth, they flew to Thailand and, in March 2013, Grace was born. At the time of writing, she has recently gained a brother using the same egg donor but born from an Indian gestational surrogate in Nepal.

This story was told to me by a friend of the couple and represents my introduction to transnational surrogacy. I was fascinated and, with the men's permission, was able to follow the different stages as their quest for parenthood unfolded (all identifying details have been changed).

To all intents and purposes theirs is a happy story, an illustration of how far some societies have come in terms of sexual equality. But there were many aspects that I found disturbing. I was astonished that a woman's eggs and idealized profile could be listed for sale. Also, how did the Caucasian stereotype described in the 'catalogue' relate to the very different profile of the other, brown woman, thousands of miles away, into whom those eggs, once fertilized, would be implanted? How would she, the so-called surrogate, feel about growing someone else's baby inside her, only for it to be handed over to a third party, the commissioning or intended parents, and never seen again?

I wanted to know how this particular trend in human reproduction had come about and, most importantly, how it affected the individual women hired to provide the body parts – what Swerdlow and Chavkin refer to in the opening chapter of this book as the 'biological bits and processes' – needed to create a child outside the 'natural' process of sexual intercourse. As an editor working in the child-centred field of adoption and fostering, I was also concerned about how the reality and/or knowledge of having developed and been brought into the world via transnational commercial surrogacy might affect the resulting offspring.

I had so many questions: What is driving the rising demand for surrogacy services? Who gains most from this global market in reproduction – and who, if anyone, loses? How far is the market regulated? Can challenging the ethics of gestational commercial surrogacy be reconciled with supporting equality for same-sex partnerships that often include a shared desire for parenthood? What has been the response of health and human rights advocates? How do feminist scholars and activists frame the debate?

I soon learned that academics from the fields of law, medicine, anthropology, philosophy, sociology and others had been questioning, researching and analysing scientific and commercial developments in human reproduction for more than three decades. In fact, the prospect that global expansion could lead to a new 'baby market' involving the exploitation of impoverished women had been seized upon by radical feminists as early as 1985. In the much cited words of Gena Corea (1985: 215):

Once embryo transfer technology is developed, the surrogate industry could look for breeders – not only in poverty-stricken parts of the United States, but in the Third World as well. There, perhaps one tenth of the current fee could be paid women.

From reading the academic literature, I began to understand some aspects of the web of economic, gender, class and racial inequalities that have enabled the explosion of the global infertility trade of which transnational commercial surrogacy has become a key component. I also read blogs from egg donors and intended parents, newspaper and magazine articles (often triggered by scandal) and, most prolific of all, the soft-focus advertising copy of commercial surrogacy agencies promising to 'make your dreams of parenthood come true'.

I started to think about producing a book that would draw together some of these strands, not only through personal stories and academic discourse but also through the views and experiences of feminist organizations in countries such as Israel, India, Greece, Australia, Sweden, Mexico, Romania and the US, who are researching and campaigning in this area – some focusing on greater regulation and/or the abolition of commercial (but not 'altruistic') surrogacy, others like the Swedish Women's Lobby shouting an emphatic 'No' to surrogacy practices in any form.

With this in mind, in August 2014 I attended the International Forum on Intercountry Adoption and Global Surrogacy in The Hague where, among the eighty or so scholars, activists and researchers who took part, I was lucky enough to meet many of the contributors to this volume.

The Forum was initiated and hosted by Kristen Cheney and the International Institute of Social Studies (ISS) of Erasmus University Rotterdam. The main aim of juxtaposing intercountry adoption and global surrogacy was to develop existing policy processes concerning challenges and good practices related to The Hague Convention on Intercountry Adoption, and to consider whether a new convention might be needed to tackle the exploitation of women and the status of children born via transnational surrogacy arrangements, a question addressed by Sonia Allan in the final chapter. But the depth and breadth of discussion went far beyond issues of regulation. This book seeks to capture and develop some of that Forum debate, without which this book might never have seen the light of day.

Miranda Davies
August 2016

INTRODUCTION

Miranda Davies

New family structures, advances in assisted reproductive technologies (ARTs) and the spread of global capitalism have led to unprecedented changes in the ways in which relationships are formed and babies made. Growing public acceptance of gay partnerships and single parenthood, cohabitation and divorce mean that, at least in western societies, the traditional heterosexual unit of a married couple with biological children is no longer the only norm. Add the development of in vitro fertilization (IVF) and egg freezing techniques against a backdrop of rising infertility, and it is not surprising that for journalists, scholars, rights activists, would-be parents and indeed anyone interested in the evolution of humankind in the twenty-first century, the popularity of transnational surrogacy has become something of a 'hot topic'.

A lot of important work on surrogacy has been published over the years spanning many disciplines: e.g. sociology and anthropology (DasGupta and Dasgupta, 2014; Hochschild, 2009; Pande, 2009, 2010, 2014; Ragoné, 1994); psychology (Golombok *et al.*, 2004, 2011; Jadva *et al.*, 2012; van den Akker, 2007); bio-ethics (Macklin, 1994); economics (Spar, 2006); and human rights and the law (Ergas, 2013; Gerber and O'Byrne, 2015; Trimmings and Beaumont, 2013). While this collection is firmly grounded in the literature, it seeks to offer a fresh approach to the complex ethical questions surrounding this increasingly recognized method of procreation. Rather than focusing on any one country or any one aspect of 'outsourcing the womb', it takes a wide-ranging, international and, as far as possible, 'bottom-up' perspective, prioritizing the concerns and experiences of the women, men and children most directly involved. It uses academic discourse but also highlights the work of national feminist organizations such as Sama Resource Group for Women and Health and the Centre for Social Research (CSR) in India, Grupo de Información en Reproducción Elegida (GIRE) in Mexico, Generations Ahead and Our Bodies Ourselves (OBOS) in the US and the Swedish Women's Lobby.

As noted in the Preface, the book's development grew out of my participation in the International Forum on Intercountry Adoption and Global Surrogacy in 2014. This groundbreaking event was led by

Kristen Cheney of the International Institute of Social Studies (ISS) in The Hague and triggered by the work of The Hague Conference on International Private Law (HCCH) in response to the rise of global surrogacy practices. Following two reports analysing issues of parentage in the context of international surrogacy arrangements (HCCH, 2014a, 2014b), Cheney saw an opportunity to gather activists, practitioners and scholars together with the aim of establishing 'an evidence base for international adoption and surrogacy problems and/or best practices' (Cheney, 2014: 2). In addition, as she notes in a later summary of her Forum report (Cheney, 2016: 8), she and other surrogacy experts felt that the HCCH documents had:

> insufficiently emphasised women's rights – their vulnerability to exploitation, lack of independent legal representation and medical, psychological and social implications – while other participants were concerned about the perceived marginalisation of the child in most surrogacy arrangements.

It was a seminal meeting, subsequently summarized in six reports, several of which (notably Cheney, and Darnovsky and Beeson, 2014) are drawn from in the following pages.[1]

When I invited some of the leading scholars and activists writing and campaigning around transnational surrogacy to contribute to this book, I asked them to try to ground their chapters in practices related to their own countries. So, writing from Israel, Hedva Eyal, Etti Samana and Carmel Shalev discuss the fallout from the Nepalese earthquake of April 2015 when pregnant Indian surrogates, intended parents from Israel and babies found themselves stranded in Kathmandu (Chapter 3). Enikő Demény looks at the politics and practices surrounding surrogacy in Romania, a nation still adapting to changes since the collapse of socialism in the aftermath of the 1989 revolution (Chapter 7). Isabel Fulde and Regina Tamés from GIRE, a Mexican NGO that has been campaigning for women's reproductive rights since 1991, explore how a largely unregulated landscape opened the way for a steady increase in surrogacy services in parts of their country (Chapter 14). Sally Whelan and Ayesha Chatterjee from OBOS write about their current project: in collaboration with the Center for Genetics and Society and partners in Asia, Africa, Latin America, Europe and the Middle East, this long-established feminist NGO is using surveys to collect information and raise public awareness of surrogacy practices among the wider population (Chapter 12).

What unites these and other contributors from India, the US, Australia, Greece, Sweden and the UK is a commitment to exposing some of the human implications of allowing new reproductive technologies, and specifically transnational commercial contract pregnancy, to become part of a billion-dollar industry that often places financial interests above the health and welfare of people. Consequently, the role of surrogates is primarily explored in the context of socio-economic deprivation and/or inadequate regulation, not only in the global south but also in European countries such as Greece and Romania, whose economies are weak and where wages are often cripplingly low. Although several authors come from the US, relatively little attention is paid to the specific surrogacy practices that currently thrive in a minority of US states, most notably California, where commercial arrangements are common and highly regulated, and clinics tend to recruit surrogates from middle-income families such as military wives (Howard, 2015; Twine, 2015: 1–2). Rather they look at the wider picture, such as the historical links between racism, bio-capitalism and fertility regulation discussed by France Winddance Twine (Chapter 6), specific instances where children have been left temporarily stateless (Chapter 10) and the reproductive justice movement here represented by Generations Ahead (Chapter 15).

Again, as was strongly reiterated at the Forum, contributors are not only concerned about the potential exploitation of women arising from inequalities of power and wealth between the contracting parties, but also the welfare and status of children born of surrogacy arrangements: the unknown physical and/or psychological impact of being carried in a stranger's womb, the danger that they might become stateless citizens or grow up wishing to know unrecorded details about their biographical and genetic heritage.

Before looking further at some of the realities and arguments surrounding transnational surrogacy, it helps to have some historical context.

A new era in human reproduction

Surrogacy itself is not a new phenomenon. The practice of using a substitute 'mother' to conceive, carry and give birth before handing over the child to its 'intended' parents can be traced back to Chapter 16 of the book of Genesis in which Sarai, finding herself infertile, suggests that her husband Abram 'visit' her Egyptian slave, Hagar, who duly provides the couple with a son and heir before her mistress's jealousy sees her cast into the wilderness. A similar scenario is described in

Chapter 30, where Rachel declares to her husband Jacob: 'Here is Bilhah, my maidservant. Sleep with her so that she can bear children for me and that through her I too can build a family.' Again, the arrival of a 'special son' triggers jealousy and recriminations, this time from the many brothers whom Jacob has already fathered.

Louise Brown, 'Baby Cotton' and 'Baby M' The precedent of the more powerful controlling the reproductive choices of poor, often enslaved women may have been set long ago but the ways in which surrogacy arrangements are executed have of course moved on. The current practice of hiring the womb of a relatively impoverished woman to create a baby for a childless couple or individual, usually from a more privileged class, stems from the development of IVF. Early attempts at artificial insemination are said to date back to the 1700s (Almeling, 2013), but none of these experiments resulted in a live birth until the delivery of Louise Brown in Oldham, England, in 1978. Ms Brown (who recently published her autobiography as the world's first 'test-tube baby') was conceived using her parents' eggs *and* sperm, mixed together in a glass tube or petri dish and inserted into the mother's womb. The unprecedented success of this procedure opened the way for the development and commercialization of ARTs that soon led to the first known cases of a woman being paid to carry and give birth to a child for another couple. These separate landmark incidents concerned the birth of two children, 'Baby Cotton' and 'Baby M', and like the stories of Hagar and Bilhah, both ended in drama and recriminations.

'Baby Cotton' involved a transnational arrangement spanning Sweden, the UK and the US. After registering with a commercial surrogacy agency in England, in 1985, British citizen Kim Cotton gave birth to a baby for a Swedish couple based in the US, using her own eggs and the sperm of the intended father. At this stage, commercial surrogacy had not even been acknowledged in law so no ban was in place in the UK. However, on hearing about the financial nature of the arrangement the authorities immediately made 'Baby Cotton' a ward of court. The press got hold of the story, vilifying Ms Cotton. This prompted widespread condemnation from the public and a legal battle that culminated in a new law, the Surrogacy Arrangements Act 1985 discussed by Marilyn Crawshaw and colleagues (Chapter 9). Eventually the (anonymous) commissioning parents were able to take the baby back to the US on the basis that she would never have any contact with her birth mother. To this day, Kim Cotton has no knowledge of the whereabouts of her daughter or the identity of her legal parents.

A year later, the 'Baby M' case featured another commercial surrogacy arrangement, this time in the US state of New Jersey. After giving birth, the surrogate, Mary Beth Whitehead, could not bear to relinquish 'Baby M' to her intended parents, William and Elizabeth Stern; she wanted to forsake the fee and keep the child to whom she was genetically related, again having used her own eggs inseminated with the sperm of the intended father. The Sterns sued. Eventually a Supreme Court invalidated the surrogacy and called the designated payment 'illegal, perhaps, criminal, and potentially degrading to women'. After a two-year battle the court granted custody to the Sterns on the basis that this was in the best interests of the child, but with visitation and parental rights awarded to Ms Whitehead. Again, this story gripped a nation – so much so that it spawned a four-hour docudrama on primetime TV.

Introducing gestational surrogacy Both the above cases involved *traditional* surrogacy whereby the woman who gives birth uses her own eggs or gametes and therefore has a genetic link to the child she carried. This differs from the *gestational* surrogacy practices that form the main topic of this book. Here a woman is hired, or in some cases agrees without payment, to gestate a fetus grown via embryo transfer and to which she has no genetic tie. Like the original experiment that led to the birth of Louise Brown, this IVF procedure entails removing a woman's ova and fertilizing them with sperm in a laboratory before implanting them into the uterus. Depending on the nature of the intended parents' infertility, or indeed their sexuality, gestational surrogacy may involve the use of eggs purchased from a 'donor' or extracted from the intended mother, in both cases using the would-be father's sperm. The demand for donors is growing, driven by an increase in infertility and a rise in the numbers of gay men seeking parenthood.

The recent escalation of gestational surrogacy has been greatly helped by the improvement of egg freezing techniques, together with progress in the modern use of ultrasound imaging to harvest the eggs under conscious sedation rather than the type of keyhole surgery employed before. As Ari Laurel describes in her personal account (Chapter 16), prior to retrieval the 'donor' is subjected to ovarian hyperstimulation, meaning she has to take various hormonal drugs that stimulate the ovaries to produce multiple mature eggs during one menstrual cycle. Once the eggs have been extracted, freezing allows for them to be stored for future use as well as for more than one embryo to be implanted in the uterus at any one time. The potential short- and long-term risks to the woman from these procedures constitute one of the many health aspects of surrogacy discussed in detail by Diane Beeson and Abby Lippman (Chapter 5).

Alongside these technological developments there have been significant changes in what Laurel Swerdlow and Wendy Chavkin refer to as 'the ways people live their most intimate lives', especially in wealthier societies (Chapter 1). In addition to new family formations, the growing acceptance of lesbian and gay parenthood and rising infertility, features of this demographic shift include: far greater opportunities for women to take control of their own reproduction through access to contraception and abortion; women's increased entry into the workforce; delayed childbearing; and growing longevity in the populations of more developed regions. Less salient, yet surely still relevant in relation to the unprecedented demand for surrogacy arrangements, has been a recent decline in intercountry adoption in Europe and the UK (Mignot, 2015; Selman, 2015).

These changes have unfolded alongside the global expansion of capitalism and with it the accelerating circulation of goods, people, money, information and ideas across national borders and cultural boundaries that characterizes transnationalism (Vertovec, 2009). Facilitated by the internet, this freeing up of markets and unparalleled linking of people across borders has led to the growth of new services, among them a flourishing reproductive tourism industry of which commercial surrogacy has become an increasingly lucrative part – particularly in parts of Europe, the US and India. While the US stands out as the only country that is 'both a common source and destination country for global surrogacy arrangements' (Bromfield and Rotabi, 2014: 125), low-cost services, a lack of regulatory infrastructure and a pool of impoverished female labour, together with a thriving privatized medical sector, have enabled India to lead the way (e.g. Centre for Social Research, Chapter 13). As many observers point out (e.g. DasGupta and Dasgupta, 2014; Sama Resource Group for Women and Health, 2012), the absence of regulatory and monitoring mechanisms since the legalization of surrogacy in 2002 makes it impossible to ascertain exact figures. However, comparisons over the years suggest that before the government of Narendra Modi unexpectedly introduced a ban on non-Indian nationals seeking surrogacy towards the end of 2015, the services some doctors refer to as 'maid business' constituted a significant proportion of India's billion-dollar medical tourism industry.[2]

Not only did India's liberalizing governments provide the necessary technical and socio-economic infrastructure, but also the common usage of English by doctors, lawyers, clinic staff and others (not usually surrogates) meant a welcome lack of a language barrier for many intended parents coming from abroad. More saliently, as both Amrita Pande (Chapter 19) and France Winddance Twine (Chapter 6) reiterate, the country also has a history of 'enforced fertility regulation embedded in colonial and post-colonial histories', which has helped to pave the way for the reproductive exploitation of poor and working-class women. As Pande explains so succinctly, this is despite the paradox of promoting 'pro-natal technologies in an anti-natal state' – in other words, encouraging the development of the latest IVF techniques, only available to a relatively wealthy elite, while enforcing contraception, including sterilization, on the poor who make up the majority of the population.

Surrogacy today: the main actors

The three main parties in transnational commercial surrogacy are the intended parents,[3] the surrogate and the child. In an interesting analysis of the parallels and differences between global commercial surrogacy and intercountry adoption, Rhoda Scherman and colleagues (2016) point out that the relationships involved share much in common with members of the adoption triangle: (1) commissioning and adoptive parents; (2) the surrogate and the birth mother; and (3) the children born of surrogacy and adopted. But while adoption necessitates the protective services of social care, legal and sometimes medical professionals, surrogacy tends to entail a far greater but less legitimate cast of characters, from the providers of the genetic material, to doctors, recruiters, agents, insurance brokers, travel agencies, taxi drivers, guides and other intermediaries employed in the surrogate's country to ensure that the whole process runs as smoothly as possible. The role of these unregulated intermediaries is discussed in depth by Sarojini Nadimpally and Anindita Majumdar, who draw from the narratives of two 'agent-facilitators' to show how, in a system devoid of oversight or regulation, Indian surrogates were recruited and then trained to recruit other women within their communities (Chapter 4).

Intended parents Although there have been cases of potential criminal intent,[4] the motives of the intended parents are by and large straightforward: to take home a child with whom they are genetically related. Their stories can be found in so many blogs, memoirs and other media that it did not seem necessary to give them much prominence in this book. However, one group specifically merits attention, partly because they are specifically targeted by surrogacy clinics online but also because of the ways in which this publicity deliberately sets out to shape the nature of their desires. Further, they represent one of the major ways in which our ideas of parenthood have shifted and are being reconstructed (Dempsey, 2013; Marsiglio et al., 2013; Murphy, 2015).

After examining twelve websites aimed at gay men seeking parenthood, Damien Riggs and Clemence Due found that not only do they 'potentially respond to the existing desires of some gay men to become parents, but they also shape the forms that such desires take by emphasizing particular factors that are deemed salient to gay men's reproductive decisions' (Chapter 2). Websites such as Circle Surrogacy, Baby Joy, Surrogacy Cancun and others speak to one of the driving forces of surrogacy: men's desire for genetic relatedness to their children.

Surrogates At the heart of every surrogacy arrangement is the surrogate 'mother': she who gives birth.[5] As Darnovsky and Beeson (2014: 24) write, a variety of terms are used to describe her:

> many if not all of [which] reflect a bias either in favour or opposed to such arrangements. Some terms such as 'birth mother' and 'gestational mother' explicitly acknowledge the maternal aspect of the woman's role. Others, such as 'gestational carrier', make her maternity and even her personhood less visible ...

In other words, as Laurel Swerdlow and Wendy Chavkin discuss in their opening chapter, the availability of ARTs has had far-reaching implications for 'the meaning of motherhood and the social understanding of biological connection'. If it can take up to five people (two commissioning parents, egg and sperm providers and surrogate) to create another human being, where does this leave the 'mother'? A more overtly political option might be to call the women who carry and give birth to the baby 'reproductive labourers' (Baylis, 2014; Pande, 2014).

The majority of arguments for and against surrogacy focus first and foremost on the position of these women – their motivations, agency and how much their usually subordinate socio-economic position is being exploited. How far do they understand the potential consequences of signing the surrogacy contract? To what extent are they putting themselves physically and psychologically at risk? Again, as Darnovsky and Beeson (2014) state in their report of discussion at The Hague Forum, the answers differ greatly according to the social contexts in which the arrangements are made. Mexico and Greece offer just two examples.

Compared to their counterparts in India, Mexican surrogates do not come from the poorest sectors of society. A significant number have migrated from other Latin American countries in search of better opportunities; others have fled from the violence in parts of Mexico. They tend to be single mothers seeking income to help bring up their own children and share a basic common language with the agencies, clinics and lawyers in charge of the surrogacy arrangement. However, as the activists from GIRE have discovered from their interviews with surrogates in Tabasco, Cancun and Mexico City, this by no means guarantees informed consent or protection. Most women are merely given a brief verbal explanation with no attention paid to whether they have understood the terms. If they do have questions, no one is available to answer them. One surrogate reported being told by a lawyer: 'You have to obey the doctors. If you don't like it, don't sign.'

Apart from the known risks from medical procedures, the former openness of some Mexican states towards gay men seeking parenthood brought with it another, less predictable hazard: in a television documentary on Mexico's baby business recently broadcast in the UK (Channel 4, 2015), a Mexican surrogate, Alejandra Mendiola, told a reporter that she had been implanted with the sperm of a man carrying the HIV virus. When challenged, Lily Frost, Director of the California-based agency Surrogacy Beyond Borders, which had brokered the arrangement, claimed the sperm had been 'scrubbed clean of HIV' though she admitted this wasn't 'ideal'. It also turned out that Alejandra, by then five months' pregnant, had not even signed a contract.

Greece, which so far only allows fertility treatment for heterosexual couples (married or unmarried) and single women, provides another scenario. While neither the intended mother nor the surrogate has to be a EU citizen, one of them must be 'a permanent resident of Greece; the other may have a temporary residence'. As Konstantina Davaki points out (Chapter 8), this relatively new legislation has attracted criticism:

> first, it officially opens the door to reproductive tourism; second, it creates circumstances conducive to the trafficking of women from poorer countries for surrogacy services; third, it can create

problematic situations, for instance, when the legal conditions for maternity are different between Greece and the intended mother's country of origin ...

Another specific feature of the surrogacy landscape in Greece is the percentage of surrogates who are either family members or 'best friends' of the intended parents. In a survey cited from Hatzis (2010), these so-called friends were mostly women from Eastern Europe, 17 per cent of whom were already known to the intended mother through their employment as domestic workers. This raises important questions, not only regarding the blurred nature of the financial arrangement but also whether the data reveal altruistic behaviour or constitute the expression of a new form of 'bodily labour'.

As in the term 'reproductive labourers' referred to earlier, this points to Amrita Pande's compelling arguments surrounding the intersections between reproduction and production. During the course of her lengthy ethnographic study into the lives of surrogates in India, Pande came to the conclusion that commercial surrogacy is a form of work that should be subject to labour laws and protections, including strictly regulated contracts and follow-up health care after the birth (Pande, 2014; also see Darnovsky and Beeson, 2014: 26). Consequently any future legislation in this area should take place under international labour law.

Pande's work is also important in that it positions Indian surrogates outside the realms of exploitation by describing the strategies that some women have used to retain a degree of control over the surrogacy process, including the toll it takes on their bodies. For example, in *Wombs in Labor* she quotes Razia, a 25-year-old mother of two, whom she met straight after she had delivered a baby by c-section for a couple from California (Pande, 2014: 122):

> I told her [the intended mother] that I want to rest for six months because of the operation. I also told her that I don't want to go home but rest at the clinic. And since we don't have extra money, I want them to pay for the extra months. They are very nice people, they agreed. With my own children I had to go back to backbreaking work almost the day they out. *This time I can make it different* [emphasis added].

Thus, in her contribution to this anthology, Pande cautions against framing the surrogacy industry through the lens of 'morality' or 'commodification' and calls for a nuanced analysis that takes into account 'intersecting layers of structural, economic, political and cultural domination' that shape the choices of women engaged in this market (Chapter 19).

Children By and large, it is the women who give birth who occupy the centre of the big 'to ban or not to ban' surrogacy debate. But what about the offspring, the babies they have gestated and who will grow into autonomous adults? Aside from widespread analysis of the many reported cases of 'stateless babies' arising from weak or poorly executed legislation, with the exception of several contributors to this book, few scholars writing on the legal aspects of surrogacy have paid much attention to the psychological implications of being born this way. For this reason, I have devoted three chapters to the interests of the children and the grown-ups they will become.

While Marilyn Crawshaw and colleagues (Chapter 9) and Marsha Tyson Darling (Chapter 10) focus mainly on social work and legal perspectives pertaining to the 'best interests' of the child, Deborah Dempsey and Fiona Kelly explore donor-conceived people's desire for knowledge about their origins and the role of the internet in their search (Chapter 11). Extensive research into identity development in relation to adoption has revealed the importance for adopted people of knowing about their birth family and the circumstances of their birth and the damage that can be done from only finding this out in later life (Brodzinsky, 2005; Harris, 2006). But apart from the work of Susan Golombok and her team (2004, 2011, 2015) and Jadva and Imrie (2014),[6] studies of surrogacy disclosure and outcomes are still few and far between. To my knowledge, these have also been limited to domestic arrangements in the UK.

As donor-assisted conception and transnational surrogacy become more common so will the demand for genetic and gestational origins, making it all the more crucial that details of the surrogate's and egg provider's name, date of birth, nationality, how they were recruited, fees paid and any advice or counselling given be recorded for safekeeping.

As Sonia Allan explains in her concluding chapter, in addition to its potential importance for people born via surrogacy, such information is needed as evidence whenever transfer or recognition of legal parentage has to occur. Amrita Pande, too, argues for the need for transparency – legal, financial, medical and in terms of relationships – if the interests of surrogates as well as the children they give birth to are to be genuinely respected.

Can transnational surrogacy ever be ethical?

Most of the issues addressed in this anthology, whether to do with the socio-economic, political, medical, psychological or legal implications of outsourcing pregnancy, lead back to matters of consent and agency. To quote again from Darnovsky and Beeson's excellent report of the findings and concerns expressed by participants at The Hague Forum (2014: 25):

> To what extent do women enter into these contracts as an expression of personal autonomy, with full understanding of the potential consequences of their action? To what extent are they motivated by structural conditions such as poverty, economic equality, and gender equality; influenced by unethical recruiting practices and/or lack of adequate information about risks and potential side-effects; or subjected to family pressures and cultural and industry discourses that present contract pregnancy as a form of altruism and simultaneously a way to a better life? Does the combination of these influences constitute coercion?

These questions, in turn, lead to the big dilemma: Can transnational surrogacy ever be ethical? As Emma Maniere demonstrates in her contribution mapping feminist views on commercial surrogacy (Chapter 18), unless like Kajsa Ekis Ekman and the Swedish Women's Lobby you are an avid abolitionist (Chapter 17), there is no straightforward answer. The complexity of arguments surrounding surrogacy is evident in some odd alliances, for instance in Romania and Greece where the Church, radical and socialist feminists, pro-life associations and supporters of the traditional family all tend to align themselves against surrogacy on bio-ethical grounds. Other arguments centre on the tension between reproductive rights and reproductive justice, as discussed by the women of colour and Indigenous women who gathered together to debate the implications of reproductive technologies on their communities in 2008 (Chapter 15).

By and large, most of the contributors to this anthology refrain from recommending a full ban and opt for a reformist approach based on careful analysis but also driven by the urgent need for coherent policies and far greater regulation. All would probably agree that transnational surrogacy practices have grown too far and too fast and in so doing allowed the spurious concept of the 'right to a child' to eclipse the fundamental human rights of the children and women most at risk.

Notes

1 In addition to Cheney's *Executive Summary*, other reports focus on findings from the Forum's five thematic areas: *HCIA Implementation and the Best Interests of the Child*; *Intercountry Adoption, Countries of Origin and Biological Families*; *Intercountry Adoption Agencies and the HCIA*; *Force, Fraud and Coercion*; and *Global Surrogacy Practices* – all available from: <http://repub.eur.nl/col/9760#filter=all:Global surrogacy>.

2 As this book prepares to go to press, the Indian government has just approved the introduction of the Surrogacy (Regulation) Bill, 2016 in Parliament. In addition to a bar on foreigners, unmarried couples, single parents, live-in partners and gay men, the Bill stipulates that the surrogate must be a 'close relative' of the couple seeking a child – in other words, introducing a highly regulated form of 'altruistic surrogacy' alongside the prohibition of commercial surrogacy arrangements in any form (*The Times of India*, 2016).

3 Throughout this book, the main clients in the surrogacy arrangement are referred to interchangeably as 'intended' 'intending' or 'commissioning' parents. As a law scholar, Sonia Allan prefers the term 'commissioning persons'.

4 Two such cases emerged around the time of The Hague Forum. First came the Baby Gammy scandal where Australian intended parents abandoned a boy with Down's syndrome with his Thai surrogate mother, taking his twin sister home; it was later discovered that the husband whose sperm had been used was a convicted sex offender against girls as young as 5 years old (Pearlman, 2014). Soon afterwards, news broke that, in the course of one year up to June 2014, a 24-year-old Japanese billionaire had fathered sixteen babies with thirteen Thai surrogates in Bangkok (Rawlinson, 2014).

5 Most of the contributors to this book use the term 'surrogate' or 'surrogate mother', often interchangeably. An alternative, preferred by Ayesha Chatterjee and Sally Whelan of OBOS, is 'gestational mother'.

6 Jadva and Imrie (2014) have also looked at the experiences and perceptions of the children of surrogates in the UK. Although this area clearly merits attention, I have not found enough sources to include it in this book. One reference to this during The Hague Forum reported the 7-year-old son of an Indian surrogate asking her not to take the money but instead to 'keep my brother' (Rotabi, cited in Darnovsky and Beeson, 2014: 24).

References

Almeling R (2013) *Sex Cells: The Medical Market for Eggs and Sperm*. Berkeley, CA: University of California Press.

Baylis F (2014) Transnational commercial contract pregnancy in India. In: Baylis F and McLeod C (eds) *Family-Making*. Oxford: Oxford University Press, pp. 265–86.

Brodzinsky DM (2005) Reconceptualizing openness in adoption: implications for theory, research and practice. In: Brodzinsky D and Palacios J (eds) *Psychological Issues in Adoption: Research and Practice*. New York: Greenwood, pp. 145–66.

Bromfield NF and Rotabi KS (2014) Global surrogacy, exploitation, human rights and international private law: a pragmatic stance and policy recommendations. *Global Social Welfare* 1: 123–35.

Brown LJ (2015) *Louise Brown: My Life as the World's First Test-Tube Baby*. Bristol: Bristol Books.

Channel 4 (2015) Mexico's baby business. *Unreported World*, 13 November.

<http://www.channel4.com/programmes/unreported-world/on-demand/60446-015>

Cheney KE (2014) *Executive Summary of the International Forum on Intercountry Adoption and Global Surrogacy*, Working Paper 596. <repub.eur.nl/pub/77408/wp596.pdf>

Cheney KE (2016) Preventing exploitation, promoting equity: findings from the International Forum on Intercountry Adoption and Global Surrogacy 2014. *Adoption & Fostering* 40(1): 6–19.

Darnovsky M and Beeson D (2014) *Global Surrogacy Practices*. ISS Working Paper Series/General Series 601: 1–54. <http://hdl.handle.net/1765/77402>

DasGupta S and Dasgupta SD (eds) (2014) *Globalization and Transnational Surrogacy in India: Outsourcing Life*. Lanham, MD: Lexington Books.

Dempsey D (2013) Surrogacy, gay male couples and the significance of biogenetic paternity. *New Genetics and Society* 32(1): 37–53.

Ergas Y (2013) Babies without borders: human rights, human dignity, and the regulation of international commercial surrogacy. *Emory International Law Review* 27: 117–88.

Gerber P and O'Byrne K (eds) (2015) *Surrogacy, Law and Human Rights*. Aldershot: Ashgate.

Golombok S (2015) *Modern Families: Parents and Children in New Family Forms*. Cambridge: Cambridge University Press.

Golombok S, Murray C, Jadva V, MacCallum F and Lycett E (2004) Families created through surrogacy arrangements: parent–child relationships in the 1st year of life. *Developmental Psychology* 40(3): 400–11.

Golombok S, Readings J, Blake L, Casey P, Mellish L, Marks A and Jadva V (2011) Families created through surrogacy: mother–child relationships and children's psychological adjustment at age 7. *Developmental Psychology* 47(6): 1579–88.

Harris P (ed.) (2006) *In Search of Belonging: Reflections by Transracially Adopted People*. London: BAAF.

Hatzis A (2010) *The Regulation of Surrogate Motherhood in Greece*. Working Paper, Social Sciences and Research Network. University of Athens.

HCCH (Hague Conference on International Private Law) (2014a) *The Desirability and Feasibility of Further Work on the Parentage/Surrogacy Project*, Preliminary Document No. 3B. The Hague: HCCH. <www.hcch.net/upload/wop/gap2014pd03b_en.pdf>

HCCH (2014b) *A Study of Legal Parentage and the Issues Arising from International Surrogacy Arrangements*, Preliminary Document No. 3C. The Hague: HCCH. <www.hcch.net/upload/wop/gap2014pd03c_en.pdf>

Hochschild A (2009) Childbirth at the global crossroads. *The American Prospect*, 19 September. <http://prospect.org/article/childbirth-global-crossroads-0>

Howard S (2015) US army wives: the most sought-after surrogates in the world. *Daily Telegraph*, 7 May. <www.telegraph.co.uk/women/mother-tongue/11583541/US-army-wives-the-most-sought-after-surrogates-in-the-world.html>

Jadva V and Imrie S (2014) Children of surrogate mothers: psychological well-being, family relationships and experiences of surrogacy. *Human Reproduction* 29(1): 90–6.

Jadva V, Blake L, Casey P and Golombok S (2012) Surrogacy families 10 years on: relationships with the surrogate, decisions over disclosure and children's understanding of their surrogacy origins. *Human Reproduction* 27(10): 3008–14.

Macklin R (1994) *Surrogates and Other Mothers: The Debates Over Assisted*

Reproduction. Philadelphia, PA: Temple University Press.

Marsiglio W, Lohan M and Culley L (2013) Framing men's experience in the procreative realm. *Journal of Family Issues* 34(8): 1011–36.

Mignot JF (2015) Why is intercountry adoption declining worldwide? *Population & Societies*, 519. <https://halshs.archives-ouvertes.fr/halshs-01326717/document>

Murphy D (2015) *Gay Men Pursuing Parenthood through Surrogacy: Reconfiguring Kinship*. Sydney: NewSouth Publishing.

Pande A (2009) 'It may be her eggs but it's my labour': surrogates and everyday forms of kinship in India. *Qualitative Sociology* 32(4): 379–405.

Pande A (2010) 'At least I am not sleeping with anyone'. *Feminist Studies* 36(2): 292–312.

Pande A (2014) *Wombs in Labor: Transnational Surrogacy in India*. New York: Columbia University Press.

Pearlman J (2014) Surrogacy case: the history of sex offences of the Australian accused of leaving surrogate baby in Thailand. *Daily Telegraph*, 6 August. <www.telegraph.co.uk/news/worldnews/australiaandthepacific/australia/11015898/Surrogacy-case-the-history-of-sex-offences-of-the-Australian-accused-of-leaving-surrogate-baby-in-Thailand.html>

Ragoné H (1994) *Surrogate Motherhood: Conception in the Heart (Institutional Structures of Feeling)*. Boulder, CO: Westview Press.

Rawlinson K (2014) Interpol investigates 'baby factory' as man fathers 16 surrogate children. *Guardian*, 23 August. <www.theguardian.com/lifeandstyle/2014/aug/23/interpol-japanese-baby-factory-man-fathered-16-children>

Sama Resource Group for Women and Health (2012) *Birthing a Market: A Study of Commercial Surrogacy*. New Delhi: Sama. <www.communityhealth.in/~commun26/wiki/images/e/e8/Sama_Birthing_A_Market.pdf>

Scherman R, Misca G, Rotabi K and Selman P (2016) Global commercial surrogacy and international adoption: parallels and differences. *Adoption & Fostering* 40(1): 20–35.

Selman P (2015) *Key Tables for Intercountry Adoption Receiving States of Origin 2003–2013*. <www.hcch.net/index_en.php?act=publications.details&pid=5891&dtid=32>

Spar D (2006) *The Baby Business: How Money, Science and Politics Drive the Commerce of Conception*. Cambridge, MA: Harvard Business School Press.

The Times of India (2016) Government proposes complete ban on commercial surrogacy, 24 August. <http://timesofindia.indiatimes.com/india/Government-proposes-complete-ban-on-commercial-surrogacy/articleshow/53844035.cms>

Trimmings K and Beaumont P (eds) (2013) *International Surrogacy Arrangements: Legal Regulation at the International Level*. Oxford: Hart Publishing.

Twine WF (2015) *Outsourcing the Womb: Race, Class, and Gestational Surrogacy in a Global Market*, 2nd edition. London: Routledge.

van den Akker O (2007) Psychosocial aspects of surrogate motherhood. *Human Reproduction Update* 13(1): 53–62.

Vertovec S (2009) *Transnationalism*. Abingdon: Routledge.

PART ONE
RECONSTRUCTING PARENTHOOD

PART ONE
RECORD INJECTION TAX METHODS

1 | MOTHERHOOD IN FRAGMENTS: THE DISAGGREGATION OF BIOLOGY AND CARE

Laurel Swerdlow and Wendy Chavkin

In western societies the definition of motherhood was once grounded in biology, such that the woman who delivered a child was considered that child's mother. If the child was then adopted by another family the woman who gave birth was still identified as the 'birth mother' in acknowledgement of their biological connection. Except in cases of adoption, maternal figures who provided children with care, but had not given birth to them, were rarely regarded as 'mothers'. Biological mothers who outsourced childcare to nannies maintained complete maternal status, regardless of their level of engagement in nurturing work. Thus, while motherhood consisted of both biological and caregiving components, primacy was afforded to biology.

The social preference for biology in establishing motherhood certainly reflected the denigration of care that feminist scholars have highlighted for decades, but it presumably also stemmed from the relative simplicity of assessing biological connection. Whereas a child could have multiple caretakers, the biological components of motherhood were, until recently, fixed, easily identifiable and limited to one person. Biological reproduction required one male and one female and relied on their ability to produce viable gametes, to effectively combine those gametes to conceive an embryo, and on the intended mother's ability to carry a fetus to term. Fecundity, the ability to reproduce, was constrained by a biological window. A woman's ability to become pregnant and successfully carry to term begins to decline by her late twenties and drops very sharply after the mid-thirties (Dunson *et al.*, 2002; Frank *et al.*, 1994). Women who wanted to be mothers but were incapable of biological reproduction, or had outrun the biological clock, were left without recourse.

The biological constraints of reproduction have become increasingly socially problematic over the past fifty years, as a growing number of women throughout the world are choosing to delay childbearing in pursuit of educational and career opportunities. However, these women no longer necessarily miss the boat for motherhood. Rather, global market forces and new technological developments offer couples enticing solutions that promise the aspirational fulfilment of both career and familial ambitions. Assisted reproductive technologies (ARTs), adoption and the market for migrant nannies all provide ways for couples with sufficient financial means to attempt to circumvent the limitations of biology, the undesirable components of care, or both, in their quest for parenthood. Increasing reliance on this 'assistance' has propelled the disaggregation of motherhood (biological) and mothering work (care), along with the subsequent fragmentation of both components. Today, the processes of biological and social reproduction may involve a cast of players in addition to the intended or commissioning parents, complicating our existing understanding of parenthood.

The availability of ARTs in particular has had dramatic implications for the meaning of motherhood and the social understanding of biological connection. ARTs come in various shapes and sizes, offering perceived fixes for whatever cog in the reproductive process is malfunctioning, expired, inaccessible or undesirable. Today, biological reproduction could incorporate half a dozen people or more, including the commissioning parents, egg and sperm providers, surrogate, and even a cytoplasm donor, in addition to facilitating parties in the fields of business, medicine and law. The availability of ARTs has thus allowed the fragmentation of the biology of reproduction into multiple elements. When assigning maternal status, we can no longer grant primacy to the biological component of motherhood because biological motherhood, as a *de facto* construct, no longer exists.

Rather, we witness the social ascription of mothering worth to each biological component. The value afforded to the various fragments is rife with contradictions, is not scientifically grounded and is dependent on the wishes of the individuals with power in any given reproductive transaction. While this disaggregation of motherhood, and the attribution of meaning to the respective components, is manifest with all types of ARTs, transnational surrogacy provides the extreme, the ultimate example. The social construction of motherhood inherent in transnational surrogacy in some ways reiterates the familiar narrative of biology trumping care but this time, as we discuss in this chapter, the biological role of gestation is misconstrued as care, resulting in its subsequent denigration. In the context of surrogacy, the disaggregation of motherhood becomes a complicated story that riffs on conventional hierarchies but also incorporates new types of contradictions and seeming inconsistencies.

The backdrop

A variety of forces sets the stage for the disaggregation of motherhood discussed in this chapter. As we consider the emergence of transnational surrogacy, we highlight the roles played by the 'second demographic transition', globalization and technological advances. By also including the often neglected discussion of the associated medical and public health concerns, we underscore how the meanings attributed to the disaggregated components and processes of motherhood do not align with the scientific evidence, but rather reflect political and social constructions.

Demand for ART emerged on the heels of a constellation of socio-economic changes that demographers term the 'second demographic transition'. In the last third of the twentieth century in higher-income countries, dramatic changes happened in the ways people live their most intimate lives. Many women deferred marriage and childbearing and entered the workforce. The incidence of single parenthood increased, as did the rate of divorce. Death rates declined, people lived longer and birth rates dropped below the level needed to replace the population. While the details vary within and between countries, the general patterns hold true for those that are highly developed. Similar changes are now taking place in many developing countries as well, with thirty-two already having birth rates below replacement levels (United Nations, 2013), including Armenia, Myanmar and Vietnam (World Bank, 2013).

The decline in birth rates has led to many positive changes on both societal and individual levels. Countries have experienced economic growth as a result of women's entry into the work force. Lower fertility rates have not only improved women's health and life opportunities, but also benefited the health and educational prospects of children. However, these demographic trends do not necessarily signify that women have unencumbered reproductive choices. Women continue to face job segregation, a substantial wage gap and inadequate work–family policies in the public sphere, while still shouldering the brunt of domestic work and caregiving at home. Therefore, women's decisions to delay and/or limit childbearing often reflect their need to make 'rational choices' in the face of having to balance disproportionate burdens of economic and social insecurity. This phenomenon is most visible when we consider childbearing trends among women whose incomes are necessary but insecure, and who lack spousal and/or governmental support. McDonald (2000), Castles (2003) and others suggest that especially low birth rates among women in such circumstances reflect the increased 'opportunity costs' of having children while carrying the burdens of both employment and domestic care without sufficient support for social reproduction from men or the state.

As mentioned above, delayed entry into childbearing leaves women with a truncated window of biological opportunity to become pregnant. While the data on the female biological clock are incomplete, they indicate that the probabilities of pregnancy for women aged 35 to 39 are about half those of women aged between 19 and 25 years (Dunson et al., 2002; Frank et al., 1994). There is thus a discordance between women's recently achieved employment trajectories and their biological capacity for reproduction. A rapidly rising number of couples are trying to resolve this discordance by turning to adoption, the technological fix of ARTs and increasingly to transnational surrogacy.

Individuals or couples who turn to ARTs have a spectrum of options at their disposal, ranging from simpler interventions that promote fertilization, such as artificial insemination and ovarian stimulation, to merging sperm and egg in the laboratory (including in vitro fertilization and intra-cytoplasmic sperm injection). In addition to procedures that facilitate the reproduction of one couple using their own bodies and body parts, the advent of gamete donation and surrogacy has provided opportunities for reproduction using others' biological bits and processes. In the ultimate expression of biological reproductive outsourcing, women for whom childbearing is either impossible or undesirable, same-sex couples and single men can now turn to other women for gestation, using gametes that they provide and/or procure from others.

These technologies have become readily available thanks to the processes of globalization, defined here as the increased interconnectedness of production and communication with reduced barriers to trade, the increased movement of people for trade and work, the rise of transnational corporations and of the involvement of supranational actors and economic institutions in national social policy formation (Chavkin, 2010). Globalization has enabled individuals to travel abroad for health care services that are unavailable, regulated and/or more expensive at home, a phenomenon referred to as 'medical tourism'. ARTs are among the most popular services offered in this global market (Patients Beyond Borders, 2014). To facilitate these transactions, internet advertisements for ART clinics and procedures offered in low-income countries target 'reproductive tourists' from near and far. The information advertised often blurs the lines between factual information and consumerist imagery, reflecting and shaping notions of biological and social relationships (Chavkin, 2010). SurrogacyIndia, for example, advertises that they have the largest selection of 'Diva Donors', who they define as 'donors who are educated, good looking, [or] may be from higher socio economic strata' (SurrogacyIndia, 2010). In creating the 'Diva Donor' category, they highlight those egg donor characteristics they believe commissioning parents deem important, and simultaneously imply that they are heritable.

The constant movement of people, products, body parts, technologies and ideas across borders has curtailed effective government regulation. Such fluid national borders mean a country's policy decisions regarding reproduction are constrained by and implicate the global landscape of ARTs. Austerity policies and welfare state cutbacks foster the availability of babies for adoption, push women from developing countries to migrate abroad in search of work as nannies and lead to the global recruitment of women into selling their gametes and bodies as surrogates. Concurrently, women who take advantage of these new markets often do so to cope with the social and economic pressures of modernity. While women in many countries have entered the labour market, neither women nor men receive sufficient social or employee benefits to enable them to balance effectively their work and family lives during their fecund years (OECD, 2011). As a result, many couples in higher-income countries choose to delay childbearing until they are more financially established, often seeking assistance for both biological and social reproduction within a two-career household.

Globalization thus encourages women in high- and middle-income countries to delay childbearing, while simultaneously offering apparent solutions in the form of adoptable babies, cheaper and unregulated ARTs and associated body parts, and caregivers for the resulting babies. To acknowledge these simultaneous 'push' and 'pull' factors does not imply that the interaction reflects comparable pressures on both groups of women. The globalization of motherhood perpetuates gender-associated limitations for both, although neither equally nor similarly (Chavkin, 2008). Despite the economic and domestic burdens still shouldered by women in higher-income countries, they have made clear progress towards gender equity in both employment and domestic responsibilities, in part because of economic and gendered inequities confronting other groups of women. A woman from Guatemala who migrates to the United States as a nanny sends remittances home to her family, while her employer's wages still fall short of those of her male colleagues. Both women strive to support their family within gendered labour markets, and give their children less direct mothering as a result. Yet, the earnings, benefits and status that the US woman garners rely on the care provided by her children's nanny, who reaps far less reward. Parallel examples of reproductive transactions in the context of transnational surrogacy highlight the social inequities as well as the public health ramifications that result from these new global reproductive relationships.

Public health ramifications

There has been considerable debate regarding the implications of socio-economic and racial discrepancies between consumers and purveyors of reproductive body parts, and the obvious potential for exploitation, much of which will be discussed in subsequent chapters. Many have considered the commodification of reproduction and how inequities of power and need play out in global surrogacy transactions. In addition to discussing the social and political attribution of meaning to the fragmented pieces of biological motherhood, we will focus on the lack of scientific underpinning and take a look at some of the proven and potential medical and public health risks associated with the use of in vitro fertilization (IVF), third-party gametes and surrogates.

ARTs were made widely available before data were disseminated about their efficacy and safety, and decades after their mass distribution, both parameters are still understudied and appear worrisome. The risks associated with IVF are among the best documented of all ART procedures. A growing body of evidence indicates that the IVF procedure contributes to an increased risk of birth defects. After controlling for maternal age and ethnicity, several studies have found that an IVF baby's odds of birth defects are roughly two to four times greater than that of a naturally conceived infant (American Academy of Pediatrics, 2012). Malformations of the eye, heart and genitourinary system are among the most common birth defects observed. Furthermore, complications for babies born as a result of IVF include increased rates of preterm delivery, low birth weight and perinatal death (Evans *et al.*, 1995; Gleicher *et al.*, 2000), and women who conceive through IVF are more likely to carry twins and higher order multiple pregnancies, which are in turn at heightened risk for all of the above. Follow-up studies of long-term survivors of very low birth weight and multiple births indicate neurological and cognitive deficits for both.

Providers who offer IVF are increasingly combining the procedure with intra-cytoplasmic sperm injection (ICSI), in which a single sperm,

sperm head or nucleus is retrieved from a man and inserted directly into the cytoplasm of a mature egg. ICSI was originally intended for men who had very few retrievable sperm (a controversial practice given that such low sperm counts are often associated with heritable conditions), but it has now become a widespread practice even in cases without male-factor infertility (National Center for Chronic Disease Prevention and Health Promotion, 2014). The mainstreaming of ICSI is problematic due to its demonstrated association with an increased rate of neurodevelopment disorders, especially autism and mental retardation, and other birth defects, which are more prevalent among children conceived using both ICSI and IVF (Bonduelle *et al.*, 2005; Sandin *et al.*, 2013). All of these procedures may be performed using fresh or frozen gametes, despite disputes among medical experts regarding the safety and efficacy of cryopreservation (Kopeika *et al.*, 2015).

Women who carry multiple gestation pregnancies, a common result of several ART procedures, have been shown to face increased risks of complications. Women undergoing the hormonal stimulation required to make ova and uteri ready for egg harvesting and/or IVF face documented short-term risks (Klemett *et al.*, 2005; Klip *et al.*, 2003). While sophisticated medical treatment can remedy these shorter-term risks, we know very little about the long-term implications of hormonal stimulation for women's health (Evans *et al.*, 1995; Gleicher *et al.*, 2000). Given the biologically plausible reasons for concern, it is troubling that we lack data on medical procedures that are already pervasive on a global scale.

Ultimately, pregnancy puts women at risk. More than a quarter of a million women die annually of pregnancy related complications in the developing world (WHO, 2013). Women serving as surrogates – particularly in places with high levels of maternal mortality and poor pregnancy outcomes – must therefore be understood to face significant risk, even before considering the ways that the procedures associated with surrogacy further threaten their health. In addition to the documented and postulated risks of the hormone stimulation required for IVF, surrogates who use third-party embryos have an increased likelihood of gestational hypertension and preeclampsia (Klatsky *et al.*, 2010). They frequently undergo multiple embryo transplants, followed by selective reduction when multiple pregnancies ensue.

Sharmila Rudrappa (2014: 299) reports:

The Delhi surrogate mother working for James and Scott from Melbourne faced such a situation, when four embryos implanted in her started to grow into fetuses. The doctor contacted the intended fathers, saying she had to reduce the fetuses to two. [The fathers] were heartbroken because fetal reduction went against their beliefs, and they mourned what felt like the death of their two babies.

Rudrappa's interviews shed light on a common practice. In cases of multi-parity pregnancy, abnormal prenatal diagnosis or a change of heart on behalf of the commissioning party, decisions surrounding pregnancy termination are often made by the commissioning couple, not by the woman in whose body these events are taking place. Indeed, commissioning parties and the clinics that represent them assume control over the majority of medical decisions involving the surrogate, including the mode of delivery. For example, it is commonplace for Indian surrogates to deliver by scheduled c-section, putting them at risk of complications from surgery, in order to accommodate commissioning parties who must travel long distances to attend the delivery (Rudrappa, 2014), or based on a misguided belief that surgical intervention is superior to vaginal delivery.

Contradictions and inconsistencies

ARTs reflect the splintering of biological reproduction into multiple fragments, with gestation and organs and gametes and intracellular ingredients and genetic components now separable (Chavkin, 2010). As a result, couples who reproduce using ART manage multiple biological mothering fragments and are faced with the prospect of ascribing mothering worth to each. As was the case pre-ART, biology is still considered highly determinative of mother status. But when we consider the various possible ART transactions, it becomes evident that what one construes as biology is highly varied, contextual and replete with contradictions.

A woman who uses a purchased egg to create an embryo, which she then gestates, deems gestation to be determinative of motherhood. Conversely, couples who combine their gametes in vitro and contract with a gestational surrogate ascribe primacy to their genetic contributions. In the case of cytoplasmic or mitochondrial transfer, nuclei containing the genetic material from one woman's eggs are suctioned out and replaced with nuclei from a 'donor' and mothering worth is ascribed to cellular nuclei. Contradictions accumulate when we consider that even within ART transactions, biology is not necessarily afforded primacy. In cases where an opposite-sex couple provides sperm to a traditional surrogate (a procedure in which the surrogate's egg is used, making her the genetic mother), the commissioning woman's relational status to the sperm provider, combined with her intention to provide care to the resulting child, establishes her role as mother. Ultimately, as was the case prior to the advent of ART, we find that each fragment of biology and care is elevated or denigrated according to the will of the party that holds political power.

As illustrated by Rudrappa (2014), these power relations may dictate decisions regarding the surrogate's control over her body. When commissioning parents decide that the surrogate should abort or insist on her continuing a pregnancy, they do so assuming that their role as contractors gives them ownership and decision-making rights over her body – an assumption that contradicts the very principles underlying reproductive freedom that many users of ARTs espouse. In a highly publicized 2013 case in the US, commissioning parents demanded that their surrogate undergo an abortion after an ultrasound revealed that the fetus had multiple anomalies. Opposed to terminating the pregnancy, the surrogate fled across the country in order to carry the pregnancy to term and subsequently relinquished the baby for adoption (Dolak, 2013). This surrogate went to great lengths to exert control over her body; surrogates elsewhere may have no recourse. Rudrappa (2014: 297) described one couple who 'mentioned that they chose India because the surrogate mothers there had little, or no rights over the baby they gestated'. These assertions of control over surrogates' decisions about their bodies collide with the notions of bodily integrity and female autonomy that justify legal abortion.

The ways that power obscures science and dictates the hierarchy of biological meaning is reflected both in the terms used to describe the transnational surrogacy process and in the birth certificate. A child born of gestational surrogacy has at least three 'mothers': the woman who provided the ova, the surrogate and the commissioning party. Yasmine Ergas (2013) emphasizes that the language used to describe the roles played by each woman indicates a clear ladder of social value. The surrogate is frequently referred to as a 'carrier' who has 'rented out her womb', reflecting her attributed status as both manual labourer and landlord, thereby ignoring her biological contributions as well as the maternal and fetal risks associated with surrogacy. The provider of the ova, on the other hand, assumes the role of 'egg donor', a label that also strips her of any maternal reference, placing her colloquially on a par with a sperm donor, despite the comparatively more arduous and riskier process of 'harvesting' eggs. Meanwhile, the couple, who either provided the sperm or simply contracted for the entire operation, assumes the role of 'parents' and are so inscribed on the birth certificate.

A birth certificate has always had both social and medical meaning, but in the age of ART it has been transformed into an exclusively social document. Most adoptees are first issued an original birth record that includes the name of the relinquishing mother and then receive an amended certificate that records the adoptive parent(s). In jurisdictions with open adoption, those wishing to trace their biological mothers can identify them from the original birth certificates. Conversely, in many commercial surrogacy transactions, commissioning parties ensure that they are the only ones recorded on the original birth certificate, erasing the gestating mother from the document that allegedly provides a record of the child's birth (Chavkin, 2010: 10). This erasure not only alters the meaning of the document, which historically served an important purpose in enabling public health surveillance and analysis, but now exclusively conveys the familial and national associations of the commissioning parents. Given the growing evidence that children born through ART have an increased need for perinatal and infant interventions, our inability to track gestation not only compromises the epidemiological record, it may additionally undercut best medical care for the child.

Commissioning parties generally make considerable efforts to oversee the surrogacy process, in part to secure healthy babies, yet they appear to disregard inconvenient data. Consider, for instance, the primacy ascribed to gametes over gestation – a ranking based on scientifically unfounded attributions of meaning to these components of reproduction. Would-be parents select gamete donors based on qualities that may or may not be heritable (Jordan, 2006), yet exhibit relative disregard for the health or circumstances of surrogates abroad, despite substantiated evidence that the 'gestational environment' can be as determinative of a child's future health as his or her genes. A host of maternal health conditions (hypertension, diabetes, obesity, malnutrition, etc.) and exposures affect blood flow to the placenta, fetal growth, and are associated with birth defects. Furthermore, we are learning how the gestational environment alters a fetus's genetic expression by altering its epigenome – the complex of molecules that surround DNA, activating and inactivating genes – in a process referred to as epigenetic inheritance (Xin et al., 2015). A fetus born through gestational surrogacy therefore has an epigenome that includes (at minimum) material from three parties and will presumably impart this conglomerate DNA to future generations.

Transnational surrogacy is thus the ultimate example of the ART-driven obfuscation of biology and kinship. In the disaggregation of biological and social reproduction, that which is considered to be biological is elevated as the determinative factor of motherhood status. In the context of surrogacy, genetic contributions are categorized as biological, while the biological contributions of gestation are deemed irrelevant, ignored or even reframed as care. As Vora (2009: 12) reports from fieldwork at the well-known Akanksha clinic in Anand, Gujarat:

> The analogy most surrogates use to explain what they are doing is that the womb is like a spare room in a home, where someone else's baby will stay and grow. The baby is a guest – separable from rather than part of the woman's whole body, and thus distinct from the surrogate as a subject.

As the uterus is considered analogous to a room, the surrogate conceives herself (and is conceived by commissioning parties) as a caretaker to its contents and her role as mother is erased. Commissioning parties assert complete parental status, ignoring the biological mothering contributions of the surrogate in a manner that harkens back to the invisibility of domestic caretakers. In doing so, they pick and choose scientific findings. While commissioning parties go to great lengths to secure 'white eggs' from western university graduates with high test scores, they disregard the ethnicity, education and even health of their surrogates, despite data which indicates the inescapable impact of gestation. As with many ART transactions, the commissioning parties choose to ignore the health risks that surrogacy poses to the resulting, longed-for children, as well as to the surrogate.

Guiding principles moving forwards

Thus far our discussion has highlighted the inequities and risks that underlie the disaggregation of biological motherhood. Yet, perhaps we could also think imaginatively about the opportunities this fragmentation might afford. Social acceptance of new familial formations certainly signals the potential for progress among single parents and queer populations, whose suitability for parenting has been historically contested, regulated and denied. Similarly, because women's reproductive capacity and social assignment for childrearing and domestic maintenance have been centrally connected to their subordination across cultures and time, reproductive technologies might have great liberatory potential. The contradictions of the disaggregation of motherhood indicate the rigidity of certain assumptions about biological and social relations, and the concurrent plasticity of others. How might we identify creative possibilities for biological and social reproduction that promote the health, relationships and dignity of everyone involved?

There are individual and public health risks implicated in the fragmentation of biological motherhood, many of which remain understudied and unknown. As with many questions regarding the health ramifications of new technologies, the precautionary principle, which states that caution should be taken in the face of scientific uncertainty, may serve as a guiding framework in the process of vetting the safety and efficacy of the ART procedures used in transnational surrogacy. Thus far, experimentation with reproductive technologies has coincided with their dissemination, revealing substantial hubris, or perhaps indifference, among scientists and corporations who make unfounded positivist assumptions regarding the safety and efficacy of their innovations. Experimental rigour and caution are necessary to safeguard women and children throughout the world, and should not be overlooked in attempts to meet consumer desire or corporate profit.

The technologies discussed in this chapter generate new types of relationships. No matter how you slice it and dice it, people are involved in the creation of every child. What once required two people may now incorporate a cluster, but we urge social recognition and respect for the relationships inherently established between each contributor. As it stands, the relationships between the surrogate and the contracting party, and between the surrogate and the fetus she gestates, are often erased. How might we creatively acknowledge and strengthen these relationships in ways that reflect their meaning and worth?

As we seek solutions for the individuals involved in transnational surrogacy, can we also shift our focus towards the structural forces that shape each of their situations? We need laws and policies that tackle those underlying factors that prompt women in higher-income countries to delay childbearing and address the gender wage gap associated with occupational segregation by gender throughout the world. Given that these structural forces implicate global inequities, is it even possible to protect the health and autonomy of transnational surrogates within the practice? Yet, Pandora's box is open; the fragmentation and technologies exist. How might we construct motherhoods in ways that unleash the liberatory potential of reproductive technologies while simultaneously advancing the agency and autonomy of women across the globe?

References

American Academy of Pediatrics (2012) In vitro fertilization linked to increased risk for birth defects. <https://www.aap.org/en-us/about-the-aap/aap-press-room/pages/In-Vitro-Fertilization-Linked-to-Increase-Risk-for-Birth-Defects.aspx>

Bonduelle M, Wennerholm UB, Loft A, Tarlatzis BC, Peters C, Henriet S and Sutcliffe AG (2005) A multi-centre cohort study of the physical health of 5-year-old children conceived after intracytoplasmic sperm injection, in vitro fertilization and natural conception. *Human Reproduction* 20(2): 413–19.

Castles F (2003) The world turned upside down: below replacement fertility, changing preferences and family-friendly public policy in 21 OECD countries. *Journal of European Social Policy* 13(3): 209–27.

Chavkin W (2008) Biology and destiny: women, work, birthrates, and assisted reproductive technologies. In: Elliott C (ed.) *Global Empowerment of Women: Responses to Globalization, Politicized Religion and Gender Violence.* New York: Routledge, pp. 45–56.

Chavkin W (2010) The globalization of motherhood. In: Chavkin W and Maher JM (eds) *The Globalization of Motherhood: Deconstructions and Reconstructions of Biology and Care.* London and New York: Routledge, pp. 3–15.

Dolak K (2013) Surrogate mother flees halfway across U.S. to save baby from intended parents. *ABC News.* <http://abcnews.go.com/US/surrogate-mother-flees-halfway-us-save-baby-intended/story?id=18668498>

Dunson DB, Colombo B and Baird DD (2002) Changes with age in the level and duration of fertility in the menstrual cycle. *Human Reproduction* 17(5): 1399–1403.

Ergas Y (2013) Babies without borders: human rights, human dignity, and the regulation of international commercial surrogacy. *Emory International Law Review* 27: 117–88.

Evans ML, Littmann L, Louis L, LeBlanc I, Addis J, Johnson M and Moghissi K (1995) Evolving patterns of iatrogenic multifetal pregnancy generation: implications for the aggressiveness of infertility treatments. *Obstetrics & Gynecology* 172: 1750–5.

Frank O, Bianchi P and Campana A (1994) The end of fertility: age, fecundity and fecundability in women. *Journal of Biosocial Science* 26: 349–68.

Gleicher N, Oleske DM, Tur-Kaspa I, Vidali A and Karande V (2000) Reducing the risk of high-order multiple pregnancy after ovarian stimulation with gonadotropins. *New England Journal of Medicine* 343: 2–7.

Jordan ER (2006) An awful alternative to work-study. *Columbia Daily Spectator.* <http://columbiaspectator.com/2006/11/20/awful-alternative-work-study>

Kahn LG and Chavkin W (in press) ARTs and the biological bottom line. In: Michel S, Ergas Y and Jensen J (eds) *Bodies and Borders: Negotiating Motherhood in the 21st Century.* New York: Columbia University Press.

Klatsky PC, Delaney SS, Caughey AB, Tran ND, Schattman GL and Rosenwaks Z (2010) The role of embryonic origin in preeclampsia: a comparison of autologous in vitro fertilization and ovum donor pregnancies. *Obstetrics & Gynecology* 116(6): 1387–92.

Klemett R, Sevon T, Gissler M and Hemminki E (2005) Complications of IVF and ovulation induction. *Human Reproduction* 20(12): 3293–300.

Klip H, Leeuwen FEV, Schats R, Burger CW and for the OPG (2003) Risk of benign gynecological diseases and hormonal disorders according to responsiveness to ovarian stimulation in IVF: a follow-up study of 8714 women. *Human Reproduction* 18(9): 1951–8.

Kopeika J, Thornhill A and Khalaf Y (2015) The effect of cryopreservation on the genome of gametes and embryos: principles of cryobiology and critical appraisal of the evidence. *Human Reproduction Update* 21(2): 209–27.

McDonald P (2000) The 'toolbox' of public policies to impact on fertility: a global view. *Low Fertility, Families, and Public Policies.* Seville: European Observatory on Family Matters.

National Center for Chronic Disease Prevention and Health Promotion, American Society for Reproductive Medicine, Society for Assisted Reproductive Technology (2014) *Assisted Reproductive Technology National Summary Report.* Atlanta, GA: US Dept of Health and Human Services. <http://www.cdc.gov/art/pdf/2012-report/national-summary/art_2012_national_summary_report.pdf>

OECD (Organization for Economic Co-operation and Development) (2011) *Doing Better for Families.* <http://www.oecd.org/els/soc/doingbetterforfamilies.htm>

Patients Beyond Borders (2014) Medical tourism statistics and facts. <http://www.patientsbeyondborders.com/medical-tourism-statistics-facts>

Rudrappa S (2014) Conceiving fatherhood: gay dads and Indian surrogates. In: Inhorn M, Chavkin W and Navarro JA (eds) *Globalized Fatherhood.* New York: Berghahn Books.

Sandin S, Nygren KG, Iliadou A, Hultman CM and Reichenberg A (2013) Autism and mental retardation among offspring born after in vitro fertilization. *JAMA* 310(1): 75–84.

SurrogacyIndia (n.d.) Egg donor process. <http://www.surrogacyindia.com/Egg-Donor-Process.html>

United Nations, Department of Economic and Social Affairs, Population Division (2013) *World Population Prospects: The 2012 Revision, Key Findings and Advance Tables.* Working Paper ESA/P/WP.227. <http://esa.un.org/unpd/wpp/Publications/Files/WPP2012_HIGHLIGHTS.pdf>

Vora K (2009) Indian transnational surrogacy and the disaggregation of mothering work. *Anthropology News*, February. <www.aaanet.org/pdf/upload/50-2-Kalindi-Vora-In-Focus.pdf>

WHO (2013) *Trends in Maternal Mortality 1990 to 2013: Estimates Developed by WHO, UNICEF, UNFPA, The World Bank and the United Nations Population Division.* Geneva: WHO. <http://apps.who.int/iris/bitstream/10665/112682/2/9789241507226_eng.pdf?ua=1>

World Bank (2013) Statistics. <http://data.worldbank.org/indicator/SP.DYN.TFRT.IN>

Xin F, Susiarjo M and Bartolomei MS (2015) Multigenerational and transgenerational effects of endocrine disrupting chemicals: a role for altered epigenetic regulation? *Seminars in Cell & Developmental Biology* 43: 66–75. <http://dx.doi.org/10.1016/j.semcdb.2015.05.008>

2 | CONSTRUCTIONS OF GAY MEN'S REPRODUCTIVE DESIRES ON COMMERCIAL SURROGACY CLINIC WEBSITES

Damien W Riggs and Clemence Due

Introduction

In this chapter we explore the ways in which clinic websites advertising commercial surrogacy services to gay men potentially shape, as well as are shaped by, the desires of gay men not only to become parents but also to conceive genetically related offspring. The websites we examine primarily target reproductive travellers, namely gay men who are unable to access surrogacy services in their own countries due to legislative restrictions. These are men who on the one hand may be viewed as 'reproductive exiles' (Inhorn and Patrizio, 2012; Riggs, 2015a) in that they must leave their country of residency in order to access fertility services, yet on the other hand may be viewed as what Kroløkke and Pant (2012) refer to as 'repropreneurs', a term they coin to describe the role of neoliberalism in the decision-making of those who are depicted as active agents in their reproductivity.

In examining the websites, we seek to identify the types of 'subjects' they produce. In other words, we suggest that not only do the websites potentially respond to the existing desires of some gay men to become parents, but they also shape the forms that such desires take by emphasizing particular factors that are deemed salient to gay men's reproductive decisions. To establish a framework for our analysis of the websites, we begin by providing a brief overview of previous research that has examined gay men's desire for parenthood in the context of commercial surrogacy. After discussing our findings, we conclude by exploring the implications of the types of reproductive desires emphasized within the websites in terms of other individuals (and specifically women who act as surrogates) who are interpellated into the logic of repropreneurship within the context of commercial surrogacy.

Previous research

A small but growing body of research has focused on the desires expressed by gay men when they enter into commercial surrogacy arrangements. Such desires often appear to centre upon the role of a yearning for genetic relatedness in regards to gay men's decisions about family formation. For example, research by Dempsey (2013) with six Australian male couples who had children through surrogacy arrangements found that, while the participants often attempted to downplay genetic relatedness in discussions about their families, that concern nevertheless remained. This focus was most evident in relation to an expressed desire for 'equality' in the chances of conceiving a child, with the privileged role of becoming a genetically related father evident in practices such as alternating who donated sperm.

Other research has produced similar findings. For example, Murphy (2015) reports that participants in his study indicated that they felt that being genetically related to children born through surrogacy arrangements would lead to a more 'complete or "authentic" kinship link' (p. 135). Thus, they expressed their desire to reproduce as something based on a sense of 'naturalness' (p. 137).

As such, research has indicated that gay men are frequently drawn to commercial surrogacy precisely because of the desire for a potential genetic relationship with their child/ren – a relationship that other modes of family formations (such as foster care or adoption) do not provide. Berkowitz and Marsiglio (2007) have similarly commented on gay men's 'fathering desire' – typically predicated on a genetic relationship – as triggering what they term gay men's 'procreative consciousness'. Lewin (2009) argues that such a fathering desire is shaped by normative 'signs' of relatedness or kinship ties such as physical resemblance. Specifically, she argues that surrogacy provides intended parents with the possibility of '"see[ing] something" of themselves in their child' (Lewin, 2009: 68).

In terms of previous investigations of clinic websites, although not focusing specifically on gay men, Hawkins (2012) reports on an analysis of the content of 372 US fertility clinic websites. He notes that the websites in his sample frequently focused primarily on emotional rather than informational content, often using images of (typically white) babies and words such as 'dream' or 'miracle'. This type of content, Hawkins suggests, tended to supersede information that might be considered as critical to decision-making, such as success rates. Hawkins's findings highlight the pivotal role that harnessing desire may play in gay men's decisions to enter surrogacy arrangements, desire that tends to be promoted and (re)produced on surrogacy clinic websites, as our analysis now demonstrates.

Method

For the purposes of this chapter we performed a Google search in order to identify the websites of fertility services that explicitly provide commercial surrogacy services to gay men. Using the search terms 'gay' and 'surrogacy' we initially identified five websites. We then performed another set of searches using these same terms in addition to the names of countries where it was, at the time, legal for gay men to commission a commercial surrogacy (i.e. Mexico, the US and Nepal). This resulted in the identification of seven further websites, giving a total sample of twelve. A summary of these websites is presented in Table 2.1.

Given our specific focus here on gay men, and given that most of the websites include extensive information about the surrogacy process

TABLE 2.1 List of websites identified for analysis

Business name	Location	Website
Baby Joy	Nepal	http://www.babyjoyivf.com
Centre for Surrogate Parenting	California and Maryland	http://www.creatingfamilies.com
Circle Surrogacy	Boston	http://www.circlesurrogacy.com
Growing Generations	Los Angeles, New York, Wheeling	http://www.growinggenerations.com
Mexico Surrogacy	Cancun	http://www.mexicosurrogacy.com.mx
Northwest Surrogacy Center	Portland and San Francisco	http://www.nwsurrogacycenter.com
Surrogacy Cancun	Cancun	http://www.surrogacycancun.com
Surrogacy Center Mexico	Nayarit	http://www.surrogacymexico.com
Surrogacy Nepal	Nepal	http://surrogacycenternepal.com
Surrogate Alternatives	San Diego	http://www.surrogatealternatives.com
The Fertility Institutes	Los Angeles, New York, Mexico	http://www.fertility-docs.com
Viva Family	Los Angeles	http://viva-family.com

which could be subject to analytic scrutiny, we made the decision to concentrate solely on the page(s) on each website that specifically addressed gay men and surrogacy. These pages were collated and subjected to a thematic analysis following the tenets outlined by Braun and Clarke (2006). This involved us both repeatedly reading all of the collated materials and noting key themes that stood out. We then compared our readings and identified the most salient themes, drawing on our knowledge of the literature on gay men and surrogacy as well as on our interest in identifying any novel themes.

Our analysis identified two themes that mirror those found in the literature on gay men and surrogacy: (1) the desirability of genetic relatedness; and (2) surrogacy services as evoking the neoliberal consumer. We also identified a third theme, which although it to a certain degree mirrors broader narratives about surrogacy was also relatively novel – namely the idea that the desire to have a child is universal and that parenthood marks a transition into family life. We now examine in more detail each of these themes.

Results

While we identified twelve websites, the amount of information specifically related to gay intending parents was relatively limited. As such, the following analysis includes all of the extracts pertaining to each theme. Although for the purposes of our analysis we did not scrutinize the images contained on the websites, we would note that on all but one website (Growing Generations) the men featured are light-skinned as were the children, thus reflecting Hawkins's findings in relation to images of white babies on fertility clinic websites.

'Having it your way': the neoliberal consumer The title of this first theme comes from the Growing Generations website. The opening phrase on the page that specifically speaks to gay men is 'Having it your way'. These words encapsulate the neoliberal framing of commercial surrogacy for gay men across many of the websites. Specifically, the phrase frames gay men's desires to become parents as something that should rightfully be tailored to gay men's lives. This idea of surrogacy services being targeted to suit gay men was evident on two other websites:

> Our expert level of care goes beyond equality – as we push forward to meet our LGBT patient's individual needs in a legal and warm locale. We help simplify same-sex couples on their

family building journey by offering services that are not only accessible to them, but structured with them in mind. (Surrogacy Mexico)

We are well aware of the patient 'run-around' aspects encountered by hopeful new parents when dealing with many other providers of similar services. To assure that our patients do not have to endure the non-centralized hardships encountered with most centers offering surrogacy services, our center incorporates all aspects of the gay surrogacy process into one centralized location. (The Fertility Institutes)

In the case of Surrogacy Mexico, surrogacy services are 'structured with [gay intending parents] in mind', and on The Fertility Institutes website a contrast is made between other clinics that allegedly give intending parents the 'run-around' and The Fertility Institutes which 'incorporate all aspects of the gay surrogacy process into one centralized location'. We would suggest that to a certain degree the information outlined on this website provides an answer to the implied 'structuring' that gay intending parents are presumed to desire, namely ease of access. This presumption that what gay intending parents want are surrogacy services that are simple and straightforward is also emphasized on other websites:

In addition, surrogacy is fast, has an extremely high success rate and gives intended parents a high degree of choice and control. (Northwest Surrogacy Center)

As gay intended parents, third party reproduction offers a more convenient parenting option to building tomorrow's families today. Often gay intended parents may have considered adoption as a possible option, but realize the difficulty being gay can pose on their ability to adopt. (Surrogacy Alternatives)

The Northwest Surrogacy Center website perhaps demonstrates the construction of potential clients as neoliberal repropreneurs at its most obvious, in the offer of a 'high degree of choice and control', along with the promise of an 'extremely high success rate'. These statements are paired, we would suggest, given that the good neoliberal citizen would clearly choose a clinic that is successful in delivering the promised service (i.e. a child). Similarly, Surrogacy Alternatives interpellates the neoliberal repropreneur who wants 'convenience' (the paired contrast being with adoption, which is positioned as being either less convenient or indeed inconvenient). The following and final extract in this theme demonstrates the neoliberal framing of gay men's parental desires in arguably its most blatant form on any of the websites:

> It's summer time. While the biggest worry for some of us is where to spend the next vacation, or to limit those ice cream dosages so that the bathing suit will stay intact, I would like to share with you the concern of my very proud, gay-dads-to-be friends, who have begun the journey of gay surrogacy. (Viva Family)

In this blog entry on the Viva Family website, the plans of a gay couple to have a child through commercial surrogacy are listed along with forms of consumption such as choosing a vacation spot. While the author may have not intended to pair a child with decisions about holidays (although they may well have, given Kroløkke's (2015) work on a similar pairing with regard to egg donors), the presentation of these decisions together relies upon a neoliberal logic of consumption in which vacations, children and indeed how much ice cream to eat are all indeed 'choices' to be weighed up and decided upon by the neoliberal consumer.

Across the extracts in this theme, then, gay men's reproductive desires are framed by a neoliberal logic in which there is an injunction upon gay men to desire services that are 'centralized', 'structured', 'fast', 'controlled', 'convenient', and perhaps most importantly, from which they can 'choose'. This type of logic is reflected more broadly in the literature on surrogacy (e.g. Kroløkke and Pant, 2012; Markens, 2012; Riggs, 2015b; Rudrappa, 2010), which suggests that the narrative of choice is problematic when compared with the limited 'choices' often available to women who act as surrogates (a point we turn to in our discussion).

Furthermore, and as we have previously argued drawing on interview data with Australian gay men who undertook a commercial surrogacy arrangement in India, the neoliberal language of 'choice' is problematic in that it may fail to prepare gay men adequately for the potential *lack* of choice they may experience (Riggs *et al.*, 2015). Our point here, of course, is not that gay men do not make agentic choices, nor that they are not consumers within a neoliberal marketplace. Rather, our point is that positioning them as such fails to acknowledge that in some contexts certain decisions (such as being present at the birth or being supported in the face of a pregnancy loss) are denied to gay men in the context of commercial surrogacy arrangements. We suggest, therefore, that while the framing of gay men's desire to become parents through the lens of neoliberalism is an accurate representation of the operations of repropreneurship, it nonetheless overwrites or renders invisible the ways in which this can fail some gay men.

Desirability of genetic relatedness This second theme highlights a concern that has been repeatedly raised in the literature on gay men and surrogacy (e.g. Dempsey, 2013; Murphy, 2013), namely the complex relationship that gay men have to normative discourses of genetic relatedness. This relationship is complex, it has been suggested, because while gay men are located outside the norm of reproductive heterosex, they are nonetheless interpellated into a norm in which genetic relatedness is privileged over other forms of kinship. This is not to say that a desire for genetic relatedness is the only factor driving some gay men to enter into commercial surrogacy arrangements, but it certainly appears to be a factor that shapes the decision-making of some of them. Consequently, the emphasis on genetic relatedness on clinic websites is not surprising, as is evident in the following examples:

> Many of our LGBT clients choose surrogacy over adoption because it allows them to have a genetic relationship with the baby. (Northwest Surrogacy Center)

> With the assistance of an egg donor and a gestational surrogate mother, gay intended parents are provided with the ability to have children biologically related to them, as well as to be recognized as the rightful and legal parents under California surrogacy and egg donation laws ... By choosing the same egg donor, sharing fertilization and transferring an embryo biologically related to each male into your surrogate mother, your dream could come true together. (Surrogacy Alternatives)

The Northwest Surrogacy Center treats a desire for genetic relatedness as a taken for granted fact. Here a paired contrast is made between adoption and surrogacy, with the latter treated as preferable because of the potential for a genetic relationship, a distinction found in other research that reports on the accounts given by parents who have had children through commercial surrogacy (e.g. Riggs, 2015a).

The Surrogacy Alternatives website takes this emphasis upon genetic relatedness a step further by not only emphasizing the fact that surrogacy allows for genetic relatedness, but also by proposing the idea that both men could fertilize eggs from the same donor and so both experience a genetic relationship to a child. While this practice is likely to be known among gay parenting communities (see Lewin, 2009), we would suggest it is notable that the Surrogacy Alternatives website specifically promotes it as a desirable option for gay intending parents, thus tapping into the idea that genetic relatedness *should* be desirable.

The following extract, although it does not specifically address the topic of genetic relatedness, implicitly supports the assumption that an *approximation* of genetic relatedness is considered desirable:

> Many gay intended parents choose an egg donor who has physical characteristics similar to the partner who is not contributing genetic material. Some look for an egg donor who shares their ethnic background. (Circle Surrogacy)

This extract suggests that an intending parent who will not be genetically related to the child might desire a physical resemblance that stands in for a genetic relationship. This mirrors the findings of Mamo (2005), who indicates that lesbian couples may similarly select a sperm donor who resembles the woman who will not be genetically related to the child. As Mamo suggests, such an approach to making decisions about genetic material is complex, as it both complicates how we understand relatedness in terms of physical appearance, and reinforces the desirability of visual similarities as a presumed representation of genetic similarity. This idea of 'matching' intending parents who will not be genetically related with the characteristics of donors of genetic materials also potentially serves to render invisible the role of donors themselves (i.e. by making it appear as though the child is the product solely of the two parents). This point about rendering invisible the role of egg donors is highlighted in the final extract included in this theme:

> The surrogate or egg donor will not be present on the birth certificate unlike the few other global destinations that allow surrogacy for singles and gay couples which makes Tabasco the most appealing destination anywhere for gay surrogacy. (Surrogacy Cancun)

Again, while this extract does not specifically speak to genetic relatedness, we believe it is important to include as it highlights how the potential drive to approximate the norm of two genetically related parents plays out in the context of gay men and commercial surrogacy. In this extract the Surrogacy Cancun website uses the fact that neither women who act as surrogates nor egg donors will appear on the birth certificate, a fact that is treated as a selling point. That this should make the Mexican state of Tabasco 'the most appealing destination' says much about what is seen as desirable by the clinic (and, potentially, gay intended parents), namely that the reproductive labour of women who act as surrogates and egg donors will not be recorded in the child's legal documents. This is a concern that we will return to in our discussion.

Universality of the desire for a child as a marker of family In this third and final theme we focus on two ideas that are frequently paired on the websites: that the desire to have a child is universal and that families only come into existence when adults have a child. Certainly the idea that having a child is a normative feature of the life course of gay relationships is evident in the literature on gay parenting (e.g. Lewin, 2009). What is relatively novel about this theme, however, is that it introduces the idea that a family is only made through adults having children.

In terms of the websites, the first set of extracts below demonstrates the ways in which the desire to have a child is naturalized:

> We strongly feel that the desire to have a child is a universal emotion and should not be treated with bias on the basis of ethnicity, geographical boundaries or sexual orientation.
> (Baby Joy)

> Mid-thirties, Dave is a lawyer and Jonathan is a high school teacher. They met, fell in love, decided they wanted to live happily ever after, did the thing all couples do – got married, and lived their life just like everyone else. Some days super happy, other days grumpy. It's called life. At some point they decided it was time to turn from a couple to a couple with a baby. A family.
> (Viva Family)

> Northwest Surrogacy Center, LLC helps gay intended parents create the families they have dreamed of – and the grandchildren their parents have dreamed of! (Northwest Surrogacy Center)

In these extracts the desire to have a child is depicted as 'a universal emotion', a 'dream' and as part of a normative relationship life course. Although these types of claims are perhaps understandable given that the websites are aimed at attracting new intended parents, the websites also function as a form of homonormativity (Duggan, 2002) by suggesting that gay men, 'just like everyone else', should experience the desire to have a child as a 'universal emotion'. This implies that gay men who do not desire to have a child are somehow either incomplete or not 'just like everyone else'. This form of exclusion is further exemplified in the following extracts:

> A family starts with a baby. It's everyone's dream to have a baby of their own genetic relationship. Surrogacy Center Nepal (SCN) is committed to making dreams come true. SCN will treat the couples who are living together and waiting to fulfill their dream of having babies of their own. (Surrogacy Center Nepal)

> Having children should be a right, and not a privilege, for everybody wanting to start a family ... For many in the gay men community, surrogacy is their best option if they are looking for a fulfilling family experience. (Mexico Surrogacy)

The first extract reinforces claims about desire made both within this theme and the previous one (i.e. that having a child is 'everyone's dream' and specifically a child that is genetically related), in addition to making the claim that 'a family starts with a baby'. This presumption is similarly made in the second extract, which positions having children as a 'fulfilling family experience'. Again, while it is not at all surprising that these websites would normalize the desire for children (given that is what they are selling), in the process they exclude or marginalize families of choice that *do not* involve children (Weston, 1991). In some ways similar to our earlier point about the possible failures associated with surrogacy and how these websites may ill prepare gay men for them, the claims examined in this theme also potentially set some gay men up for failure. In other words, if 'family starts with a baby' and having a baby is 'everyone's dream', then what happens to those gay men who, for various reasons, may be unable to have a child through surrogacy despite that being their desire (i.e. due to a pregnancy loss, infertility or economic reasons)? Furthermore, what does it mean that gay men's 'dream to have a baby of their own genetic relationship' is dependent upon the reproductive labour of others?

Discussion

Mirroring previous research by Kroløkke and Pant (2012), the findings reported in this chapter suggest that commercial surrogacy clinic websites typically position gay men as neoliberal repropreneurs making active choices concerning having children. Also mirroring previous research, our analysis indicates that the websites often emphasized the desirability of the genetic relationship provided by surrogacy (e.g. Dempsey, 2013; Murphy, 2015). It is notable that a focus on gay men's desire was such a prominent feature of the websites reviewed (thereby supporting the work of Hawkins (2012) in relation to the emotive aspects of fertility websites). Finally, while Lewin (2009) has previously suggested that having children is seen by some gay men as part of a normative life course progression, our findings extend this argument by highlighting the ways in which some of the clinic websites further emphasized the idea that a family can *only* be achieved through having a child.

Having provided a critique of the type of neoliberal repropreneur evoked by the websites, it is nonetheless important to acknowledge the broader contexts shaping gay men's desire to have children. Specifically, and as we have argued elsewhere (Riggs, 2015a; Riggs and Due, 2010), a desire to have genetically related children is likely the product of living in western nations where particular forms of kinship are privileged over others; that is, where genetic relationships are privileged over other forms of kinship. For gay men specifically, this investment in genetics may be further exacerbated by the effects of heteronormativity, which function both to close down the range of options deemed viable by gay men wishing to start a family, as well as endorsing a very narrow (i.e. neoliberal, nuclear) version of family to which gay men are expected to subscribe. Indeed, our findings reported in this chapter provide further evidence of this in relation to promoting genetic relatedness as the normative and most desirable mode of kinship.

Nevertheless, and as noted throughout our analysis, this focus on gay men's desires and the emphasis upon normative modes of kinship (that is, the privileging of genetic relationships) is problematic, not least for the ethical issues it poses in relation to the role of women who act as surrogates. In particular, such women are open to commodification – a point taken up in a now significant body of literature that examines the potential constraints on choice experienced by women acting as surrogates as compared to intending parents (Kroløkke and Pant, 2012; Markens, 2012; Riggs, 2015b; Rudrappa, 2010). As such, it is important for gay men intending to undertake surrogacy to engage in a praxis that explicitly connects surrogacy to both a critique of the commodifying effects of commercial surrogacy, and to the role of so-called 'developed' nations in the perpetuation of global inequalities, which result in the production of (particularly non-western) women's bodies as available for commodification.

As a counter to the problematic conflation of kinship with genetics and following Vora (2009), we would note the importance of considering multiple forms of kinship relationships, especially in the context of transnational surrogacy. Vora suggests that women who act as surrogates may be woven into the kinship narratives of intending parents and their families. Obviously claims to kinship with women acting as surrogates have the potential to be taken up in ways that assert inclusion, when in reality they function to feign kinship when really it is not desired. At the same time, however, emphasizing the relationship between intending parents and women who act as surrogates (as well as egg donors) may go at least some way towards encouraging recognition of the global context in which transnational surrogacy occurs, and in which intending parents most often stand to benefit. Taking on a sense of relationship (either at a distance through sharing photos, through the stories that are told about the family formation, or in building a relationship between the parties if desired by each one) may help intending families to recognize the privileges that they hold, and may also help to address issues of commodification.

Furthermore, and again in relation to claims to genetics and kinship, it is important to consider the logic in play when genetics are foregrounded in one instance (i.e. for intending parents) but not in another (i.e. when emphasis is placed upon the woman who acts as the surrogate having no genetic relationship to the child, as mentioned previously in relation to a desire to ensure that no mention of the surrogacy arrangement is recorded on the child's birth certificate). If genetics are made to matter, and if they are seen as central to family formation in some instances, then both gay men and surrogacy clinics must be prepared for the fact that genetics will potentially be made to matter across a range of contexts and relationships, sometimes in ways that work against a desire for a nuclear family. While not likely their intent, the websites analysed in this chapter thus highlight the complexities surrounding commercial surrogacy, specifically with regard to the intersections between desire, agency and kinship.

References

Berkowitz D and Marsiglio W (2007) Gay men: negotiating procreative, father and family identities. *Journal of Marriage and Family* 69(2): 366–91.

Braun V and Clarke V (2006) Using thematic analysis in psychology. *Qualitative Research in Psychology* 3(2): 77–101.

Dempsey D (2013) Surrogacy, gay male couples and the significance of biogenetic parenting. *New Genetics & Society* 32: 37–53.

Duggan L (2002) The new homonormativity: the sexual politics of neoliberalism. In: Castronovo R and Nelson DD (eds) *Materializing Democracy: Toward a Revitalized Cultural Politics*. Durham, NC: Duke University Press, pp. 175–94.

Hawkins J (2012) Selling ART: an empirical assessment of advertising on fertility clinics' websites. *Indiana Law Journal* 88: 1147–79.

Inhorn MC and Patrizio P (2012) The global landscape of cross-border reproductive care: twenty key findings for the new millennium. *Current Opinion in Obstetrics and Gynecology* 24(3): 158–63.

Kroløkke CH (2015) Have eggs, will travel: the experiences and ethics of global egg donation. *Somatechnics* 5(1): 12–31.

Kroløkke CH and Pant S (2012) 'I only need her uterus': neo-liberal discourses on transnational surrogacy. *NORA: Nordic Journal of Feminist and Gender Research* 20(4): 233–48.

Lewin E (2009) *Gay Fatherhood: Narratives of Family and Citizenship in America*. Chicago, IL: University of Chicago Press.

Mamo L (2005) Biomedicalizing kinship: sperm banks and the creation of affinity ties. *Science as Culture* 14(3): 237–64.

Markens S (2012) The global reproductive health market: U.S. media framings and public discourses about transnational surrogacy. *Social Science and Medicine* 74(11): 1745–53.

Murphy D (2013) The desire for parenthood: gay men choosing to become parents through surrogacy. *Journal of Family Issues* 34(8): 1104–24.

Murphy DA (2015) *Gay Men Pursuing Parenthood through Surrogacy: Reconfiguring Kinship*. Sydney: New South Publishing.

Riggs DW (2015a) '25 degrees of separation' versus the 'ease of doing it closer to home': motivations to offshore surrogacy arrangements amongst Australian citizens. *Somatechnics* 5(1): 52–68.

Riggs DW (2015b) Narratives of choice amongst white Australians who undertake surrogacy arrangements in India. *Journal of Medical Humanities* [Epub ahead of print].

Riggs DW and Due C (2010) Gay men, race privilege, and surrogacy in India. *Outskirts: Feminisms along the Edge* 22. <www.outskirts.arts.uwa.edu.au/volumes/volume-22/riggs>

Riggs DW, Due C and Power J (2015) Gay men's experiences of surrogacy clinics in India. *Journal of Family Planning and Reproductive Health* 41: 48–53.

Rudrappa S (2010) Making India the 'mother destination': outsourcing labor to Indian surrogates. *Research in the Sociology of Work* 20: 253–85.

Vora K (2009) Indian transnational surrogacy and the commodification of vital energy. *Subjectivity* 28(1): 266–78.

Weston K (1991) *Families We Choose*. New York: Columbia University Press.

PART TWO

GLOBAL BABIES: WHO BENEFITS?

3 | TRANSNATIONAL SURROGACY AND THE EARTHQUAKE IN NEPAL: A CASE STUDY FROM ISRAEL

Carmel Shalev, Hedva Eyal and Etti Samama

In April 2015, an earthquake hit Nepal. Dozens of Israelis who were in Kathmandu as parents and children born from transnational surrogacy arrangements were stranded amid the disaster. A few dozen women from India were also there as surrogate mothers and caught in the devastation, as well as some women from South Africa who were in Nepal to provide egg cells for potential surrogacy arrangements. Under favourable media coverage and the warm support of public opinion, the drama became the focus of a heroic national rescue operation and immigration procedures were relaxed to allow the immediate travel of the newborns. But at the same time some government officials, feminists and social activists raised concerns about reproductive trafficking. This chapter discusses the dynamics of the transnational surrogacy practices that came to light during these dramatic events.

The earthquake

On Saturday morning, 25 April 2015, the earth shook in Nepal. An earthquake measuring 7.8 on the Richter scale killed thousands of people and many others were rendered homeless. It was followed by several aftershocks that caused great anxiety, and on 12 May another powerful earthquake hit.

Thousands of miles away, in Israel, a different kind of earthquake was felt by the transnational surrogacy brokerage agencies operating in the country. At the time, dozens of surrogates from India were in Kathmandu, on behalf of these agencies, some of them with children or husbands, at various stages of fertilization and pregnancy or after c-section delivery. Young women from South Africa were also there to undergo egg cell retrieval. In addition, there were several dozen Israeli civilians: intended parents, family members and newborn babies, some of them preterm.

The event led to intensive media coverage. Parents described how they evacuated infants from the hospital to find improvised shelter in cars (Zeveloff, 2015) and called upon the government to undertake a rescue operation, since many of them were in Nepal because of legal restrictions on access to surrogacy inside Israel, which is confined to married heterosexual couples. When the second earthquake occurred, a couple anxious for the safety and health of their preterm twins, a son and a daughter, posted a selfie video in which they cried desperately, 'Get us out of here!' (Ynet, 2015).

Government officials at the Ministries of Health, Foreign Affairs and Interior held emergency consultations and decided to facilitate the speedy rescue of the parents and infants through relaxing normal immigration procedures, such as the requirement of a genetic test to ascertain a parent–child relationship (Kamin, 2015). As a matter of course, Israel joined the international humanitarian effort, but its delegation also included neonatal intensive care physicians, nurses and incubators for the care of the infants. Intended parents in Israel awaiting the birth of their children asked to extend the rescue effort to include expectant mothers in advanced stages of pregnancy and immigration officials, in principle, agreed.

However, the Ministry of Justice expressed concern about trafficking in women and insisted that the surrogates should be able to come only of their own free will. Eventually this turned out to be a moot point since the Indian women had travelled to Nepal overland and none of them had passports, without which they could not fly to Israel. Feminists, who were already engaged in the debate on transnational surrogacy, also voiced criticism.

Before exploring the dynamics of the transnational surrogacy practices that came to light during these extraordinary events, we explain the background of the regulatory debate on transnational surrogacy in Israel. We then describe the rescue effort undertaken by Israel's government, the regulatory background to the presence of Israelis in Kathmandu for surrogacy at the time of the earthquake, the agencies' response to the emergency, the experience of one client (intended parent) and the Justice Ministry's concern about trafficking in women. We conclude with some thoughts on bio-piracy.

Methodology We systematically reviewed the widespread coverage of the earthquake in Hebrew-language news media (including Ynet, Mako, Nana, Walla and *Ha'aretz*). We held in-depth interviews with three individuals who were involved: a principal actor in Israel's transnational surrogacy market, one of his clients and a policy-maker.

Two of the interviewees were people with whom we had professional relations in the context of parliamentary debates, policy and academic discussions, and similar public activities. We contacted the third interviewee via Facebook, introducing ourselves to her as researchers and public interest activists. We explained that the interviews would last for no more than two hours, and scheduled them for a time and place at their convenience. At the beginning of the interviews we explained the purpose of the research and after obtaining informed consent we tape-recorded them. We started by asking the interviewees about their general involvement in transnational surrogacy and their particular experience during the earthquake. Otherwise the interviews were unstructured and open-ended. Interviewees were guaranteed anonymity and their names are pseudonyms.

All the quotations in the text come from either media reports or the interviews. What we learn about the women involved in transnational surrogacy arises from these narratives.

Regulatory background

Of all the countries that allow surrogacy, Israel is the most highly regulated. In 1996, the country's parliament enacted a surrogacy law, Surrogate Mother Agreements (Approval of the Agreement and Status of the Child) Law 1996 – hereafter referred to as the Law – which was the first of its kind to allow commercial surrogacy. In essence it requires all surrogacy arrangements to be approved prior to conception by a statutory committee, whose task is to verify numerous conditions designed to clarify the parentage of the child-to-be and protect the rights of the women who carry the pregnancies.

Israel has a liberal jurisprudence that recognizes a constitutional right to parenthood, regardless of marital status and sexual preference. However, according to the Law, only married couples are eligible to enter a surrogacy agreement (as a rule, with single women), while there are legal barriers to access for singles and gay couples. As in other countries, these restrictions, together with a low 'supply' of women willing to act as surrogates in-country, have given rise to transnational surrogacy practices.

Gay rights activism through legal action and political lobbying was a major factor in the appointment of a professional public commission in 2010 (the 'Mor-Yosef Commission'), which published its report in 2012 (Ministry of Health, 2012). The Commission was split as to whether the criteria of eligibility for commercial surrogacy should be extended indiscriminately. The majority view was to maintain the restriction of in-country commercial surrogacy for heterosexual couples only and to answer gay couples' needs through altruistic surrogacy within Israel as well as cross-border arrangements under special regulation. The minority view was to change the Law so that surrogacy would be accessible universally, including for gay couples and single women and men, but only on an altruistic, non-commercial basis.

Consequently, in 2014, after twenty years of closely controlled in-country surrogacy, Israel's government presented a legislative bill that adopted the Commission's majority view and proposed to regulate transnational surrogacy unilaterally through the licensing of local intermediary agencies and the accreditation of medical facilities abroad, on condition that they prove that their activities accorded with the domestic law of the country of destination.

A coalition of feminist organizations had opposed the government's legislative initiative for several reasons (e.g. Lipkin and Samama, 2010). They argued that the bill did not give adequate protection to the human rights of third-party women who are involved in transnational surrogacy as either surrogate mothers or egg cell providers, such as guaranteeing the safety and quality of the medical procedures they undergo. There is ample data from Israel to indicate that surrogate mothers are normally more vulnerable than the intending parents, and in intercountry settings global structural inequalities enhance their vulnerability. However, the government bill left these matters to be settled in a standard contract that would be approved as a precondition for issuing a licence to agencies. In other words, the bill laid down a double standard regarding the rights and interests of the surrogate mothers. Critics also suggested that regulation should follow the intercountry adoption model and that agencies should be not-for-profit organizations acting under central coordinating authorities within the framework of bilateral arrangements between countries of origin and destination.

The legislative process was interrupted in November 2014 when general elections were announced for the following March, and parliament dispersed without changing the current law. Meanwhile the practice of transnational surrogacy was growing rapidly, first in western countries, especially the US, and in recent years in low-income countries such as India and Thailand where the costs are far lower, both for medical services and the payment given to the surrogates. In Israel alone, over 500 children have been born in the last four years via transnational surrogacy (more than the overall number of in-country surrogacy children throughout the twenty-year period since the Law's enactment).

Until 2012, India was the preferred destination for Israelis seeking transnational surrogacy arrangements, but in January 2013 India changed its law to prohibit surrogacy for intended parents who were not married heterosexual couples. Some Israeli agencies moved their activity to Thailand, but soon that country also closed its doors and their operations moved to Nepal. It was here that surrogate mothers and egg cell providers, intended parents and newborn infants, together with other relatives and agency staff (translators, doctors, nurses and other on-the-ground employees) found themselves when the earthquake struck.

The rescue effort

The total number of individuals involved in transnational surrogacy in Kathmandu at the time of the earthquake is not known. According to media reports at least two Israeli agencies were operating there (Zeveloff, 2015). The agent we interviewed for this chapter told us that he could account for over 100 surrogates and family members (children and husbands), eleven women from South Africa who had come to provide eggs for prospective surrogacy pregnancies, twenty to thirty local staff members and approximately fifty Israeli intended parents and family members (grandparents and children) with fifteen newborn infants, including two pairs of premature twins born after thirty-two weeks of pregnancy on oxygen support at the hospital. At least one of the surrogates was in hospital recovering from a c-section delivery. The others, most of them pregnant, were living in shared homes in the city.

The earthquake constituted not a single event but several tremors. After the first tremor people left the hospital in search of a safe place outdoors. One of the parents described the situation at the hospital (Zeveloff, 2015):

The day after the first earthquake the physicians left. The nurses were the only ones around, continuing their watch. A few of the parents decided to take shelter in a car near the hospital. The car became a kind of big incubator, inside there were babies and supplies of oxygen.

News travelled fast via social media and the drama of the babies and their families soon hit the headlines in Israel. Captions on online news sites Ynet and Maariv online included: 'Israelis in Nepal with one-week old babies: "Total chaos"'; 'Parents and babies in a tent at the embassy in Nepal: "Hoping the nightmare will be behind us"'. And when the second quake occurred: 'We tore the tubes with our teeth and ran away' (quoting the parents of twins born after only thirty-two weeks of pregnancy). Reports abounded on the parents' fear and panic and the babies' distress. Public opinion instantly embraced the babies as 'ours'.

Politicians in Israel rose to the challenge of an emergency. Search and rescue efforts for Israelis caught in natural disasters are standard procedure, in addition to sending medical and humanitarian aid for local populations. Only half a year earlier, such efforts had been made to find some forty trekkers caught in an avalanche on the Annapurna range in Nepal. Now, within less than twenty-four hours rescue efforts were underway. Furthermore, Israel's Minister of the Interior announced that the immigration authority would waive regulatory formalities normally required to bring the children into the country, such as DNA tests to establish a parent–child relationship (and to rule out trafficking in babies in contravention of intercountry adoption law).

Early on Sunday morning, a rescue team flew out with professional personnel and equipment and tents for taking care of the babies. *The Times of India* (2015) reported: 'Israel to airlift 25 infants from Nepal born to surrogates.' The agent we interviewed described the government effort as the best he could have hoped for:

> The rescue effort was incredible ... We're good at that, at getting our act together and bringing in airplanes ... They were just wonderful. The media were with us also and we had a direct line to the Foreign Ministry, usually we don't speak to them directly.

By afternoon, the headlines on Walla News were announcing: 'After the quake: surrogates from Nepal will be allowed to come to Israel to give birth.'

The agents also petitioned the Minister of the Interior on behalf of intending parents who were expecting babies, to extend rescue activity to include pregnant women and allow them to come to Israel to give birth under safe and hygienic conditions. Early on 27 April, the Minister gave an interview on a leading political talk show and said he had been in personal contact with the expectant couples, and would allow eight women who were eight to nine months pregnant to come under special visas, because 'when the lives of fetuses are in danger there is no bureaucracy'. A spokesperson for the Foreign Ministry, also interviewed, acknowledged concern about twenty women in the late stages of pregnancy.

However, under the Law, only women resident in Israel can act as surrogates and women cannot be 'imported' into the country for such a purpose. Also, the Foreign Ministry was sensitive to diplomatic relations with India, since the pregnant women were Indian nationals who had crossed into Nepal overland legally, but if any stage of the surrogacy procedure had taken place at home, it would have been illegal. Moreover, the Ministry of Justice said it was essential to verify that the women wanted to come of their own free will, or else airlifting them might amount to 'trafficking in women' (Ynet, 2015) – the first official mention of such concern (as opposed to earlier debates on 'commerce' in egg cells).[1] Eventually, however, it transpired that the women did not have passports as they didn't need them to travel overland from India to Nepal.

Media coverage focused on the plight of the babies. There was no concern about the condition of the surrogates who gave birth either before or after the earthquake and were still in Kathmandu.

Inside the business

The offices of the agency where we interviewed the surrogacy agent (Daniel) are in an apartment in a prime residential location in the centre of Tel Aviv. This is where they hold evening workshops or 'classes' for prospective parents more or less at the same stage of expectancy. Meetings deal with 'remote control' pregnancy, and offer participants instruction on using baby slings, bottle-feeding and first aid. The interior design is minimal and on the walls there are mounted blown-up photos: for example, a group of couples sitting with their babies around the pool of a hotel in India, fifteen babies arranged in carriers in a circle on the floor and twenty Indian women with eight children posing on the steps of their home in Kathmandu with a white man, the agency representative, perching one of the children on his knee.

There were five such homes for the women, each with a caretaker responsible for their needs. The women were free to come and go. They were recruited in Bihar, the most impoverished and backward state in the subcontinent, which borders on Nepal to the southeast of Kathmandu. Many of the women were illiterate. They spoke a local dialect and had no English. Daniel described them as 'girls living scattered like Bedouin without a normal address'. An Indian partner in Delhi pays local agents Rs.50,000 (approximately US$750) for each woman recruited; Daniel didn't know exactly how.

The women were invited to come to Nepal with their husbands and children. Approximately half brought one or two small children, leaving older ones at home; few of the husbands had accompanied them. The women received their payment (US$7,000) either directly or to a 'family' bank account. There were bonuses for twins (US$2,000) and also for c-sections (US$1,500), which the staff ob-gyn doctor presented as the 'best way' to give birth. The result was a c-section rate of 100 per cent: 'It's the doctor's decision ... the women don't really have a choice.'

After Daniel and his partner had a child of their own via surrogacy in the US, they opened the agency in 2008 to seek and establish a more affordable route for others, first in India. When that country closed its doors to gay couples the business moved to Thailand and then to Nepal. At the time there were several IVF clinics in Nepal, but the standard of care was poor. Daniel partnered with a former finance minister who invested money in a new state-of-the-art facility. When transnational surrogacy in Thailand ceased at the end of 2014, in the wake of public outrage at the Baby Gammy case – when a newborn boy with Down's syndrome was abandoned by his Australian intended parents – (Ynet, 2014), he speeded up the opening of the Kathmandu facility. The clinic staff there included an IVF specialist from Germany and an ob-gyn from India, as well as a lab technician trained specially by the agency. But since Nepal does not allow Nepalese women to be surrogates, the women were brought from Bihar, travelling overland by public transport.

At the time of the earthquake, women were at different stages of pregnancy, some awaiting impregnation. Because of intended parents' concern for the well-being of the fetuses and pregnant women, Daniel sent a team of nine with tents and equipment to find the surrogates. The homes were standing, but three had been damaged and needed to be evacuated. Daniel also hired a local doctor with an ultrasound device who went from home to home to examine the women. As it happened, in the earthquake's aftermath, there was an unusually high rate of premature births; this partly explains the high number of such births affected by the second quake, when another rescue operation took place.

There was also a need to take care of the young women from South Africa. But first we need to explain why they were there in the first place. Gay couples pursuing surrogacy require women to provide them with egg cells and like surrogacy there is a large transnational market for their procurement. White South African women are one source of supply because of the preference of western couples for Caucasian offspring.

In principle, the egg cells could be fertilized in the women's country of residence (with sperm transported from the intended parents' country of origin), frozen after fertilization and the resulting embryos transported to the destination country for the surrogate pregnancy. Or the egg cells could be transferred after vitrification (i.e. being frozen). However, freshly procured egg cells are assumed to be more effective than frozen ones in terms of rates of fertilization and freshly fertilized embryos are likewise more effective than frozen ones in producing pregnancies. Recently it has been shown that frozen egg cells and embryos are not necessarily inferior, but it is less costly and more convenient from a business point of view – hence more 'efficient' – for providers to travel to the country of destination and undergo the egg cell extraction procedure there.

According to the agency's scheme, potential providers begin the hormonal treatment that induces super-ovulation in South Africa and travel to Nepal a few days later. On arrival, they receive ultrasound follow-up; optimally the egg cells would mature and be extracted within a few days. All the egg cells from any one cycle are promised to the intended couple who chose the 'donor' as 'theirs'.

Daniel told us that he usually worked with a turnover of ten to fifteen women at any one time. 'Once the egg cells are fertilized, there are always multiple surrogate mothers available for embryo implantation.' He also described an option of 'parallel pregnancies' for intended parents: gay couples often want to have two children, related genetically to each one. 'In our animal side everyone wants their own genetic child,' he said. Most couples do not want to know which is whose, and the woman is impregnated with one embryo from each, which might explain the unusual number of twins or 'twiblings' in gay families. But those who do want to know for sure whose child it is might employ two surrogates at the same time. This was forbidden in India but allowed in Nepal.

At the time of impregnation the women do not know who the intended parents are. Pregnancies are normally carried up to week 38 when a c-section is scheduled, allowing the intended parents to plan for the arrival of the baby. They usually meet the surrogate mother for the first time just before delivery in a café at the clinic. The egg provider is anonymous, unless the intended parents wish to know her identity and she agrees. As a general rule, there is no legal obligation to keep medical records of the egg cell providers and surrogates (including for the children to know) or of the procedures they undergo, and Daniel was the only person who had any information about the women.

In addition to the trauma of the earthquake, the young women needed urgent medical care since they had begun hormone treatment and were at risk of ovarian hyper-stimulation, a potentially life-threatening condition, if the egg cells were not extracted. However, the IVF facility in Nepal had been damaged and the procedure could not be carried out safely there. Two days after the quake, Daniel arranged for the women to fly to a clinic in Thailand, with which he presumably had a connection stemming from when he used to do business there. Owing to the new regulations, the egg cells could not be fertilized in Thailand so they were vitrified instead in the hope that they could be successfully fertilized later.

A client's experience

Most of the Israeli agencies' clients are gay couples, and their views – that the women do it for the money but it is a 'sacred' gesture – are well represented in the political debate around transnational surrogacy. We chose to interview one intended parent, Netta, who was a single woman and might have a different perspective. Her child was born prematurely two months ahead of time, with low birth weight and in need of intensive care, and she had to fly out to Nepal immediately, arriving just before the earthquake.

She said her experience with the agency (i.e. Daniel) had been 'excellent', referring to them as 'hi-tech go-getters'. But in general, she was angry. For example, at the preparation workshop they had talked about 'remote control' pregnancy and some people had been worried about what the women eat and drink, while what she experienced was lack of control. Likewise, she had not been prepared for a premature delivery and never imagined that the baby would need intensive care or that its life might ever be in danger.

She was also angry because she had not been told that all the women gave birth by c-section, until a meeting with the agency lawyer, himself the father of triplets from two surrogates, who said that 35 weeks was the customary time of delivery. This gave her moral qualms:

> The matter of the c-section troubled me a lot. ... I was angry
> they didn't tell me. I heard about it by the way from the lawyer

... They said there were many risks, they're not so good at giving birth naturally, there are all sorts of complications in the hospitals there. You know, somehow there aren't a lot of options. You can stand on your hindquarters, I might have said [something] but it's as if the machinery is sort of well greased. ... The c-section – that's where I felt it wasn't moral. Perhaps if I were more radical in my orientation I would have made a deeper investigation of these points and said it's not for me.

Her first meeting with her surrogate, Mukta took place in public, in the maternity ward at the hospital. It was also the first time they talked. She described the meeting as an emotional experience of mutual appreciation and gratitude, as if she were meeting a long-lost sister or falling in love. But it was also a difficult situation and she had to ask the translator to tell the other women to leave them alone:

The whole meeting with the surrogates, not just with Mukta, was not simple. You see women sitting in front of the TV, waiting for a couple to come from Israel, or after meeting them. Even if you go to the ob-gyn department at Tel Hashomer [one of Israel's largest hospitals] it's not a simple sight. They all look miserable.

She was uncomfortable to learn that Mukta had left one of her children behind in India and was also concerned about exploitation:

When I met Mukta it was clear to me that she and I were not in the same situation. Of course, there's a gap, we're not [of the same] socio-economic status; she's from a very weakened population. She was 26 years old but she looked very fragile and childish ... It was hard for me. She was after a cesarean operation. And she's just a girl. And she gave me a hand and hugged and didn't let go. At first, it was very powerful and moving and I felt as if, you know, [I was meeting] a lost sister. It was very powerful and all the time I told her thank you and I cried.

Netta raised money (anonymously – 'people knew why but not for whom') to compensate Mukta for an unforeseen complication of gestational diabetes. But the love affair ended after Mukta begged her for financial support, saying, 'I brought you a daughter, and I have a daughter who I want to send to university. I want you to give me money.' Netta felt uncomfortable with the pressure, which started to be a nuisance. The translator, an agency employee who also had the job of escorting the women, told her that they compare what they receive as tips from parents and make demands. She advised Netta: 'Don't give her your details, that's a recipe for problems ... our experience has proven it's not good.'

The relationship was abruptly severed by the earthquake. The baby was not well; there had been complications in her care and the Israeli doctor who arrived with the rescue team told Netta to get her out of Nepal as soon as possible.

Reproductive trafficking

There is a thin line between commercial surrogacy and selling babies. Israel's supreme court drew it in a recent judgment, *Anonymous v. Ministry of Welfare and Social Services* (Israel Supreme Court, 1 April 2015), as requiring a genetic relationship between the person who commissions the arrangement and the child. If not, it amounts to commerce in children in contravention of the law on international adoption. Selling babies is also prohibited under the criminal law on human trafficking, which was amended in 2006 to include 'commerce in human beings' for the purpose of 'bearing a child and removing it' (Israel Penal Law, 1977, section 377A).

Yet trafficking in children is one thing and trafficking in women another. Trafficking in women for prostitution had been on the agenda of Israel's Ministry of Justice since the mid-1990s, but more recently officials became concerned about pieces of information they were receiving on transnational surrogacy. In 2012, they submitted a position paper to the 'Mor-Yosef Commission' (Ministry of Justice, 2012). The paper analysed three contracts (two from India and one from Armenia) which had been submitted for the immigration authority's approval, and expressed alarm about women's vulnerability to exploitation, and the 'extreme' objectification, negation of autonomy and degree of control to which, as surrogates, they were subjected.

When we interviewed Maya, a senior official at the Ministry of Justice with both academic and professional expertise in sexual trafficking, she explained that the penal law defines 'commerce in human beings' as 'selling or buying a person or performing some other transaction in a person, whether or not for consideration' (Israel Penal Law, 1977, section 377A). In other words, trafficking occurs when a transaction is performed 'in' rather than 'with' a person. Israeli courts of law ruled, in the context of prostitution, that whether a contract existed or the woman received payment was irrelevant. What mattered was whether she had been treated as a piece of property. Likewise, the cross-border transfer of women as part of the deal is a sign of potential trafficking in human beings.

The position paper indicated several aspects that might amount cumulatively to trafficking. Was it clear that the woman was a party to the transaction or was it her husband? At what stage did she sign the contract, before or after becoming pregnant? In the case of a multiple pregnancy, who decided? Were the risks disclosed and had she understood them? Is she obliged to pay compensation in the case of abortion? Is her payment conditional on giving birth? Is she transferred across borders? Does she have direct contact with the intended parents? Do they know how much money she receives from the large sums they pay the agency? To what degree does she exercise control over her person? Contracts contained sweeping prohibitions against sexual activity and travel, as well as using cosmetics and close control of nutrition and exercise. Some required the women to give notice of any change in address for up to eighteen years. Where they are subject to 24/7 surveillance, clearly they are not free.

Thoughts on bio-piracy

The earthquake in Nepal led to a secondary earthquake in the public debate about transnational surrogacy in Israel that exposed details of the practice. All those involved in such arrangements seem to have a common aim of trying to improve their lives, but there are moral costs to allowing the formation of families in this way. The technology deconstructs the holistic experience of women as people who are active reproductive agents and breaks them down into parts that can be tweaked and controlled and transferred across borders. Rather than treating them as individuals, their bodies are used in bits and pieces, as if they are mere functions for the propagation of the species. Women's fertility has served the needs of others since the dawn of history and they have been instrumentalized as childbearers in the service of economic and political interests. But when progressive medical technology is harnessed to treat women as things, servile bodies fragmented into parts and functions, we have to raise questions of ethics and morality.

Our study shows the agency as a slick operation that worked in the interstices of the law and used a sophisticated business model typical of a hi-tech culture of efficiency and creative problem-solving to satisfy client demand and desire, that includes technology transfer and staff training to establish a facility that answers western standards. The industry controls the women's lives for the duration of the surrogacy procedure (before, during and after pregnancy) under close medical supervision without any degree of autonomy. They and the egg cell providers are removed from their natural environment and support systems and transferred to a strange country where they do not speak the language. At the time of impregnation the surrogates do not know who the intended parents are. They have no say in the medical procedures – the intended parents make those decisions – and it is unlikely they are informed adequately about what to expect. They do not have a common language to communicate with intended parents and have no power to determine what degree of contact or kind of relationship they would like to have with them and the children after birth. And the agency advises its clients not to share any contact information.

The idea that there is freedom of contract serves the market well, but it preserves pre-existing power relationships and imbalances that are enhanced in intercountry settings characterized by structural global inequity. When Mukta asked Netta to support her child's education, she was challenging the structure of the relationship, trying to create a discourse of equality and mutuality based on their shared motherhood. But Netta was afraid of being taken advantage of and the agency translator told her not to cooperate.

The transnational surrogacy industry operates as a grey market that shops for opportunities and takes advantage of loopholes in domestic laws, shifting rapidly between jurisdictions as their regulations are tightened. If surrogacy for gay intended parents is illegal in India, the law is circumvented by recruiting women there and transporting them to Nepal. If surrogacy is illegal in Nepal for Nepalese women, again, the law is circumvented by using women from India. If transnational surrogacy is no longer legal in Thailand and egg cells provided by the South African women cannot be fertilized there, they are simply vitrified and returned to Nepal in a frozen state.

Maya at the Ministry of Justice expressed concern that, if countries continue to restrict transnational surrogacy practices within their jurisdictions, the procedures might eventually be performed on ships outside any territorial waters – like piracy, 'an act resembling robbery on the high seas'. The women are robbed of their personhood within a grey global market that like the high seas is essentially lawless.

As for the element of assault or attack normally associated with piracy, the lawlessness of the market allows a double standard of medical care and a disregard for clinical ethics, including standard practices of informed consent and medical record-keeping for people undergoing invasive interventions. The women, however, are not viewed as patients since they are in the service of the client 'parents' and controlled to that end. Taking advantage of their naiveté, giving birth by c-section is falsely misrepresented as a procedure that would be 'spoiling' them with the best medical technology that would otherwise be outside their reach – a symbol of the kind of lives they might only glimpse in the movies.

Israel is one of many countries whose nationals take advantage of the growing global 'fertility' market. The disaster in Nepal revealed the concrete workings of the baby business and its complexities, all wrought with deep emotions. National public opinion empathized with the gay couples who had become fathers and viewed the rescue effort as heroic. The government turned a blind eye to the tricky circumstances that had resulted in the families being in Nepal in the first place, for the sake of saving the infants' lives. As Maya commented, 'In times of trauma we don't split hairs.' The detailed exposure of the drama in the media seemed to be good for business, normalizing and legitimizing gay families as equal with others.

Meanwhile, in August 2015, the Nepal Supreme Court ordered a stop to transnational surrogacy, pending a decision on a petition to ban commercial surrogacy in the country. Agencies in Israel told the press that 100 children had been born there since the beginning of 2014 and there were ninety currently pregnant women in Kathmandu, but these arrangements would not be affected by the court order (*Ha'aretz*, 2015). Only one month later, a product placement item in the Hebrew-language media announced: 'The Far East closes – Mexico becomes the destination for surrogacy' (Nana10, 2015).

Note

1 The word for 'trafficking' in Hebrew (*sa'khar*) can also be understood as 'commerce', but in the context of surrogacy the sense of 'trafficking' is accurate.

References

Ha'aretz (2015) Nepal has frozen surrogacy for foreigners: only the United States remains open to same-sex couples in Israel. 27 August. <www.haaretz.co.il/news/education/.premium-1.2717273>

Israel Supreme Court (2015) Judgment of 1 April, Administrative Appeal Motion 1118/14. *Anonymous v. Ministry of Welfare and Social Services*.

Kamin D (2015) Israel evacuates surrogate babies from Nepal but leaves the mothers behind. *Time*, 28 April. <http://time.com/3838319/israel-nepal-surrogates>

Lipkin N and Samama E (2010) *Surrogacy in Israel: Status Report 2010 and Proposals for Legislative Amendment*. Haifa: Isha L'Isha – Haifa Feminist

Centre. <http://isha.org.il/wp-content/uploads/2014/08/surrogacy_Eng001.pdf>

Ministry of Health (2012) *Report: The Public Commission on the Legislative Regulation of Fertility and Reproduction (Known as the Mor-Yosef Commission).* Jerusalem: Ministry of Health. In Hebrew at: <www.health.gov.il/English/News_and_Events/Spokespersons_Messages/Pages/20052012_1.aspx>

Ministry of Justice (2012) *Problems and Troublesome Signs in Transnational Surrogacy Cases.* Jerusalem: Ministry of Justice, Office of the National Anti-trafficking Co-ordinator.

Nana10 (2015) Far East closes: Mexico becomes the destination for surrogacy. 25 September. <http://news.nana10.co.il/Article/?ArticleID=1149795>

The Times of India (2015) Israel to airlift 25 infants from Nepal born to surrogates. 26 April. <http://timesofindia.indiatimes.com/world/south-asia/Israel-to-airlift-25-infants-from-Nepal-born-to-surrogates/articleshow/47061640.cms>

Walla News (2015) After the quake: surrogates from Nepal will be allowed to come to Israel to give birth. 26 April. <http://news.walla.co.il/item/2848873>

Ynet (2014) Prohibition of surrogacy in Thailand: no baby factory. 28 November. <www.ynet.co.il/articles/0,7340,L-4597301,00.html>

Ynet (2015) The Israeli delegation to Nepal: flying the premature babies. 12 May. <www.ynet.co.il/articles/0,7340,L-4656498,00.html>

Zeveloff N (2015) Where do Israeli babies come from? Nepal. But after quake, for how long? *Forward*, 27 April. <http://forward.com/news/israel/306944/where-do-israeli-babies-come-from-nepal-but-after-quake-for-how-long>

4 | RECRUITING TO GIVE BIRTH: AGENT-FACILITATORS AND THE COMMERCIAL SURROGACY ARRANGEMENT IN INDIA

Sarojini Nadimpally and Anindita Majumdar

Sama, a Delhi-based resource group working on women's and health issues, has been engaging with ARTs for more than eight years, raising concerns around gender and health rights emerging from the unchecked proliferation of these commercialized technologies including, more recently, surrogacy. Research initiatives by Sama on these issues have contributed to uncovering the social, medical, ethical and economic implications of ARTs on the lives of women accessing them, as well as the role of these technologies as part of a globalized industry. The group's findings and conclusions have located discussions and debates on ARTs within the framework of women's health, women's rights and social justice in India, and have contributed to the consolidation of existing knowledge and analysis of the reproductive tourism industry. This chapter combines findings from the organization's highly influential study on surrogacy, *Birthing a Market* (Sama Resource Group for Women and Health, 2012), with ethnographic data collected during Anindita's doctoral fieldwork on commercial surrogacy and kinship.

Background

Commercial surrogacy in India occupies a terrain of furious debates around ideas of reproductive rights, families and the ethics of technology. These debates emerge from the practice of employing Indian women to fulfil the role of gestates in a technologically induced arrangement involving the donated gametes of commissioning couples and/or that of anonymous donors of sperms and eggs. Enmeshed within such debates are questions regarding the value of the child born from the arrangement, as well as the manner in which the surrogate's contribution is 'measured'. The horror accompanying the commoditization of intimate relationships is seen in how ethics have been framed within public discourses on the commercial surrogacy arrangement (Majumdar, 2014).[1] Yet, the transaction is marked by the way in which the contract is used to control participation in the arrangement, as much as the ways in which the entire process is managed by agent-facilitators (Deepa et al., 2013).[2]

In addition to the clinics that are engaged in providing and promoting ARTs, including surrogacy, the industry in India includes several other actors. These include a wide array of organizations and personnel catering to a national and international clientele: health care consultants, various bodies associated with the hospitality industry, travel agencies, law firms, surrogacy agents, tourism departments and surrogacy hostels. These actors have sprung up to provide diverse kinds of support services to the ART and surrogacy industry. Among them are the recruiters or agents who are central to this chapter

The recruitment process in commercial gestational surrogacy in India follows a set of interconnected chains within a network of agents, surrogates, couples and IVF specialists. Sama's (2012) study found a multi-layered network operating primarily via word of mouth and sometimes through advertisements in local newspapers. Part of this process involved the transition whereby the surrogate becomes a recruiter for other surrogates. Entering the arrangement also followed the trajectory of being an egg donor or attempting egg donation before opting for surrogacy. This helped the women who were considering surrogacy to familiarize themselves with the medication and injection process.

Local networks were used to recruit surrogates; many of those who had successfully undergone the process went back to their neighbourhoods with this purpose in mind. The focus of this chapter is on the process of recruitment that creates a situation of vulnerability for surrogates who otherwise form the core of the arrangement.

Many who have studied the marketing of surrogacy and ARTs (Qadeer and John, 2009; Sama Resource Group for Women and Health, 2010, 2012) have pointed out that the evolution of this competitive service environment has led them to focus on two of the important marketing decision variables: success rate and costs. The process of using the internet as well as mass media to market ARTs, based on these variables, has created a strange paradox: on the one hand, these processes have been normalized and almost routinized (where it no longer seems odd that in the section for advertisements in the fortnightly women's magazine *Woman's Era* one often finds ads for egg donation) and on the other, the actual experience of achieving conception by women (whose bodies/body parts are the sites for most of such interventions) remains invisible.

In a recent mapping of the transnational surrogacy industry, Deepa and colleagues (2013) found that agents or middlemen were essential 'facilitators' defining the modalities of the entire surrogacy arrangement. Indeed, their importance has come to overshadow the role of the IVF specialist her- or himself. Known as 'intermediaries', 'providers of end-to-end solutions', agents are indispensable to the surrogacy arrangement in India (Bisht, 2013). They have identified themselves in the role of the 'ART Banks' as mandated by the Indian Council of Medical Research (ICMR) ART Guidelines (2010).[3] This means that clinics have been gradually outsourcing the work of recruiting surrogates, egg donors and clients to these agents.

As institutionalized biomedical ventures, IVF clinics operate within the arena of market logic or demand and supply. They are driven less by the considerations of treatment and more by the creation of demand. The market for infertility is largely dominated by private interests, the prime players being dedicated infertility/surrogacy clinics in Delhi, Mumbai, Kolkata, Chennai, Bangalore, Hyderabad and other major Indian cities (Deepa *et al.*, 2013). Corporate hospitals have entered the IVF business with specialized wings. In a metropolis like Delhi, many of the clinics are run by the IVF specialists themselves with third-party affiliates usually providing services for claims and cashless health insurance. However, in her ongoing research of surrogacy clinics and agencies in Mumbai, Bisht (2013) found that these intermediaries refer to agents or those who liaise between the clinic, client and the surrogate. In the Delhi data the agents were not specifically known as third-party affiliates (TPAs) but did work with the affiliates identified above. Primarily, the TPA or administrator's work as a conduit was different if seen as an agent, and completely different as a source of funding and investment.

To overcome or avoid negative experiences with a clinic many surrogates and couples contact agencies to make their surrogacy experience more comfortable. Agents, or 'middlemen' in common Indian-English parlance, are a ubiquitous part of Indian, South Asian everyday life. They dominate every aspect of service delivery, from bureaucratic to private, from buying railway tickets to arranging marriages. The difficulty of accessing basic services means that agents are an important part of most negotiations. Often legitimacy in complicated bureaucratic exercises is granted through them (Maunaguru, 2013).

While the medical agent has existed at various levels of treatment and access to medical care for some time, recently the 'medical tourism' agent has emerged as a conduit for patients coming from foreign countries to access health services in India. He or she (usually he) creates networks and linkages between various sectors to facilitate an easier flow of service delivery. Thus, arrangements for meeting with the doctor, hotel reservations, insurance, and so on are provided by agents.

In the case of commercial gestational surrogacy, the recruitment of surrogates is undertaken through a network of doctors, agents and local neighbourhood contacts. The surrogate, as well as her husband, also actively participates in recruiting women as potential surrogates. While the surrogacy agency remains the primary recruiter within this network, others operate in association with the agent in recruiting and disseminating information regarding surrogacy. The nature of this information and how it is circulated has a major impact on the recruitment process and the ways in which the surrogate is positioned within the arrangement.

According to Bharadwaj and Glasner (2009: 9), this is a characteristic of the intersection of the global and the local in the 'bio-crossings' that technologies and the people involved undertake. In such a situation the emergence of a liminal third space is:

> anomalous, that is unpredictable. It provides an open-ended opportunity to critique, challenge and change the state of affairs ... these spaces are both a challenge to the official governance models and to the moves to reformulate the ethical and moral controls on science within India.

While friends or relatives can act as surrogates in altruistic surrogacy arrangements, in commercial surrogacy the surrogates are generally recruited through: fertility clinics that have surrogacy programmes; surrogacy agents and websites or online recruitment links; advertisements in the classified section of magazines (English and Hindi); and voluntary advertising by individuals looking to act as surrogates. Women also hear about surrogacy through local cable TV programmes about IVF technology and clinics, or from media reports about IVF/surrogate births at specific clinics.

In our own work over the last decade we have observed that the hospitals/IVF clinics have links with agencies or independent agents. These, in turn, depend more and more on the formation of chains via word of mouth, often depending on surrogates and egg donors to locate and bring women as potential donors/surrogates to the agents, for which the women are offered a commission. This trend is increasing fast. Egg donors are also considered as potential surrogates.

The agent-facilitators tend to come from a similar socio-economic background as the surrogates and often have formal links with the hospitals, for example, as nurses, procurers of referrals or working as lab technicians. They are also employed for their social skills and for having good networks in their community.

In this chapter, we draw from the narratives of Deepal and Paromita, two such agents working at two different, yet also similar, levels of engagement within the surrogacy process. Their narratives are analysed from the perspective of how the surrogate is not only sourced, but also 'trained' to effectively contribute to the success of the arrangement. This process is far from simple, revealing class and cultural cleavages that the agent-facilitator has to navigate carefully and in which they themselves are also enmeshed.

Recruiting to survive: Deepal

By the time we spoke to him, Deepal Kumar had already arranged more than 150 cases of surrogacy in his six years as an agent. His experiences may resemble a potboiler, but in reality they are representative of the ways in which surrogacy recruitment happens through complicated and unregulated processes that exacerbate inequality and a life on the brink.

Before becoming a marketing agent in a hospital, Deepal had had a contractual job with the gas agency, Bharat Petroleum. After two years he found himself unemployed and unable to sustain himself. While living precariously, he heard about surrogacy and became involved in it 'by mistake' through friends and through his networks in different hospitals and clinics.

Deepal started by hiring his wife as his first surrogate. Initially she refused to believe him, but once she had agreed to participate, the process earned the couple Rs.4 lakhs.[4] He did not discuss the final payment they received. For Deepal, his wife's role as a surrogate helped him to reach potential surrogate clients. As he explained, 'The response is better when one gives an example. Then, slowly, people started coming. The first time, neither the couple nor the doctor gave me money.'

Despite initial squeamishness on the part of the husbands of potential surrogates (it is always preferable to target a wife rather than a daughter, according to Deepal), once they realize how much they can earn it becomes easier to convince them to agree to being part of the arrangement:

Yes, that's because they earn Rs.5,000 to 6,000 [US$74–88], they get Rs.3 to 4 lakhs [averaging US$5,000] in a year. If they are convinced properly, then there are no problems. If you convince them, they agree.

By giving his own example, Deepal was able to appeal to husbands, other male kin and women who were eligible to be surrogates. And even though it was difficult initially, he slowly began to recruit surrogates through what he called 'the chain system':

One surrogate tells others. One comes back with four to five surrogates on average. Like this one, she was nothing, but a woman staying next door did it and told her. She was motivated and has been a donor and is now doing surrogacy. She now says that she wants to tell people once hers is successful. And that will be additional income.

Deepal was paid Rs.25,000 [US$37] each time a new surrogate was introduced, and Rs.5,000 [US$74] for an egg donor. He worked freelance but was attached to a few clinics; he received commission from both the commissioning couples and the surrogate, as his narrative describes. He was very particular about the kind of 'compensation' he could seek for the surrogates and positioned himself in a way that gave him the power to make a contract, laying out the payment required:

I am getting a contract done for four people for Rs.3 lakh 70,000 [US$5,475], with diet, conveyance and all. If you say Rs.5,000 for the diet, then it is Rs.55,000 [US$814] for 11 months. People give diet for only nine months. When you deliver, it's not like it is over. She has to return to the normal state, like she was when I first take [her for surrogacy]. I take medicines from the couple, whatever is needed after delivery also, for the next two, two-and-a-half months. Other people take Rs.4–5 lakh from the couple and then give Rs.2–2.5 lakh [US$3,000] and keep the rest. They don't care about whether the surrogate is taking medicine. Surrogate lives in her home. Is she resting, is she working? They don't care. No care from their side.

Initially, Deepal didn't know that he could charge a commission for arranging a surrogacy, but as his cases grew he began to ask for a 10 per cent commission on each one to avoid getting into haggling over his price:

> I did not know that people take money! Then I told the doctor that one to two cases are done and I have not received any commission. On top of that I was blamed that 'he took commission'. I was angry. They said he's given us this much and kept the rest. Now each couple has different demands, they have their budget. They say we can pay this much, if you want to, do it. So then I started and whatever amount was fixed, 10 per cent was mine. So if it's Rs.4 lakh [US$5,900] then Rs.30,000 [US$440] I keep.

However, Deepal had worked out a way in which he did not have to seek a commission from the surrogate and could also retain a considerable amount from the entire arrangement. Because he reiterated that taking a commission from the surrogate was something unsavoury, he had prefixed the amount he would give her from the entire process. Thus:

> If there is a package of Rs.15–20 lakh [US$22,000–$29,500], it is decided that I take so much from the couple. Then I will give Rs.3.5 or 4 [lakh] to the surrogate. The couple has nothing to do with that. Suppose they agree to Rs.20 lakh, then the surrogate may be given Rs.4 lakh. She'll sign for Rs.4 lakh. This is better. Since taking commission from them [surrogates] is wrong. So I just write the amount on the agreement.

The positioning of his role as a facilitator for the surrogate was part of the overriding theme in his interview. Deepal was helping women and their families by introducing them to surrogacy. He emphasized repeatedly how he did not charge the women but asked for a fraction of their earnings in a staggered manner: 'From surrogates, I don't take payment like that [similar to the way he charges couples], so say the diet is of Rs.8,000, then I give her Rs.5000. That is how. So they don't feel it.'

Deepal's supposed goodwill enabled him to build a network of surrogates. Thus, he mentions how he started recruiting by employing women who had come as surrogates to source other potential candidates:

So when a surrogate came, I told her, 'Tell other women around you,' then I used to say, 'Introduce me.' Then surrogates themselves said they know others – 'Then what will we get?' I said, I will give you something from what I get.

Deepal had to work through different sets of clients to make the arrangement work. Thus, he would pay an amount to the staff of the hospital including the nurse, receptionist and others to facilitate the correct administration of medication to the surrogate, and proper care.

And does the doctor pay you or do you pay the doctor?
Neither pays the other. Doctor does not have any role. They take surrogates from us to develop their business. And I supply. So no give and take there. But there is some with staff.

Staff?
The people who sit outside ... at the reception. If you need to get your work done quickly, you have to give them. I have so many cases, I need to get work done, want appointments. They recommend and do things in our favour. With the doctor, I have a personal touch [sic] but outside, despite a long queue, our work gets done. The medicine, credits and all, I can pay as I want.

How much is given to the staff?
Between Rs.10,000 to 25,000 [US$148–370] ... not monthly but per case. Only one person is paid from the staff ... for the rest there are parties ... all are involved including the doctors. So, for instance, food would be ordered from a restaurant ... especially when the ET[5] is successful, or the surrogate delivers. One box of sweets, food from a restaurant and wine for the male staff.

Supervision of the surrogate during the pregnancy was an important part of Deepal's duties, which he fulfilled by seeking to position each surrogate against the other:

To supervise, I just reach their homes anytime, all of a sudden. Also, jealousy works for us very well – and women are jealous. If one surrogate stays next to the other, they give information about each other.

However, Deepal had also worked out an informal system with a neighbourhood grocer where the surrogate lived, suggesting that he not sell her certain types of food. Such indirect surveillance was carried out through a network of relations and people, leaving Deepal with more time to handle the other modalities within the arrangement.

Navigating couples was another important part of Deepal's task, including taking into consideration their various requests and demands. Most of the commissioning parents he arranged for were non-resident Indians coming from Canada and the US. Indian couples in particular had all kinds of requests regarding the surrogate, including her looks, living conditions and caste affiliation. However, Deepal's primary tasks lay with her, including explaining the arrangement and sustaining her involvement throughout the whole process.

Recruiting to train: Paromita

Paromita's daily rounds included a trip to Clinic A with the surrogates for their check-ups, ETs and other necessary medical tests. She would often take some of the pregnant women for their ultrasounds to another clinic close by (which was run by one of the visiting doctors at Clinic A). On one such occasion, a few of her pregnant surrogates had registered a low Beta hcG test count. When asked about what it meant, she gave a rudimentary idea of the test:

> I am unaware of the technicalities of what the test means, but it usually signifies the health of the embryo-fetus. A '50' on the Beta test means pregnant – after which a 500+ count means that the embryo is growing and is healthy. Both our surrogates have a very low count of 250.

Paromita admonished the surrogate Rubina for the low count, 'Embryo *ko toh khana hain, usko* grow *karna hain… . isiliye khana dena hain*' (The embryo has to eat … it has to grow … that is why you have to give it food). Within a week Rubina had started bleeding and aborted spontaneously.

Paromita knew where the surrogate was positioned within the arrangement. She made sure that they and their husbands understood that the pregnancy was a responsibility (*zimmedari*) that they had been entrusted with. Yet navigating this terrain was difficult, especially when the 'sense of responsibility' on the part of the surrogate and her family was fuelled by financial considerations. She felt that she could empathize with them from her position as a mother of a 7-year-old. In being more 'sympathetic' towards the surrogate and her family's experience of the pregnancy, Paromita insisted that she should live in her own home:

> I want my surrogates to stay in their own homes. But if there is a request for a separate home, we can arrange for it ... but we try to convince our clients that it is best that they stay with their families.

Yet, 'surprise visits' were the norm and included checking up on their living conditions, hygiene, etc. Entry into the surrogacy programme at the Building Futures agency with which Paromita was associated was open only to healthy, married women with one live child. But blood tests and scans often were more important than her marital status or where she lived or her age. 'Only if the doctor says "OK" we recruit the surrogate.'

Although the doctors' perception of the health of the surrogate was the primary marker, interestingly the eligibility of a woman to be a surrogate traversed socio-medical notions of suitability. This was a subjective judgement that created divisions between agent-facilitators and IVF doctors. We discussed one such case with Paromita, recorded in our field notes for 2 August 2011:

> It seems that one of the surrogates I had met earlier, Cheena, had been rejected by the doctor because of her 'appearance'. Referring to her case, Paromita did not think that this was a very good idea as the surrogates had no contribution whatsoever to make to the baby. Neither genes nor looks – they were mere carriers. So this concern for the 'right looking' surrogate seemed to be a little out of place. Paromita noted that the IVF specialist refused to cooperate with the surrogate because she was worried that the couple may not like their child being carried by this woman. [Cheena had buck teeth and was extremely emaciated. The day I met her she had come from her home in a hurry without having had the time to make herself look 'presentable'.] Paromita felt that this kind of objection fell flat because after all it was 'they' [the agency] who were dealing with the couple-clients and not the IVF doctors. So this concern for the couple's sensibilities seemed misplaced. Paromita had retained Cheena for later.

The fetus was important; it was not however the 'baby' but an organism growing in her body that she needed to nurture because she had undertaken to do so contractually. Paromita wanted to stress the responsibility of the pregnancy without creating any emotional linkages or sense of ownership to the fetus. When Building Futures experienced a setback with two of its four surrogates suffering an early miscarriage, Paromita was visibly upset. The kind of money that clients/intended parents invested in the arrangement meant that nothing could be taken for granted.

On the other hand, Paromita was the 'field person'; she recruited surrogates, kept a track of their health and administered prescribed medication during the IVF process. After unsuccessfully trying to recruit women through advertisements in newspapers and social networking websites, Paromita and Kripa (Paromita's associate at the surrogacy agency who liaised with the commissioning couples) decided to try word-of-mouth advertising. This worked better for them as many of their earlier surrogates themselves became 'recruiters', spreading the word among neighbours, friends and relatives in exchange for Rs.6,000 [US$88] for every successful recruitment. In May–June 2011 they had seven surrogates who were either undergoing or had undergone embryo transfers, excluding two who were pregnant with twins and triplets. Paromita outlined the selection procedure: she had to be married (unless she was divorced or widowed), had to have one living child, should live in relatively hygienic conditions and must be healthy, after which the final decision was left to the doctor who tested the women before accepting them into the surrogate programme. Blood tests were an important first step towards ascertaining the health of the potential surrogate, followed by an ultrasound. If all the tests were clear, the woman was asked to sign a contract drafted by the agency's lawyers, but translated into Hindi by Paromita and Kripa for the benefit of the women and their husbands, who were either non-literate or unable to read English. Paromita was particularly vigilant about addressing the surrogates' husbands' concerns regarding the procedure and the arrangement. A detailed explanation of the IVF-surrogacy process was given through an interactive video as well as through verbal explanations. Both the women were very careful about the legalities and illegalities of the arrangement and insisted on referring to the ICMR guidelines for every decision. This also posed a problem as the guidelines are not legally enforceable, leaving their applicability and interpretation in the surrogacy arrangement in a grey zone.

Discussion

The position that agent-facilitators occupy is essential for sustaining the surrogacy arrangement. Their part in managing the process encompasses all the stakeholders involved, including donors, doctors, couples and of course surrogates. Paromita and Deepal fulfil not only the role of recruiting and training surrogates, but also of recreating the structures of inequality that mark the arrangement. So while they manufacture the 'mother-worker' by positioning surrogates within frames of reference that draw from motherhood and in opposition to prostitution (Pande, 2010), they also support an arrangement that inherently recreates cycles of dependence and inequality. It is important to note here that Deepal and Paromita belong to differing class positions: whereas Deepal took to surrogacy as an escape from impoverishment by recruiting his wife as his first surrogate, Paromita is an educated, middle-class woman who joined an international donor agency and sees her role within the surrogacy arrangement as a career move, intended to enhance her professional prospects and deliberately distancing herself from the surrogates she recruits. In that sense, Deepal and Paromita occupy different levels of the tiered structure of recruitment that is central to the surrogacy process.

In recent writings on agents and recruiters in transnational commercial surrogacy, their presentation of their work as 'social workers' (Rudrappa, 2015) seems to help them legitimize their work to surrogates and a larger clientele. However, in the cases of Deepal and Paromita this particular rhetoric was not present. In fact, Deepal presents himself as close to the 'precariat' (Standing, 2011) and thus forced to undertake such work, while Paromita does it as a job, a

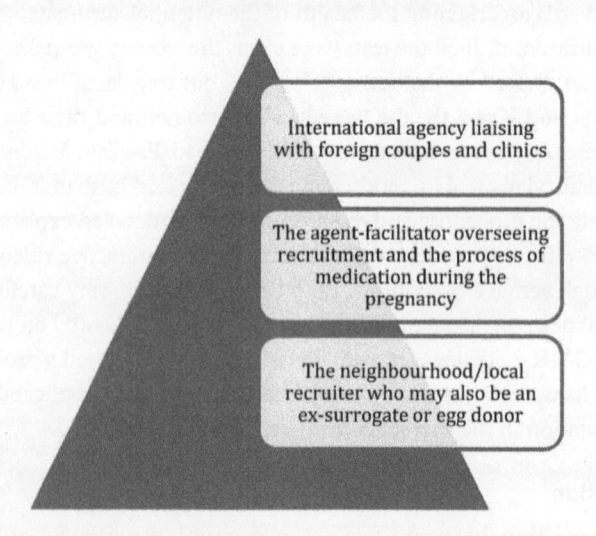

International agency liaising with foreign couples and clinics

The agent-facilitator overseeing recruitment and the process of medication during the pregnancy

The neighbourhood/local recruiter who may also be an ex-surrogate or egg donor

4.1 The three-tiered structure of the agent-facilitators in the commercial surrogacy arrangement

professional requirement. In Deomampo's (2013) research on agents, the work of being a recruiter is a 'move up' from being a surrogate. The material transition and prosperity are a sign of having left behind the necessity of taking on surrogacy for the purpose of earning money.

Though both occupy different terrains, their role within the arrangement resurrects what Saskia Sassen (2002) calls 'counter-geographies of globalization'. In an attempt to alleviate national debt, the state creates export-oriented markets that are often played out through the bodies of women supporting a falling deskilled economy. Here, Deepal occupies a terrain wherein he himself is positioned with his surrogates, navigating an economy that has collapsed and in which he cannot find a suitable form of employment. Thus, he too forms and in turn feeds into a feminization of survival, 'because it is increasingly on the backs of women that these forms of making a living, earning a profit and securing government revenue are realized' (Sassen, 2002: 258). And while Sassen writes of the feminization of survival in relation to sex trafficking, the surrogate agent is also part of this circuit. He enlists the help of ex-surrogates and himself convinces them based on reasoning that helps to create cycles of dependence.

In that sense, Deepal and Paromita also have the power to legitimize the arrangement – by controlling the minutiae involved, both can secure documents, medicines and processes that may otherwise seem problematic. So, for instance, Paromita exercises extra-medical authority (akin to extra-judicial authority) to repudiate the doctor's rejection of a candidate for surrogacy. Similarly, Deepal uses his own experience of being a surrogate's husband to convince others to participate effectively. He reaches out to husbands and uses his experience and authority to draw them in.

The husband's consent is pivotal, making it mandatory in the arrangement. One of the agents we interviewed noted how he approached husbands first. Once convinced of the asexual nature of the arrangement, they would then convince their wives to participate (as evident in an earlier quotation). However, the man may be reluctant to begin with. As one agent notes:

Some people say that this is *do number kakaam* [illegal work]. We say it is not like that. Nobody gets to know whose sample [sperm] it is, so it's OK. So, sometimes gents [husbands] say that we will come along. I take them and show them there is no such problem.

In this way, the agent-facilitator controls the kind of ideology discourse that needs to be shared in recruitment. In Pande's (2014) research it was the idea of the 'good mother'; in the case of Paromita it was a sense of *zimmedari* or responsibility. Whichever worked better, the ex-surrogate as recruiter had already been socialized into it. Thus, she was the best choice for Deepal. In the tapping of local networks for recruiting surrogates a sense of familiarity and trust is clearly helpful.

Hence, a pool of women who are willing to take up this work and look out for other women is created. Some of the surrogates we interviewed spoke about how recruiting other women for egg donation and/or surrogacy was a means of additional income for them. Surrogates were also paid a commission for 'identifying' and 'introducing' other egg donors and surrogates to agents. One of the agents said that she paid approximately Rs.1,100–1,200 [US$16] in the case of egg donors and Rs.25,000–40,000 [US$370–590] to surrogates for 'introducing' other surrogates. This was reiterated by at least three surrogates who stated that they had received commissions for identifying and introducing donors and surrogates to agents. One woman described her plans after returning to her hometown from Delhi, where she had moved for surrogacy: 'When I go back to Indore, I know a lot of women. I will explain it [surrogacy] to them properly since we are on good terms.' Being on good terms is an important aspect of reaching out and talking to women about something intimate and stigmatizing such as surrogacy. This was why whispers regarding surrogacy began to get louder. Some surrogates came to know about it because someone in the family, in the neighbourhood or in the village had been a surrogate or had donated eggs. 'Ladies get to know about such things from each other ... I used to hear of this from everyone where we stay.'

Some of the surrogates we interviewed in Delhi heard about the practice from their local community primarily because the agents operated in localities within neighbourhoods. Agents would help surrogates relocate to areas in their neighbourhoods to facilitate close contact and monitoring of the pregnancy. One of the surrogates interviewed was introduced to the arrangement by her sister-in-law, who had previously been a surrogate herself. Her positive experience stemmed from reassurances she had been given by the agent and the remuneration and care.

Conclusion

Reproductive tourism is clearly a burgeoning trend among ART clinics in India. In recent years, the sharp growth in commercial surrogacy has drawn much attention and raised several concerns. The tendency to market ART abroad has also expanded and shifted to include clinics located in smaller cities and towns with many intermediary third parties. Lower prices seem to be the guiding mantra in the marketing of services overseas. Commercial surrogacy is often portrayed as a win-win situation, seen to give 'desperate and infertile' parents the child they want and poor surrogate women the money they need. The ART industry has flourished because of global trade systems and the business of making mothers and babies. However, the human rights component of issues emerging in the contemporary encounter of globalization, technology, labour and gender requires greater attention. The Draft ART Regulation Bill 2014, in its present form, focuses only on IVF clinics and ART banks and does not take into consideration other parties such as consultancies, clinics, hospitals, legal firms, agents, private agencies and travel agencies, involved in promoting IVF/ART techniques, egg donation and surrogacy. The present Draft Bill must acknowledge the increasing number of 'players' in the ART 'industry' and take measures to specify their role and status in light of this legislation. Complete monitoring and regulation of ARTs will not be possible without looking at this component. Further, the Draft Bill does not adequately dwell on the regulation and monitoring mechanisms for the public hospitals offering these technologies. As long as egg 'donation' and surrogacy procedures continue to be commercialized by the involvement of these agencies in the wider context of 'fertility tourism', any future legislation must take all of these elements into consideration.

Postscript

As this book goes to press, the government of India prepares to table the new Surrogacy (Regulation) Bill 2016. According to the latest news reports, the Bill allows only 'altruistic' surrogacy by a close relative for heterosexual Indian couples who have been married for five years and do not have any children. By effectively putting a bar on homosexual couples and all single persons, the state has constructed a category of people who can become parents in keeping with the wider patriarchal bias of the state and in the law. It conforms to the current legal framework that still does not acknowledge and respect the reproductive and sexual rights of most individuals, particularly the queer. According to the Union Health Minister (Ghosh, 2016):

Doctors are welcome to provide altruistic surrogacy facilities as per provisions of the Bill. The ICMR guidelines on ART treatment are independent of provision of the Surrogacy Regulation Bill, 2016. The intention of the Bill is to ensure there is no commercial surrogacy (and) violation of provision of the Act shall attract strict penal action as per relevant section of the Bill. Guidelines cannot be enforced unless there is legislation.

The ripple effects of a draft law, which awaits the Indian Parliament's approval to come into effect, have been massive and already some surrogacy centres are planning to appeal to the court against the ban.

Notes

1 Although this chapter was written before the Indian government's decision to ban all commercial surrogacy, many surrogacy centres plan to appeal; the debates are far from over.

2 Emerging literature in the area of surrogacy agents oscillates between the terminology used to identify them. Whereas some clinics in India refer to them as third-party affiliates (TPAs), in this chapter we prefer to use the term agent or agent-facilitator.

3 Clause 26 of the ART Bill of 2010 (ICMR, 2010: 20) states the following on the role of ART banks:

'(1) The screening of gamete donors and surrogates; the collection, screening and storage of semen; and provision of oocyte donor and surrogates, shall be done by an ART bank registered as an independent entity under the provisions of this Act.

(2) An ART bank shall operate independently of any assisted reproductive technology clinic.

(3) ART banks shall obtain semen from males between 21 years of age and 45 years of age, both inclusive, and arrange to obtain oocytes from females between 21 years of age and 35 years of age, both inclusive, and examine the donors for such diseases, sexually transmitted or otherwise, as may be prescribed, and all other communicable diseases which may endanger the health of the parents, or any one of them, surrogate or child.

(4) All ART banks shall have standard, scientifically established facilities and defined standard operating procedures for all its scientific and technical activities.

(5) All ART banks shall cryo-preserve sperm donations for a quarantine period of at least six months before being used and, at the expiry of such period, the ART bank shall not supply the sperm to any assisted reproductive technology clinic unless the sperm donor is tested for such diseases, sexually transmitted or otherwise, as may be prescribed.

(6) An ART bank may advertise for gamete donors and surrogates, who may be compensated financially by the bank.

(7) An ART bank shall not supply the sperm of a single donor for use more than 75 times.'

4 Current (January 2016) exchange rate for US$1 = Rs.67 approximately. A lakh in the Indian numbering system is equal to 100,000. Therefore, 4 lakh = 400,000 rupees or around US$5,900. All conversions in square brackets in the text are approximate.

5 This refers to a test to detect Essential Thrombocythemia, a disorder that can cause complications in pregnancy.

References

Bharadwaj A and Glasner P (2009) *Local Cells, Global Science: The Rise of Embryonic Stem Cell Research in India*. New Delhi: Routledge.

Bisht R (2013) Commercial surrogacy and transformations in Mumbai's birth market. Paper presented at Science, Technology and Medicine in India, 1931–2000: The Problem of Poverty, organized by the School of Community Health and Social Medicine, Jawaharlal Nehru University, and the University of Warwick, New Delhi, India.

Deepa V, Rao M, Baru R, Bisht R, Sarojini N and Murray SF (2013) *Sourcing Surrogates: Actors, Agencies, Networks*. New Delhi: Zubaan Publishing Services.

Deomampo D (2013) Transnational surrogacy in India: interrogating power and women's agency. *Frontiers* 34(3): 167–88.

Ghosh A (2016) 'Urgency to introduce surrogacy rules due to number of complaints': Health Minister JP Nadda. *Indian Express*, 3 September. <http://indianexpress.com/article/india/india-news-india/urgency-to-introduce-surrogacy-rules-due-to-number-of-complaints-health-minister-jp-nadda-3010922>

ICMR (Indian Council of Medical Research) (2010) *The Assisted Reproductive Technologies (Regulation) Bill*. New Delhi: Ministry of Health and Family Welfare, Government of India.

Majumdar A (2014) Transnational surrogacy. *Economic and Political Weekly* 48(45–6): 24–7.

Maunaguru S (2013) Transnational marriages: documents, wedding photos, photographers and Jaffna Tamil marriages. In: Palriwala R and Kaur R (eds) *Marrying in South Asia*. Delhi: Orient Blackswan, pp. 253–70.

Pande A (2010) Commercial surrogacy in India: manufacturing a perfect mother-worker. *Signs* 35(4): 969–92.

Rudrappa S (2015) *Discounted Life: The Price of Global Surrogacy in India*. New York: NYU Press.

Qadeer I and John ME (2009) The business and ethics of surrogacy. *Economic and Political Weekly* 44(2): 10–12.

Sama Resource Group for Women and Health (2010) *Constructing Conceptions*. New Delhi: Sama.

Sama Resource Group for Women and Health (2012) *Birthing a Market: A Study of Commercial Surrogacy in India*. New Delhi: Sama.

Sassen S (2002) Women's burden: counter-geographies of globalization and the feminization of survival. *Nordic Journal of International Law* 71: 255–74.

Standing G (2011) *The Precariat: The New Dangerous Class*. London: A&C Black.

5 | GESTATIONAL SURROGACY: HOW SAFE?

Diane Beeson and Abby Lippman

Introduction

Surrogacy, particularly when it spans cultures and legal jurisdictions, has raised a plethora of economic, legal, social and psychological questions. However, despite the concerns increasingly expressed by women's health and human rights activists, its safety and potential risks have received little attention, either in mass media or in policy discussions. For example, the report on global surrogacy practices from the International Forum on Intercountry Adoption and Global Surrogacy in The Hague (Darnovsky and Beeson, 2014) identified numerous problematic health issues related to these arrangements and concluded that our understanding of risks remains inadequate. Failure rates and adverse outcomes for women serving as gestational surrogates, as well as risks for the infants they bear and for the women who provide eggs, are difficult to ascertain. Individual clinic reports are poor or non-existent, and an absence of regional or national registries providing long-term reliable safety and risk information precludes truly informed consent for egg donors and gestational mothers.

In this chapter we offer an overview of some recent medical studies on health risks of the assisted reproductive technologies (ARTs) required for gestational surrogacy, in vitro fertilization (IVF) and egg harvesting, as well as procedures specific to these activities. This is not intended to be an exhaustive review, nor does it address psychological risks. Rather, it primarily draws attention to research gaps and to existing data on health issues that are often ignored by the media but are of importance both to policy-makers and to anyone considering such arrangements, especially those of a commercial nature.

We begin with a brief history of the development of ARTs and then turn to concerns about the health risks for the main parties concerned in transnational surrogacy arrangements: the women who serve as gestational surrogates. We next consider risks to women who provide the eggs that are fertilized in vitro prior to implantation in the uteruses of those who carry the embryos to term, and explore the health consequences of this new beginning of human life for the resulting fetuses, infants and children. We conclude by highlighting the health issues that seem in most urgent need of further research.

Background In 2010, some fifty years since the start of his pioneering work, Robert G Edwards received a Nobel Prize for the development of human IVF as a treatment for infertility (Nobelprize.org, 2010). Building on work done by others on rabbits, he had determined how hormones regulate the maturation process of human eggs. Importantly, but often forgotten, it was only when he and his research partner, Dr Patrick Steptoe, decided to 'follow the patient's own menstrual cycle' rather than manipulate this with hormonal drugs to cause 'superovulation' that they managed to retrieve one naturally matured egg from an Englishwoman, Lesley Brown. After being fertilized in a petri dish this was successfully implanted, as a single eight-celled embryo, into her uterus. Although she was the second woman to become pregnant via IVF without hormonal intervention, she was the first to successfully complete a pregnancy conceived in vitro, culminating in the birth of a daughter, Louise Brown, in 1978.

This strategy of following a woman's natural hormonal rhythms was demanding for patients and their physicians, requiring the surgical team to be on call around the clock (Edwards and Steptoe, 1980). It led Edwards and Steptoe to carry out further research into the complex hormonal processes of ovulation and pregnancy: they hoped to find a way to obtain larger numbers of mature eggs to compensate for subsequent failures in fertilization and implantation. They also wanted to gain greater control over the timing of the release of eggs and to avoid the destructive effects of exogenous hormones on embryos and implantation they had observed earlier.

Other fertility specialists joined these quests, experimenting with various combinations of hormones and harvesting large numbers of oocytes in the hope of fertilizing and implanting them with fewer casualties. Over time, although failure rates remained substantial, success rates did improve and growing numbers of women began to seek similar assistance to circumvent their fertility problems. The 'baby business' soon became big business (Spar, 2006).

Nearly two decades after the birth of Louise Brown, Edwards expressed concern about what had become the typical hormonal approach to ovarian stimulation and the excessive numbers of follicles brought to maturity. He called for less aggressive measures, warning that high-order ovarian stimulation 'could be injurious to women's health', and adding that 'any damage may appear only after several years'. Edwards *et al.* (1996: 918) stressed the need for simpler endocrinological approaches, 'preferably reinforcing the natural cycle and acceptable for successive cycles of mild stimulation'. Still concerned a decade later, Edwards (2007a: 267) noted that '[c]linical and scientific doubts have emerged about the safety and damage that may be caused by routine IVF'. Emphasizing that the methods used to stimulate follicle growth and ovulation were 'too extreme and too expensive', he called on his colleagues to 'rethink' routine IVF in favour of natural cycle or minimal stimulation IVF (Edwards, 2007b: 106).

Despite repeated early warnings from Edwards and others about overly aggressive hormonal manipulation of women's endocrine systems, a global industry now centres on these approaches. In commercial surrogacy today, it is increasingly common for younger women to provide eggs for fertilization and gestation by other women. The recipients include women whose own eggs are no longer viable but who wish to become pregnant, women gestating a pregnancy for others who themselves are unable to carry a pregnancy and men without a female partner.

In Europe and many countries where the sale of human eggs and commercial surrogacy are tightly regulated or prohibited, health concerns are leading to a growing use of natural cycle and minimal stimulation IVF. However, in the US and in other jurisdictions participating actively in the global commercial egg market, more aggressive, heavily drug-dependent approaches that yield eggs in greater numbers remain the norm.

Beyond their exposure to exogenous, usually synthetic, hormones used in IVF, egg providers, gestational mothers and fetuses/infants also face risks from anaesthesia and still unknown surgical and psychological effects. The size of the risks is unknown, and adequate oversight and follow-up tend to be poorest in those jurisdictions where commercial surrogacy is most prevalent. Many of the data on risks come from studies of women undergoing IVF for themselves, often in countries where practices are more closely monitored.

Risks to gestational surrogates

Gestational surrogates face all the usual risks of pregnancy, plus some of those compounded by clinical and commercial practices for IVF. Reports of death and disability associated with women carrying a pregnancy for another are not systematically collected. However, deaths associated with IVF and surrogacy have occurred in India as well as in western countries (Vorzimer, 2011). Interestingly, these cases, when they do come to light, fail to receive the mass media attention given to celebrities who build their families using surrogacy.

While known deaths associated with IVF are not fully understood, some of the poor outcomes may be related to underlying – and undetected – health problems that cause subfertility and the often older ages of the women seeking IVF. Another cause is sometimes ovarian hyperstimulation syndrome (OHSS, discussed further below). These causes may be minimized or eliminated in gestational surrogacy where the contract pregnant woman is younger. But while IVF/gestational surrogacy reduces some medical risks, it introduces new ones.

The most substantial risks related to IVF and surrogacy come from the implantation of multiple embryos. Maternal mortality rates for women experiencing multiple pregnancies are more than double those for women with singleton pregnancies (Horon, 2005: 481; Yazbeck, 2011) and in California between 2009 and 2011, multiple gestations were increased twenty-four- to twenty-seven-fold among women undergoing ART/AI compared to pregnancies conceived without medical intervention (Merritt *et al.*, 2014). This was accompanied by increased rates of c-section and related complications including higher rates of preterm labour and longer hospital stays.

Unfortunately, professional guidelines encouraging single embryo transfer are not necessarily followed in jurisdictions that permit commercial surrogacy (Kawwass *et al.*, 2013). In fact, a review of surrogacy practices in three cities in India (Mumbai, Anand and Delhi) in 2011 and 2012 found that women of all ages typically were implanted with four embryos each, the goal being to produce 'one to two viable fetuses per surrogate mother' after 'fetal reduction' (Rudrappa and Collins, 2015: 945). None of the seventy contract pregnant women interviewed had received information regarding the kinds of medical interventions they would undergo, nor were they told about the health risks of hormonal hyperstimulation. Many were unaware that they would probably deliver by c-section even though almost all had previously given birth to their own children vaginally. Moreover, none of them received postnatal care from the agencies that hired them.

Other sources of elevated risks for gestational surrogates may stem from placental abnormalities, including the pregnancy complication of placenta previa (when the placenta covers the cervix and obstructs delivery), which occurs more frequently (perhaps six times higher) in singleton pregnancies conceived by IVF than in those conceived without medical assistance. Placenta previa can lead to c-sections as well as to haemorrhaging in the second or third trimester and premature birth (Romundstad *et al.*, 2006; Rosenberg *et al.*, 2011). A more subtle consequence of IVF pregnancies also related to the placenta may be the decreased efficiency of this organ. This can potentially lead to restricted fetal growth and low birth weight (Wei *et al.*, 2015).

In contract pregnancies, unlike many other IVF pregnancies, the fertilized eggs a woman carries are not her own. Although there are few studies on the long-term outcome of pregnancies with third-party eggs, the literature conclusively demonstrates an increased risk of complications for the mother (van der Hoorn, 2010), perhaps because she is exposed to complex immunologic interactions unlike those that occur when her own egg is used. In fact, this 'immunologic theory' has been proposed to explain the increased risks for gestational hypertension and preeclampsia that some researchers found in egg donation pregnancies, despite their adjustments for maternal age and several other factors (Levron *et al.*, 2014).

Beyond the elevated pregnancy related risks when IVF and egg donation are used, numerous reports in the medical literature also suggest links between IVF and an increased risk of various cancers. Not all of these risks accrue to the gestational surrogate, however. Some, particularly those related to exposure to exogenous hormones, are transferred to, or at least shared with, the egg provider (discussed below), while other new risks are introduced.

When a woman is contracted for gestational surrogacy, her ability to obtain full and accurate information is always constrained by the absence of research data and a usual lack of independent counsel. But when commercial contracts are signed by a woman who greatly needs the income or who has limited education, as is more often the case in some jurisdictions than others, understanding the process and its risks is even more difficult. This is of special relevance since contracts may limit a woman's control over her own health care, including how she gives birth – with c-sections often encouraged merely for the convenience of the intended parents or treating physician – as well as her choices about fetal reduction, in cases of multiple pregnancies, and pregnancy termination if there are complications or unwanted traits detected in the fetus.

Finally, the woman who gives birth may receive little if any postnatal or other medical follow-up care once a child is born (Rudrappa and Collins, 2015). Moreover, in transnational surrogacy it is typical for the baby to be relinquished to the contracting parent(s) immediately after it is born, and this prevents or interrupts breastfeeding. The latter may lead to future physiological consequences for the woman who gave birth (e.g. higher prevalence of hypertension, diabetes, hyperlipidemia and cardiovascular disease) (Schwartz *et al.*, 2009, 2010) and for the infant (see below).

Risks to egg providers

Only a small percentage of women who provide eggs for commercial surrogacy are the intended mothers; more often, they are healthy young women from various countries (e.g. Georgia, South Africa, Romania, Russia, Ukraine, the US) who 'donate' or, more accurately, sell their eggs for use by others. When eggs are obtained in the US and countries where such a market in eggs flourishes, the usual harvesting practice involves bringing to maturity as many eggs as possible without causing serious injury to the woman from whom they will be extracted.

Eggs are removed surgically using a needle that is pushed through the vagina and into the ovary. Occasionally this procedure punctures an artery or the ureter, causing intra-abdominal bleeding or intestinal and other injuries. As ovaries swell to produce large numbers of maturing follicles, they may twist around a supporting ligament thereby cutting off their blood supply. This is a painful condition that may require removal of the ovary. Such injuries are said to be rare, but with reporting not required in most jurisdictions, their actual frequency remains unknown and the possibility cannot be excluded.

However, the greatest and most frequent risks for egg providers are those associated with the administration of exogenous hormones. While some protocols involve inhaled medications, most require women to self-inject a series of drugs in varying doses daily over a period of two to four weeks. These drugs, commonly including a synthetic hormone that acts on the pituitary, shut down and then stimulate an accelerated process of multiple egg maturation and release. There are individual differences in reactions to these drugs, but in general, the quantity and type of hormones given will affect the number of follicles that develop as well as the likelihood of the greatest and most frequent risk: OHSS (Guidice and Committee Members, 2007: 58). Because eggs are in great demand for reproduction and for research, and because regulation and oversight are virtually non-existent, the economic incentives to increase egg yield by giving high doses of exogenous hormones are significant.

OHSS is an exaggerated response to fertility drugs used to stimulate egg growth and, despite it generally being described as the 'most common' and 'most threatening' risk in women undergoing IVF overall (Guidice and Committee Members, 2007: 57), it is a risk only to the egg provider. Symptoms may include rapid weight gain, pain, diarrhoea, nausea and vomiting. In severe cases, blood vessels become somewhat permeable, allowing fluids to accumulate in the peritoneal cavity. This can lead to the blockage of blood vessels (thrombosis), kidney and other organ failure or, in extreme cases, death. OHSS can occur soon after egg retrieval, or it may be delayed for days, making follow-up essential.

The actual frequency of OHSS (mild, moderate or severe) in women undergoing ovarian stimulation for egg harvesting is unclear; estimates are based primarily on studies of those who are undergoing fertility treatment in an attempt to become pregnant themselves and range from 1 to 10 per cent, with most provider recruiting agencies citing the lower estimates. Because pregnancy is known to increase this risk, some claim that egg providers are actually at lower risk than the IVF patients from whom the data are drawn. However, the age of a woman also matters, with those who are younger and who have more pre-ovulatory follicles to respond to hormonal stimulation actually at increased risk. One British study concluded that, if fewer than twenty follicles are brought to maturity, the risk of OHSS is very small, whereas most non-pregnant women who developed more than twenty follicles did experience adverse symptoms, with 15 per cent of this latter group requiring hospitalization (Jayaprakasan *et al.*, 2007). Making this observation especially troubling are data for 2010 from the US National ART Surveillance System, revealing that more than twenty eggs were retrieved in 40 per cent of donor cycles (Kawwass *et al.*, 2013). Furthermore, the low estimates of OHSS provided by clinics and egg donation agencies are suspect since independent research data are sparse and US egg providers themselves regularly report having much larger numbers of eggs harvested. In one independent retrospective study of 287 egg donors, 30.3 per cent experienced medical complications and 11.6 per cent required hospitalization and/or paracentesis (Kramer *et al.*, 2009).

Fertility clinicians are under great pressure to stimulate a donor to produce the maximum number of eggs as a strategy to increase a recipient's chances of successful implantation. However, there is also sharing of eggs with more than one paying client, whether legally or otherwise, which provides an additional incentive to increase stimulation. Since overstimulation can adversely affect the lining of the uterus and decrease the chance of successful implantation (Kalfoglou and Geller, 2000: 237), there may be greater caution when the eggs will be returned after fertilization to the same woman than when a woman is providing eggs for someone else. Clearly the need for reliable and complete data is growing as the US market in human eggs expands. Women's health advocates have repeatedly called for independent registries to facilitate data gathering – essential if a woman is to provide truly informed consent. These groups also highlight the need for oversight, and for guidelines to manage conflicts of interest and conflicts of commitment by physicians and intermediaries (Blake et al., 2015).

Absence of data does not mean absence of risk

In a 2007 report, the US's Institute of Medicine (IOM) stated: 'One of the most striking facts about in vitro fertilization ... is just how little is known for sure about the long-term health outcomes' (Guidice and Committee Members, 2007: 51). Eight years later, there is still a lack of long-term follow-up research on egg providers and IVF patients in the US. Meanwhile, fertility clinics and egg donor agencies claim that 'Empirical studies have not demonstrated ... any definitive link between egg donation and infertility, cancer, or any other significant long-term health problems' (Infertility Resources, 2015). Most inappropriately, they seem to confuse an absence of data about harm with an absence of harm.

Notably, and despite limited data, the IOM report did consider two potential long-term risks associated with egg donation and IVF: cancers (breast, ovarian and endometrial) and future fertility problems. They dismissed concerns that egg harvesting might compromise future fertility, concluding that 'based on what is known about the biology of follicles over time, we do not think that even repeated donations will cause a woman to have an earlier menopause'. But they, too, confused no data with no risk, adding: 'but again there are no data that tell us that for sure. We don't really know that' (Guidice and Committee Members, 2007: 53).

Because fertility drugs affect the production of a wide range of hormones, not just those involved in pregnancy, they may influence not only the processes of ovulation, but also such functions as blood pressure, mood, general metabolism, kidney functioning, temperature, pain, hunger, sex and sleep (Kiessling, 2007: 40). The extent of these and any other changes is important information for women and clinicians, yet follow-up studies on long-term effects on women are lacking. Furthermore, without registries that monitor and track the health of egg donors, most of what we now know comes from studies that are too small and too short-term to be informative about long-term and low(er) frequency risks (Guidice and Committee Members, 2007: 25). California legislators have responded to the concerns of women's health advocates by passing a law requiring health risk warnings on ads soliciting egg donors. Unfortunately, this law and the professional guidelines that require it are often ignored (Alberta et al., 2014).

In view of the absence of longitudinal studies of women who have been exposed to fertility drugs for long enough and in large enough numbers to provide definitive findings, and the existence of some data suggesting increased overall risks of cancer (Reigstad et al., 2015) as well as higher rates of cancers of specific organs, including ovaries (van Leeuwen et al., 2011; Horlyck, 2015), breast (Pappo et al., 2008; Reigstad et al., 2015), thyroid (Hannibal et al., 2008; Pazaitou-Panayiotou et al., 2014) and the central nervous system (Reigstad et al., 2015), it would seem appropriate to follow the precautionary principle. This might include a moratorium on commercial activities that expose healthy young women to fertility drugs.

Members of the fertility industry often dismiss findings suggesting a risk of cancer, saying that such cases are probably caused not by the drugs, but rather by the underlying infertility of the women being treated. They also tend to emphasize that the increases in risks are quite small. But with some research challenging this claim and that on which reassurances are based being quite limited, or from countries where fertility treatments tend to be more conservative than is usual in jurisdictions that permit commercial surrogacy, caution would seem appropriate. Also, even if the increased cancer rates reported are even partly attributable to the underlying infertility of the women having IVF and not resulting from the drugs used in the process, current protocols often involve much higher exposures to gonadotropins than were given at the time when the women studied were treated (Brinton, 2007: 42). Moreover, while drug protocols continue to change, researchers rarely have information on specific drugs used.

One highly controversial drug widely administered as the 'drug of choice', to both women carrying a pregnancy for another and egg providers, is the potent gonadotropin-releasing hormone analog/agonist (GnRHa) Lupron (leuprolide acetate), which is also distributed under a variety of other names. This drug, which temporarily shuts down the pituitary gland, was first approved by the US Food and Drug Administration (FDA) in 1985 for the treatment of men with advanced prostate cancer and has since been approved for treatment of a few other specific conditions, including endometriosis. However, it has never been approved for use in ARTs. In fact, the FDA classifies Lupron as a 'Pregnancy category X drug', meaning that 'studies in animals or humans have shown positive evidence of fetal risk, and the risk of the use of the drug in pregnant women clearly outweighs any possible benefits'. Consequently, its use in ARTs is 'off label' – legal but questionable.[1]

The US National Institutes of Health (NIH) and the Occupational Safety and Health Administration (OSHA) also classify Lupron as a 'hazardous drug' and advise health care workers to wear protective gowns and gloves when they use it.[2] These US government agencies warn health care professionals who intend to conceive or father a child to avoid handling Lupron or other such hazardous drugs for three months before conception. In response to many requests from women who claim to have suffered serious long-term side-effects from Lupron, US women's health advocacy groups and affected women have repeatedly called for the government to investigate this drug and to fund independent follow-up research, but to no avail (Flinn, 2008). The drug continues to be widely prescribed to egg providers and IVF patients (including gestational surrogates) in the US.

Risks to embryos, fetuses and infants

Although ARTs have enabled many people to have genetically related children, these interventions continue to fail more often than succeed. Failures may occur at fertilization, implantation or at any time during a pregnancy. Even in the US, the surrogacy destination of choice for some of the world's wealthiest commissioning parents, success is very limited. In 2013, only 33 per cent of all reported ART procedures begun with the intention of resulting in a live birth actually did so (Centers for Disease Control, 2015: 3). These figures primarily reflect attempts to overcome infertility, so the age and health of the pregnant woman, and perhaps that of her partner, could partially explain these poor success rates. For gestational surrogacy, where birth mothers are younger and usually of proven fertility, and the eggs or embryos are provided by women under 35, the live birth rates are much higher. For example, 55.3 per cent of pregnancies of 'gestational carriers' resulted in a live birth when the egg/embryo-providing genetic mother was under 35, but this figure dropped to 16.2 per cent when she was aged over 43–4 (Centers for Disease Control, 2013; 2015: 41).

Transferring multiple embryos poses by far the single greatest risk to ART-conceived offspring (American Congress of Obstetricians and Gynecologists, 2005) – and the women pregnant with multiple embryos – mainly because it can lead to multiple births and the serious health consequences that typically accompany them. Multiples are more often stillborn, premature and/or of low birth weight and may experience many medical complications. In their review of US data from 1996–7, Reynolds and colleagues (2001) found that multiple embryo implantations increased the rates of multiple births, but did not improve the chances for a live birth. Reports such as this led to single embryo transfers (SET) being made the standard. But despite professional guidelines, regulations and even laws (e.g. in Sweden) promoting SET, multiple implantation persists in the US and several other countries where commercial surrogacy is increasing. Some medical experts even refer to this as an 'epidemic of multiple gestations', adding that it leads to 'enormous unacceptable human, emotional and financial costs' (Janvier et al., 2011: 413).

In 2012, the most recent year for which figures are available, 'on average, two embryos were transferred per cycle in ART procedures among women aged <35 years' in the US. Among ART births that year, twins were approximately four-and-a-half times more likely than singletons to be born preterm, and approximately six times more likely to have low birth weight (Sunderham et al., 2015).

Often, the choice of how many embryos to implant is left to intending parents making commercial surrogacy arrangements. Unfortunately, however, they are not given proper counselling and so may have little understanding of the medical risks involved with twins. Romanticized impressions of the prospects garnered from mass media may mislead them. Furthermore, commissioning parents may believe that completing their family in one pregnancy this way might also allow them to save time and/or money. In addition, because of high failure rates, clinicians in India commonly implant multiple embryos in two women simultaneously, presenting this as a kind of 'insurance' to the intended parents. In fact, it can result in their taking home two to three infants born of two different surrogate mothers (Rudrappa and Collins, 2015: 945).

All this can encourage intending parents to downplay or ignore the high risks to the pregnant woman, especially in commercial situations, probably in part because these risks are borne by someone else and in part because they are invisible. And while physicians often claim that their clients/patients insist on multiple implantations, critics question clinicians' apparent lack of fiduciary responsibility for fully informed consent.

Some have argued that the risks of implanting multiple embryos can be minimized by 'fetal reduction'. However, this claim ignores research on the 'vanishing twin' (VT) syndrome, the situation when what appears to be a singleton pregnancy actually began as twins with one embryo dying in utero. VT syndrome is 'by no means a rare occurrence' in ART pregnancies and may be associated with higher than usual rates of preterm deliveries, and low and very low birth weight neonates (Almog *et al.*, 2010). There are concerns, too, about a higher frequency of neurological consequences among such births, and researchers have proposed that this information should be provided whenever more than one embryo is transferred (Shebi *et al.*, 2008).

In light of the heavy casualty rates resulting from implanting more than one embryo, some physicians have become increasingly outspoken in support of mandatory single transfer: 'It is time for physicians to accept our responsibility to "first do no harm" in providing safe and highly effective infertility care' (van Voorhis *et al.*, 2013: 5).

Risks to singletons Unfortunately, all risks are not eliminated when only one embryo is implanted and there appear to be more adverse gestational and perinatal outcomes for ART singletons than for spontaneously conceived infants even if their risks are, in general, lower than those for ART multiples (Pinborg *et al.*, 2013). In a meta-analysis of forty-five cohort studies, Australian researchers found an overall 32 per cent increased risk of birth defects when children born following ART were compared with non-ART infants. This risk was slightly greater when singleton births were examined separately (36 per cent) to eliminate the effects of the higher risks known to be more common among multiples. The risks are as high as 42 per cent greater when the focus is on major birth defects in ART singletons only (Hansen *et al.*, 2013: 13). Finally, ART singletons also appear to require longer hospital stays following birth as well as increased risks of being admitted to hospital and of having excess medical costs during their first five years of life (Chambers *et al.*, 2014).

To control for the possibility that these problems reflect the subfertility of women having ART, a recent large California study included a group diagnosed as infertile but who subsequently became pregnant without ART/artificial insemination (AI) (Merritt *et al.*, 2014). The researchers found that the 'infertile' women who became pregnant on their own did have a significantly higher two- to three-fold fold risk of stillbirths compared with other women who had never been labelled 'infertile', but that this was lower than the four- to five-fold increase for all ART pregnancies, an indication that ARTs themselves lead to greater risk. Similar increases were found in rates of preterm labour when subgroups were compared.

Gestational surrogacy based on IVF requires the egg to be handled outside the woman's body, and eggs and sperm and embryos are exposed to the various chemicals and manipulations used in ART at a time when they may be particularly vulnerable to external disturbances. Furthermore, the increasingly common use of intra-cytoplasmic sperm injection (ICSI) in IVF has been linked in a number of studies to higher rates of birth defects, with some attributing problematic outcomes to the subfertility of the males for whom this approach, in which a single sperm is injected directly into an egg rather than exposing an egg to many sperm in a dish, is needed. Because of all the unknowns about specific causes, the American Society of Reproductive Medicine (ASRM) recently concluded that, despite trends to 'normalize' ICSI, existing data do not support its safe routine use for non-male factor infertility (ASRM Practice Committees, 2012: 1397).

Recently too, concern has been raised about potential long-term consequences of IVF conception that might result from possible epigenetic alterations in gene expression generated by the handling of gametes and their exposure to chemicals in culture media.[3] Epigenetic changes do not involve the DNA sequence *per se*, but may still alter postnatal biological and physiological functioning and lead to such consequences as cardiometabolic dysfunction. To date, higher systolic and diastolic blood pressures and triglycerides have been found in children aged 8–18 (Ceelen *et al.*, 2008) and 4–14 years (Sakka *et al.*, 2010) who were conceived after classic IVF compared to controls. These and similar findings point once again to the need for large-scale and long-term outcome studies as well as for more laboratory research, with all investigators also collecting detailed information about the culture media used in IVF and their effects.

While the undetected subfertility in a woman or a man may well explain some of the range of problems observed pre- and postnatally in children born with the use of ARTs, treatment factors themselves can be sources of damage. They include the medications used, length of time an embryo is in culture, the freezing, thawing and manipulation of embryos, altered hormonal environment at the time of implantation, or a combination of these (Chambers *et al.*, 2014; Grace and Sinclair, 2009; Pinborg *et al.*, 2013).

The idea that the human embryo is sensitive to its very early environment should not be surprising, yet uncontrolled variations in the culture media to which it is exposed in the laboratory and varying protocols for handling embryos and their manipulation abound with limited information as to their effects. Unfortunately, much of the research needed here is probably constrained because 'the precise ingredients of each culture medium are tightly guarded commercial secrets' (McLachlan, 2015: 1); many are registered company formulations and detailed protocols are not always provided. Furthermore, it is well known that human embryo development in utero is sensitive to environmental conditions, with direct and subtle epigenetic modifications prior to and after fertilization and implantation not necessarily apparent before adulthood (Grace and Sinclair, 2009). As noted earlier, these too, need further longitudinal study. There are limited data from one group of European researchers who found persistent effects on prenatal growth and birth weight of variations in the type of medium used for culturing human embryos during IVF treatment prior to implantation. Because their study ended when the children reached the age of 2, they themselves call for further long-term monitoring of the growth, development and health of IVF children (Kleijkers *et al.*, 2014). Findings that gene expression is altered by the culture medium used are also reasons for further research, since the long-term effects of these changes on children born after IVF, if there are any, remain unknown (Kleijkers *et al.*, 2015).

Surrogacy risks shared by pregnant women and infants

The possible effects of c-sections C-sections can sometimes be medically necessary and can even save lives, but they can also pose significant additional risks to both the pregnant woman and the infants born through surrogacy arrangements. In a recent California study, 41 per cent of ART/AI pregnancies ended with birth by c-section, a fourfold increase compared with naturally conceived pregnancies (Merritt *et al.*, 2014).

The association of placenta previa with ARTs and the subsequent medical need for c-sections was discussed earlier, but in transnational commercial surrogacy c-sections may not be medically indicated. More often than not, they reflect market and social pressures on the part of commissioning parents who wish either to spend as little time as possible in the surrogate's country or to make advance travel plans. They may also occur merely for the convenience of clinics and physicians. Moreover, these c-sections may be carried out even earlier than the 'normal term' range of 37 to 41 weeks of gestation, as has been reported for children born of Indian surrogate mothers (Rudrappa and Collins, 2015). This is concerning given the close association of gestational age and subsequent development: even those born at 37 and 38 weeks have significantly lower reading and maths achievement scores in the third grade than children born at 39, 40 and 41 weeks (Noble et al., 2012).

There is also evidence that children born by c-section have an increased number of chronic health problems later in life than children born vaginally. These include higher rates of childhood asthma, obesity and type 1 diabetes (Blustein and Liu, 2015). This may relate to how the first bacterial community develops in utero and during vaginal birth as well as to the quality of this colonization and its role in the child's immune system (Neu and Rushing, 2011).

Breastfeeding Breastfeeding and how infants born via surrogacy arrangements are fed has not been given sufficient research attention. At present, the World Health Organization (WHO) recommends that 'infants should be exclusively breastfed for the first six months of life to achieve optimal growth, development and health' (WHO, 2015). Feeding infants with breast milk has been shown to provide numerous benefits for babies, including lower rates of childhood obesity, decreased incidence of asthma and even better brain development. Furthermore, there is mounting evidence that skipping lactation, as women giving birth for commissioning parents are expected to do, seems to put them at higher risk for many serious health conditions, including breast and ovarian cancer, diabetes and cardiovascular disease (Harmon, 2010). Although children born through surrogacy might be bottle-fed with breast milk, obtained either from pumping by the woman giving birth or from banked milk, how often either of these occurs and what effects they may have on bonding and other relationships between the intended parent and child are unknown. More often infants will be given formula milk, which has unknown benefits or risks in ART situations.

Conclusion

Unquestionably, commercial gestational surrogacy has allowed many who could not otherwise have genetically related children to become parents. This makes enthusiasm for these developments understandable, particularly since many children of surrogacy appear to be healthy and developing successfully. Consequently, if one accepts that infertility is a problem deserving of medical attention, it is imperative that efforts at solutions not be allowed to proliferate without more systematic and rigorous attention to long-term consequences and resulting casualties.

The research currently available does not address all or even many of the potential health issues in surrogacy. Nor does it, in and of itself, lead to clear conclusions that commercial gestational surrogacy is necessarily detrimental to, or positive for, the health of women and children. Many of the adverse consequences we have discussed here occur rarely or require confirmation by other researchers. Many may be minimized by adjustments to medical protocols or industry standard practices. Perhaps the clearest conclusion one can draw about gestational surrogacy is that more systematic, independent, long-term follow-up research, on women and children whose bodies are implicated in gestational surrogacy and the technologies on which such arrangements depend, is urgently needed.

The health of IVF/ART-conceived children is of concern to many clinicians and researchers, but existing registries are inadequate for determining accurately what problems may result from the procedures and how the children born will develop in infancy, later in childhood and beyond. The complexity of ART treatments and the (mostly undocumented or reported) variations and constant changes in protocols also make the identification of specific risk factors almost impossible.

No doubt there are serious methodological challenges to determining accurate rates of health problems. For example, Hansen and colleagues (2013) explain that published data on birth defects often do not include some of the most severely affected children who die in the neonatal period, or in the first year after birth. In fact, even the use of ART may not be recorded (to allow comparisons), since the clinicians doing IVF may not be the ones caring for a pregnant woman, assisting at the child's birth or caring for sick newborns. Additionally, birth defect data derived from hospital notes are often incomplete, as are data from birth defect registries, since they rarely actively promote and seek notifications beyond the immediate birth period, or in some instances, even to the end of a pregnancy. And even were data to be accurate and generally complete, many, if not most, of the existing studies include too few women and children to yield accurate risk estimates.

For all these reasons, researchers have emphasized the importance of collecting detailed and accurate information about all treatments that couples have undergone, including their underlying causes of infertility. Imperative, too, are better means of identifying and following all children born subsequent to the use of ART procedures (e.g. via registries) so they can be followed. Until there are such valid, unbiased and reliable data, truly informed consent is not possible; counselling potential users about IVF/ART must be considered *non-evidence-based*; and application of the precautionary principle is warranted.

Given the speed with which reproductive technologies have been deployed and the lucrative nature of the 'baby business', it is essential to learn from women's prior experiences with reproductive medicine about the need for caution. ARTS are not the first interventions to be widely and enthusiastically applied for extended periods of time before their true benefits and harms were known, and there is evidence of serious and widespread health consequences from some of these earlier treatments that enthusiastic adherents were unaware of or ignored. A classic example centres on the synthetic hormone, diethylstilbestrol (DES), a drug commonly prescribed for pregnant women from 1938 to 1971 in the mistaken belief that it would prevent miscarriage. By the time it became clear that DES caused an increased risk of a virulent form of vaginal cancer in their daughters, between five and ten million women worldwide had been exposed. Subsequently, and belatedly, DES was also found to increase risks of reproductive tract abnormalities, infertility and pregnancy complications in daughters, genital abnormalities in sons and increased cancer rates in DES mothers. And the damage may even be multi-generational, something being studied in the US by tracing the grandchildren of the women given this drug to study possible effects (Centers for Disease Control, 2015).

The history of hormone replacement therapy (HRT) for menopausal women is another example where physicians used limited and weak research to encourage healthy women to take exogenous hormones to 'protect' their future health. It was decades before the harmful side-effects of these heavily prescribed medications were documented, and their use in healthy women decreased. Important in the history of both DES and HRT is that grassroots movements were needed for government-supported research to be launched.

Many now fear that ARTs will repeat this history of damage to women and children. These fears are augmented by the expansion of transnational commercial surrogacy and the adoption of neoliberal policies in which women's bodies are increasingly viewed as sites of profiteering when any of the components of commercial surrogacy occur. This context of 'a profit generating industry often values the money brought in by immediate gains of pregnancy and live birth over long-term considerations about the health of the mothers and children' (Kamphuis *et al.*, 2014: 2).

Because public 'education' about ARTs currently comprises fertility industry press releases and mass media stories glamourizing celebrities having successful outcomes, obtaining informed consent from those involved is probably impossible. Women urgently need complete, unbiased, reliable information, but repeated calls by women's health advocates for the appropriate research on a full range of risks and consequences that would provide this remain mostly unanswered (Cool, 2013; Schneider, 2008; Stern, 2015).

Increasingly physicians are sharing women's concerns. European fertility experts, in particular, are challenging conventional approaches to IVF, pointing out their high incidence of OHSS and the increased risks of maternal mortality, chromosomally abnormal oocytes, low birth weight and stillbirth associated with them. They are asking, 'Is the profitability of clinics more important than the benefit of society in general?' and call on fertility doctors to 'ensure that we do no harm to the women who are undergoing IVF treatment, regardless of whether they get pregnant, regardless of whether they have a baby, and that we consider the long-term health of the offspring born as a result of IVF treatment' (Frydman and Nargund, 2014: 1540). They propose following milder, more physiological stimulation protocols, including minimally intrusive approaches in the laboratory, including the reduced use of ICSI wherever possible, and single embryo transfer (Frydman and Nargund, 2014: 1541).

Mild approaches are being embraced by few US fertility specialists or others practising commercial surrogacy, but US perinatologists, concerned about the problems they observe in babies conceived with ART, are pointing out that 'complications occur at enormous cost compared to infants conceived naturally and born at term' (Goldstein *et al.*, 2015: 3).

In conclusion, we can only reiterate a common theme throughout this chapter – the urgent need for more evidence-based and fully independent and accessible information sources for women considering ART – and call for a greater focus on understanding and encouraging what is physiologically more appropriate (Goldstein *et al.*, 2015). Surely women and children are too important ever to be seen primarily as sources of profit, or to be treated as unaware participants in uncontrolled experiments. As Our Bodies Ourselves and other women's health activists, in addition to the National Perinatal Association, urge: we need good, proper and relevant research. Without this IV/ART may be over used and even lead to a potential 'developmental time bomb' (Kamphuis *et al.*, 2014), especially if the use of these technologies creates harmful epigenetic modifications that do not become apparent until adulthood (Grace and Sinclair, 2009). It is late, but is it too late for serious discussion of applying the precautionary principle to ARTs, and to full public debate about how this might happen in the climate of neoliberal individualism and globalization in which the 'baby business' continues to thrive?

Notes

1 See <http://www.fda.gov/Drugs/DrugSafety/ucm350684.htm>.

2 Links to multiple government sources identifying Lupron's 'hazardous' and 'reproductive and developmental toxicant' status can be found at: <www.lupronvictimshub.com>.

3 Culture media refers to the liquid or gel designed to support the growth of micro-organisms or cells.

References

Alberta HB, Berry RM and Levine AD (2014) Risk disclosure and the recruitment of oocyte donors: are advertisers telling the full story? *Journal of Law, Medicine & Ethics* 42(2): 232–43.

Almog B, Levin I, Wagman I, Kapustinsky R, Lessing J, Amit A and Azem F (2010) Adverse obstetric outcome for the vanishing twin syndrome. *Reproductive BioMedicine Online* 20: 256–60.

American Congress of Obstetricians and Gynecologists (ACOG) (2005) Perinatal risks associated with Assisted Reproductive Technologies. *The Committee Opinion.* No. 324, November. <http://www.acog.org/Resources-And-Publications/Committee-Opinions/Committee-on-Obstetric-Practice/Perinatal-Risks-Associated-With-Assisted-Reproductive-Technology>

ASRM Practice Committees (2012) Cytoplasmic sperm injection (ICSI) for non-male factor infertility: a committee opinion. <www.smru.org/uploadedFiles/ASRM_Content/News_and_Publications/Practice_Guidelines/Committee_Opinions/Intracytoplasmic_sperm.pdf>

Blake VK, McGowan ML and Levine AD (2015) Conflict of interest and effective oversight of assisted reproduction using donated oocytes. *Journal of Law, Medicine & Ethics* 43(2): 410–24.

Blustein J and Liu J (2015) Time to consider the risks of caesarean delivery for long-term child health. *British Medical Journal* 350. doi: <http://dx.doi.org/10.1136/bmj.h2410>

Brinton L (2007) Long-term effects of ovulation-stimulation drugs on cancer risk. *Reproductive BioMedicine Online* 15(1): 38–44.

Ceelen M, van Weissenbruch MM, Vermeiden JP, van Leeuwen FE and Delemarre-van del Waal HA (2008) Cardiometabolic differences in children born after *in vitro* fertilization: follow-up study. *Journal of Clinical Endocrinology and Metabolism* 93(5): 1682–8.

Centers for Disease Control (CDC) (2013) *Assisted Reproductive Technology: National Summary Report.* National Center for Chronic Disease Prevention and Health Promotion, Division of Reproductive Health. <http://www.cdc.gov/art/pdf/2013-report/art_2013_national_summary_report.pdf#page=52>

Centers for Disease Control (CDC) (2015) *DES Update: About DES.* <http://www.

cdc.gov/des/consumers/about/history.html>

Chambers GM, Lee E, Hoang VP, Hansen M, Bower C and Sullivan EA (2014) Hospital utilization, costs and mortality rates during the first 5 years of life: a population study of ART and non-ART singletons. *Human Reproduction* 29(3): 601–10.

Cool R (2013) Egg donors create support group for women and push for more safety data. Our Bodies Ourselves, 30 July. <http://www.ourbodiesourselves.org/2013/07/egg-donors-create-support-group-for-women>

Darnovsky M and Beeson D (2014) *Global Surrogacy Practices*. ISS Working Paper Series/General Series 601: 1–54. <http://hdl.handle.net/1765/77402>

Edwards RG (2007a) Are minimal stimulation IVF and IVM set to replace routine IVF? *Reproductive BioMedicine Online* 14(2): 267–70. <http://humrep.oxfordjournals.org/content/11/5/917.long>

Edwards RG (2007b) IVF, IVM, natural cycle IVF, minimal stimulation IVF – time for a rethink. *Reproductive BioMedicine Online* 14(1): 106–19.

Edwards R and Steptoe E (1980) *A Matter of Life: The Story of a Medical Breakthrough*. New York: William Morrow & Co.

Edwards RG, Lobo R and Bouchard P (1996) Time to revolutionize ovarian stimulation. *Human Reproduction* 11(3): 917–19.

Flinn SK (2008) Lupron: what does it do to women's health? *National Women's Health Network Newsletter*. September/October. <https://www.nwhn.org/lupron-what-does-it-do-to-womens-health>

Frydman R and Nargund G (2014) Mild approaches in assisted reproduction: better for the future? *Fertility and Sterility* 102(6): 1540–1.

Goldstein M, Merritt TA and Phillips RM (2015) Assisted reproductive technologies (ART) and in-vitro fertilization (IVF): has the promise been realized? *Neonatology Today* 10(9). <http://www.neonatologytoday.net/newsletters/nt-sep15.pdf>

Grace KS and Sinclair KD (2009) Assisted reproductive technology, epigenetics, and long-term health: a developmental time bomb still ticking. *Seminars in Reproductive Medicine* 27(5): 409–16.

Guidice LC and Committee Members (2007) *Assessing the Medical Risks of Human Oocyte Donation for Stem Cell Research: Workshop Report*. Washington, DC: National Academies Press. <http://iom.nationalacademies.org/Reports/2007/Medical-Risks-of-Oocyte-Donation-for-Stem-Cell-Research--Workshop-Summary.aspx>

Gundogan FD, Bianchi W, Scherjon and Roberts DJ (2010) Placental pathology in egg donor pregnancies. *Fertility and Sterility* 93(2): 397–404.

Hannibal CG, Jensen A, Sharf H and Kjaer SK (2008) Risk of thyroid cancer after exposure to fertility drugs: results from a large Danish cohort study. *Human Reproduction* 23(2): 451–6. <http://www.ncbi.nlm.nih.gov/pubmed/18065402>

Hansen M, Kurinczuk JJ, Milne E, de Klerk N and Bower C (2013) Assisted reproductive technology and birth defects: a systematic review and meta-analysis. *Human Reproduction Update* 19(4): 330–53.

Harmon K (2010) How breastfeeding benefits mothers' health. *Scientific American*, 30 April. <http://www.scientificamerican.com/article/breastfeeding-benefits-mothers>

Horlyck L (2015) IVF linked to increased risk of ovarian cancer. *BioNews*, 26 October. <http://www.bionews.org.uk/page_579635.asp>

Horon IL (2005) Underreporting of maternal deaths on death certificates and the magnitude of the problem of maternal mortality. *American Journal of Public Health* 95(3): 478–82.

Infertility Resources (2015) Risks and side-effects of donating eggs.

<http://www.ihr.com/infertility/egg-donation/for-egg-donors/egg-donor-risks-side-effects.html>

Janvier A, Spelke B and Barrington KJ (2011) The epidemic of multiple gestations and neonatal intensive care unit use: the cost of irresponsibility. *Journal of Pediatrics* 159(3): 409–13.

Jayaprakasan K, Herbert M, Moody E, Steward JA and Murdoch AP (2007) Estimating the risks of ovarian hyperstimulation syndrome (OHSS): implications for egg donation for research. *Human Fertility* 10(3): 183–7.

Kalfoglou AL and Geller G (2000) Navigating conflict of interest in oocyte donation: an analysis of donors' experiences. *Women's Health Issues* 10(5): 226–39.

Kamphuis E, Bhatacharya S and van der Veen F (2014) Are we overusing IVF? *British Medical Journal* 348: g252. <http://www.bmj.com/content/348/bmj.g252>

Kawwass JF, Monsour M, Crawford S, Kissin DM, Session DR, Kulkarni AD and Jamieson J for the National ART Surveillance System (NASS) Group (2013) Trends and outcomes for donor oocyte cycles in the United States, 2000–2010. *JAMA* 310(22): 2426–34.

Kiessling AA (2007) Human eggs: the need, the risks, the politics. *Burrill Stem Cell Report,* October: 38–45. <www.bedfordresearch.org/articles/Burrill-StemCellReport07.pdf>

Kleijkers SHM, van Montifoort APA, Smits LJM, Viechtbauer W, Roseboom TJ et al. (2014) IVF culture medium affects post-natal weight in humans during the first two years of life. *Human Reproduction* 29(4): 661–9.

Kleijkers SHM, EijssenLMT, Coonen E, Derhaag GJ et al. (2015) Differences in gene expression profiles between human preimplantation embryos cultured in two different IVF culture media. *Human Reproduction* 30(10): 2303–11.

Kramer W, Schneider J and Schultz N (2009) US oocyte donors: a retrospective study of medical and psychosocial issues. *Human Reproduction* 24(12): 3144–9.

Levron Y, Dviri M, Segol I, Yerushalmi FM, Hourvitz A, Orvieto R, Nazaju-Tovi S and Yinom Y (2014) The immunilogic theory, of preeclampsia revisited: a lesson from donor oocyte gestations. *American Journal of Obstetrics & Gynecology* 211(4): 383–5.

McLachlan S (2015) IVF culture media may influence sex of embryo. *BioNews* 795, 23 March. <http://www.bionews.org.uk/page_508825.asp>

Merritt, TA, Goldstein M, Phillips R, Peverini R, Iwakoshi J, Rodriguez A and Oshiro B (2014) Impact of ART on pregnancies in California: an analysis of maternity outcomes and insights into the added burden of neonatal intensive care. *Journal of Perinatology* 34(5): 345–50.

Neu J and Rushing J (2011) Cesarean versus vaginal delivery: long-term infant outcomes and the hygiene hypothesis. *Clinical Perinatology* 38(2): 321–31.

Noble KG, Fifer WP, Rauh VA, Nomura Y and Andrews HE (2012) Academic achievement varies with gestational age among children born at term. *Pediatrics* 130(2): e257–64.

Nobelprize.org (2010) The Nobel Prize in Physiology or Medicine. Press release, 4 October. <www.nobelprize.org/nobel_prizes/medicine/laureates/2010/press.html>

Pappo IL, Lerner-Geva A, Halevy A, Olmer L et al. (2008) The possible association between IVF and breast cancer incidence. *Annals of Surgical Oncology* 15(4): 1048–55.

Pazaitou-Panayiotou KK, Toulis S, Mandanas S and Tarlatzis BC (2014) Thyroid cancer after in vitro fertilization: a retrospective, non-consecutive case-series analysis. *Gynecological Endocrinology* 30(8): 569–72.

Pinborg A, Wennerholm UB, Romundstad LB, Loft A et al. (2013) Why do singletons conceived after assisted reproduction technology have adverse perinatal outcome? *Human Reproduction Update* 19(2): 87–104.

Reigstad MM, Larsen IK, Myklebust TA et al. (2015) Risk of breast cancer following fertility treatment: a registry based cohort study of parous women in Norway. *International Journal of Cancer* 136(5): 1140–8.

Reynolds MA, Schieve SA, Jeng G, Peterson HB and Wilcox LS (2001) Risk of multiple births associated with in vitro fertilization using donor eggs. *American Journal of Epidemiology* 154(11): 1043–50.

Romundstad L, Romundstad P, Sunde A, von Düring V, Skjærven R and Vatten L (2006) Increased risk of placenta previa in pregnancies following IVF/ICSI: a comparison of ART and non-ART pregnancies in the same mother. *Human Reproduction* 21(9): 2353–8.

Rosenberg T, Pariente G, Sergienko R, Wiztner A and Sheiner E (2011) Critical analysis of risk factors and outcome of placenta previa. *Archives of Gynecology & Obstetrics* 284(1): 47–51.

Rudrappa S and Collins C (2015) Altruistic agencies and compassionate consumers: moral framing of transnational surrogacy. *Gender & Society* 29(6): 937–59.

Sakka SD, Loutradis D, Kanaka-Gantenbein C, Margeli A et al. (2010) Absence of insulin resistance and low-grade inflammation despite early metabolic syndrome manifestations in children born after in vitro fertilization. *Fertility and Sterility* 94(5): 1693–9.

Schneider J (2008) Fatal colon cancer in a young egg donor: a physician mother's call for follow-up and research on the long-term risks of ovarian stimulation. *Fertility and Sterility* 90(5): 2016.

Schwarz EB, Ray RM, Stuebe AM, Allison MA, Ness RB, Freiberg MS and Cauley JA (2009) Duration of lactation and risk factors for maternal cardiovascular disease. *Obstetrics & Gynecology* 113(5): 974–82.

Schwarz EB, McClure CK, Tepper PG, Thurston R, Janssen I, Mathews KA and Sutton-Tyrrell K (2010) Lactation and maternal measures of subclinical cardiovascular disease. *Obstetrics & Gynecology* 115(1): 41–8.

Shebi O, Ebner T, Sommergruber M, Sir A and Tews G (2008) Birth weight is lower for survivors of the vanishing twin syndrome: a case-control study. *Fertility and Sterility* 90(2): 310–14.

Spar D (2006) *The Baby Business: How Money, Science, and Politics Drive the Commerce of Conception*. Cambridge, MA: Harvard Business School Press.

Stern JE (2015) Informed consent for egg donors won't exist unless we track egg donors' health. Our Bodies, Our Blog. 1 October. <http://www.ourbodiesourselves.org/2015/10/informed-consent-for-egg-donors-wont-exist-unless-we-track-donors-health>

Sunderham S, Kissin DM, Crawford SB, Folger SG, Jamieson DJ, Warner L and Barfield WD (2015) *CDC Assisted Reproductive Technology Surveillance – United States, 2012 Reports*, 14 August, 64(6): 1–29.

van der Hoorn ML (2010) Clinical and immunologic aspects of egg donation. *Human Reproduction* 16(6): 704–12.

van Leeuwen FE, Klip H, Mooij TM, van de Swaluw AMG et al. (2011) Risk of borderline and invasive ovarian tumours after ovarian stimulation for *in vitro* fertilization in a large Dutch cohort. *Human Reproduction*. <http://humrep.oxfordjournals.org/content/early/2011/10/19/humrep.der322.full.pdf+html>

van Voorhis B, Levens ED and Hill MJ (2013) Should single-embryo transfer be mandatory in patients undergoing IVF? *Contemporary*

OB/GYN, 1 November. <http://contemporaryobgyn.modernmedicine.com/contemporary-obgyn/content/tags/vitro-fertilization/should-single-embryo-transfer-be-mandatory-patie?page=0,0>

Vorzimer A (2011) Outsourcing surrogacy in India. *The Spin Doctor*, 22 November. <http://www.eggdonor.com/blog/2011/11/22/outsourcing-surrogacy-india>

Wei Y, Shuquiang C, Xiuying H, Sin ML, Guanghou S and Fangzen S (2015) Assisted reproduction causes intrauterus growth restriction by disrupting placental lipid metabolism. *bioRxiv*, 8 November. <http://biorxiv.org/content/early/2015/11/08/030965>

WHO (2015) World Health Organization's infant feeding recommendation. <http://www.who.int/nutrition/topics/infantfeeding_recommendation/en>

Yazbeck C (2011) Elective single embryo transfer for all patients? *Middle East Fertility Society Journal* 16(3): 182–4.

6 | THE FERTILITY CONTINUUM: RACISM, BIO-CAPITALISM AND POST-COLONIALISM IN THE TRANSNATIONAL SURROGACY INDUSTRY

France Winddance Twine

Introduction

In 2013, in their first report on pan-European altruistic and commercial surrogacy, the Policy Department for European Legal and Parliamentary Affairs revealed that '160 million European citizens have no full access to donor procedures in their own country' (Brunet *et al.*, 2013: 26). Consequently, those seeking to form a family with children who are genetically related to them are increasingly motivated to travel across national borders to procure Assisted Reproductive Technologies (ARTs) that are not legal in their native country. According to Market Data Enterprises (2013) more than 3 million babies have been born worldwide using ARTs; the US fertility services market alone, including surrogacy, produces over 50,000 babies per year in the US via 152,000 IVF procedures and is worth $3.5 billion dollars. India, which liberalized its economy in the 1990s, was, until recently, a magnet for an international clientele seeking ARTs and, at the time of writing, ranks ahead of the US as the world's largest supplier of gestational surrogates.[1] The Confederation of Indian Industry anticipated that medical tourism, including surrogacy, would generate US$2.3 billion by 2012 (Pande, 2014b: 88).

Surrogacy is a form of commercial or 'contract' labour that involves purchasing the 'reproductive' labour of a third party in order to conceive a baby and carry it to term. It constitutes a type of 'stratified reproduction', a concept introduced by the anthropologist Shellee Colen (1995: 78) to explain how:

> physical and social reproduction tasks are accomplished differently according to inequalities that are based on hierarchies of class, race, ethnicity, gender, place in the global economy ... The reproductive labor of bearing, raising, and socializing children ... is differentially experienced, valued and rewarded according to

inequalities of access to material and social resources in particular historical and cultural contexts.

Poor and/or married mothers, who need supplemental income, often sell their reproductive labour to more economically privileged individuals or couples from diverse racial, ethnic and national backgrounds.

In this chapter I draw upon several qualitative studies of gestational surrogacy in India (Krølokke and Pant, 2012; Pande, 2009, 2010, 2014a; Vora, 2009), a documentary film (*Made in India*, 2010) and critical race studies (Roberts, 1998, 2009, 2015; Smith, 2005) to consider the following questions. How can we understand commercial surrogacy as part of a larger history of fertility regulation and the reproductive injustice embedded in colonial and post-colonial histories and hierarchies? What role do neoliberal discourses and global capitalism play in the transnational surrogacy industry? How do gestational surrogates in India strategically employ their bio-capital and assert their 'constrained' agency as female contract labourers? What steps can the industry take towards reproductive justice? The chapter ends by suggesting a way forward that encourages far greater regulation together with a reproductive justice agenda that takes into account structural inequalities related to poverty, women's reproductive health and women's reproductive rights.

The fertility continuum: from sterilization abuse to surrogacy

A history of fertility regulation in the US The US has a history of sterilization abuse dating back to the late 1800s and the rise of the 'eugenics' movement, a socio-political campaign that promoted the reproduction of the 'fittest' and set out to limit reproduction of the unfit or those deemed to have 'inferior' genes. Early eugenicists embraced sterilization as a means of addressing the problems of poverty and to achieve the goals of racial regeneration of White Anglo-Saxon Protestants (WASPs) and 'improve the quality of future generations'. In 1907, Indiana became the first state to pass eugenics laws, followed by California, the largest state by population in the US, which established a eugenics programme in 1909. Initially the people targeted for sterilization were individuals who had mental and/or physical disabilities and resided in state mental institutions. However, sterilization programmes were expanded to include poor people on welfare, racial minorities, unmarried women deemed promiscuous, children who were victims of rape, people who were blind, deaf or had other disabilities, and alcoholics. Journalistic reports on coerced sterilizations (e.g. Johnson, 2013) reveal that informal eugenics programmes were still operating in California prisons as recently as 2010.

The US embrace of sterilization as a part of a eugenics programme was conceived and financed by elites before the rise of the National Socialism (Nazi) Party in Germany (Hansen and King, 2013). Between 1909 and 1964, eugenics was officially practised in thirty-three US states, including California where an estimated 20,000 people were sterilized, among them women who were considered immoral or 'bad' mothers.

This type of reproductive abuse involving controlling the fertility and reproductive labour of enslaved, colonized and later impoverished and unmarried 'free' women has been central to European and Anglo-American colonial and post-colonial projects on both sides of the Atlantic. For example, in *Conquest: Sexual Violence and American Indian Genocide*, Andrea Smith (2005), a Native American scholar, details the sterilization programmes established throughout the US in areas where Native Americans (also referred to as American Indians within their community) were concentrated. During the late 1960s when activists created the American Indian Movement (AIM), a civil rights movement that challenged the ongoing neo-colonial policies and discrimination faced by Native Americans, the US government secretly targeted Native women for sterilization (Smith, 2005: 81–2):

> Native women became targets of the population craze when Indian Health Services (IHS) initiated a federally funded sterilization campaign in 1970. Connie Uri, a Cherokee/Choctaw medical doctor, was one of the first people to uncover this mass sterilization of Native women in the 1970s after a young Indian women entered her office in Los Angeles in 1972 and requested a 'womb transplant'. Upon further investigation, Uri discovered that the woman had been given a complete hysterectomy for birth control purposes when she was 20 years old and had not been informed that the operation was irreversible. The woman was otherwise completely healthy.

Uri and other activists pressurized Congress to investigate until finally a Democratic Senator, James Abourezk from South Dakota, requested a study of IHS sterilization policies. The ensuing report, issued by the General Accounting Office in 1976, revealed that '3,001 Native women of childbearing age, or approximately 5% of all Native women of childbearing age in these areas, were sterilized between 1973 and 1976' (Smith, 2005: 81).

Against this backdrop of enforced fertility regulation embedded in colonial and post-colonial histories, ARTs and the commercial surrogacy industry must be analysed from the perspective of a holistic reproductive justice agenda that addresses 'the social reality of inequality, specifically, the inequality of opportunities that we have to control our reproductive destiny' (Ross, n.d.).

Building upon the work of distinguished North American critical race feminists, Andrea Smith and Dorothy Roberts, I argue that there is a 'fertility continuum' that sorts women into a global 'reproductive caste system'. This continuum has been central to the enforcement of post-colonial and post-socialist hierarchies of race, caste, class and gender. It includes domestic and international population control incentives to restrict the fertility of lower-income women, racial and ethnic minorities or unmarried women. Poor women can be offered access to contraception or sterilization while more economically privileged women can afford to pay for ART therapeutic treatments that enhance their fertility.

In *Killing the Black Body: Race, Reproduction and the Meaning of Liberty* (1998), Dorothy Roberts, a US Black scholar, provides a historically grounded analysis of the denial of reproductive liberty to Black women both during and after slavery. She has scrutinized the relationship between eugenics, sterilization and surrogacy, in particular the critical role of state-sanctioned White supremacist policies in the surveillance and regulation of Black women's fertility.

Describing the medical abuse of US Blacks who were diagnosed with sickle-cell anaemia, Roberts argues that where new reproductive technologies have been directed towards Blacks they have been used to restrict procreative freedom, not increase it. More than a decade later, she revised her earlier arguments and writes (Roberts, 2009: 784):

> Rather than place these [Black and White] women in opposition, I tied them together in relation to the neoliberal trend toward privatization and punitive governance. Both population control programs and genetic selection technologies reinforce biological explanations for social problems and place reproductive responsibility on women, thus privatizing remedies for illness and social inequity.

On 7 July 2013, the Center for Investigative Reporting published an article by Corey G Johnson titled 'Female inmates sterilized in California prisons without approval' (retitled when reproduced in the *Guardian* on 8 November). The reader learns that: 'Former inmates and prison advocates maintain that prison medical staff coerced the women, targeting those deemed likely to return to prison in the future.' Johnson goes on to call attention to an ongoing pattern of sterilization abuse:

> Doctors under contract with the California Department of Corrections and Rehabilitation sterilized nearly 150 female inmates from 2006 to 2010 without required state approvals ... From 1997 to 2010, the state paid doctors $147,460 to perform the procedure, according to a database of contracted medical services for state prisoners.

California lawmakers had banned forced sterilizations in 1979. Since 1994, elective sterilizations have required approval from top medical officials in Sacramento, the state capital, on a case-by-case basis. The revelation that women were being pressured to accept sterilization provoked outrage.

The history of enforced sterilization in the US has certain parallels with the state management of women's reproduction as a means of controlling certain sectors of the population of post-colonial India.

Post-colonialism and fertility regulation in India The use of state-sanctioned technologies designed to restrict and control the fertility of women is an important element in the lives of Indian women who decide to become gestational surrogates. In *Wombs in Labor*, Amrita Pande (2014a) clarifies the similarities between the control of poor women, Black women, Native Americans and others in the US and that of Indian women.

In India, in the late nineteenth and twentieth centuries the management of childbirth became a 'key issue in colonial and nationalist discourses'. Further, 'the colonial state's "concern" for maternal and infant mortality was partly also designed to legitimize colonialism as necessary for the emancipation of the vulnerable subaltern women' (Pande, 2014a: 27).

Pande goes on to provide an important discussion of the Indian government's state surveillance and control of women's fertility (pp. 29–30):

these fertility-control-driven modernization campaigns in India cannot be understood in isolation from similar movements in Britain and the United States ... These dialogues and connections among Indian and international reformers and the determined focus on birth control as a sign of modernity and rationality inevitably constructed the subaltern woman (especially those from the lower classes, lower castes, and Muslims) as backward, sexually irresponsible, and immoral. ... Regardless of the jargon used for state policies, the underlying impact of the anti-natalist ambition has been state surveillance of fertility, especially of poor and working-class women.

The enforcement of state birth control in India represents a fundamental difference between its policies and those of many countries in the global north where many women historically had to struggle for access to contraception.

In her description of what scholars have referred to as the 'revised eugenics script', Pande outlines the paradox of commercial surrogacy within the context of India's neoliberal population policies:

On the one hand, negative eugenics, targeted mainly at minorities, continue with policies like voluntary or incentivized sterilization. On the other hand, positive eugenics has appropriated the language of 'individual choices' to strategically emphasize assisted fertility options for upper-class white couples. (p. 34)

Pande (2014a: 34–5) elaborates further contradictions inherent in the very existence of 'pro-natal technologies in an anti-natal state':

The revised eugenics script is evident in the policies of the government of India. Indian scientists are investing in new reproductive technologies like test tube babies, IVFs, and surrogacy and medical tourism (especially in these assisted reproductive services) is booming. Commercial surrogacy is yet another paradox of the post-liberalization era. It is ironic that a country that has the highest absolute number of maternal deaths and only 51 doctors for every 100,000 people is focusing on providing birth-related service to international patients.

The shift from population control to 'reproductive tourism' is an important one and enables us to understand the fertility logics employed by Indian surrogates. Although their experiences may vary, they are operating in a state that has an interest in restricting the fertility of poor women. For instance, in 2003, the Supreme Court of India upheld the rights of individual states to adopt the two-child norm, which 'encourages' couples to adopt a permanent method of contraception after their second child, with disincentives for those who do not comply, a pre-condition for elected representatives (Das, 2003).

Bio-politics, neoliberalism and global capitalism

In an analysis of the development of bio-politics, Thomas Lemke (2011: 110–11) details the origins of human capital theory, which emerged after the Second World War and in which 'every individual becomes not only a capitalist but also the sovereign of him- or herself. With every action, he or she maintains his or her individual advantage'. He explains further:

> Through the lens of human capital theory, a human being is a rational actor who is constantly allocating scarce resources in the pursuit of competing goals. ... The basis of this theory is a methodological individualism, whereby a person maximizes benefits and weighs options in a marketplace in which offers and demands coexist in perpetual interplay. Becker and Schultz understand human capital to mean the abilities, skills and health ... of a person. It consists of two components: an inborn corporeal and genetic endowment, and the entirety of the abilities that are the result of 'investments' in appropriate stimuli – nutrition, upbringing and education, as well as love and care.

In his historical overview of the different meanings of bio-politics, Lemke (2011) writes about the fragility and instability of the border between 'life' and 'politics'. He argues that a rupture or transformation in the structure of capitalism has occurred and that (Lemke, 2011: 69):

> Life does not represent a stable, ontological and normative point of reference. The impact of biotechnological innovations has demonstrated that life processes are transformable and controllable to an increasing degree, which renders obsolete any idea of an intact nature untouched by human action. Biological resources are the object of juridico-political regulation, while 'nature' processes are opened up to commercial interests and potential industrial use. Nature thus becomes a part of economic discourse.

Political philosophers and theorists have argued that the structure of global capitalism changed during the late twentieth century and in the early twenty-first century has provided 'new forms of life and work' (Hardt and Negri, 2000). While debates continue between supporters of altruistic (but not commercial) surrogacy, and opponents attempt to draw a line between the two, the surrogacy industry is a 'market' in which body parts and bodies are being rented, and embodied labour sold to produce new life in exchange for economic capital.

In *Our Bodies, Whose Property?* Anne Phillips (2013) asks, 'What's so special about the body?' She writes (p. 19):

> While no one wants to be regarded as an object, many like to think of themselves as 'self-owners', like to see themselves, that is, as in a relationship of ownership to their bodies and selves. For the devotee of self-ownership, the rights we enjoy over our bodies closely parallel the rights of the archetypical owner of property over things. The right to bodily integrity, for example, can be refigured as the right to determine who has access to the body, in ways that mimic the rights a landowner has to exclude trespasses from his property.

Writing for the *Wall Street Journal* in 2010, Tamari Audi and Arlene Chang describe and problematize the ethics of the business models of transnational surrogacy agencies that produce 'global' babies for an international clientele who are 'assembled' with genetic material and rented wombs from several regions of the world:

> In a hospital room on the Greek island of Crete, with views of a sapphire sea lapping at ancient fortress walls, a Bulgarian woman plans to deliver a baby whose biological mother is an anonymous egg donor, whose father is Italian, and whose birth is being orchestrated from Los Angeles. She won't be keeping the child. The parents-to-be – an infertile Italian woman and her husband (who provided the sperm) – will take custody of the baby this summer, on the day of birth ... Prospective parents put off by the rigor of traditional adoptions are bypassing that system by producing babies of their own – often using an egg donor from one country, a sperm donor from another, and a surrogate who will deliver in a third country to make what some industry participants call 'a world baby'. They turn to Planet Hospital and handful of other companies. 'We take care of all aspects of the

process, like a concierge service,' says Mr Rupak, a 41-year-old Canadian.

In the Indian context, the procedure described above can be characterized as a form of global bio-capitalism in which Indian women, as gestational surrogates, sell their biological labour, reproductive services, to Indian nationals, non-resident Indians and non-Indian foreigners (Vora, 2009). They are reproductive service providers working in a global capitalist system. In Vora's words (p. 266):

> Because the consumers and producers of the biological and affective labor commodified in commercial surrogacy are marked by differentials of class, race and gender, Indian transnational surrogacy reproduces a disparity between where this value is extracted and where it is invested.

Drawing on research conducted in northern India in 2008, Vora argues that commercial surrogacy in India represents an expansion of 'the realms of commodification'. Furthermore, in commercial surrogacy, India's reliance upon a western medical understanding of the body has 'constructed the uterus as surplus' (Vora, 2009: 268). Like other forms of bodily and intimate labour, including sex work and domestic labour, Vora points to an important change in late capitalism (p. 267): 'The identification of affective and biological labour points to a change in the subject of capitalist production. This subject participates in not only a global commodification of labour, but also a global organization of the affective and biological production.'

One of the paradoxes here is that the impoverished Christian and Hindu women interviewed by Vora were trained to think of their uterus as an 'empty' body part, which they owned and which could be rented out to generate income. This required them to 'commodify' a certain type of biological labour. To use a term developed by Krølokke and Pant (2012) and discussed below (see also Riggs and Due, this volume), they became 'repropreneurs'.

Women who enter into commercial surrogacy contracts temporarily relinquish some forms of control over their bodies. Their bodily integrity is compromised because they can be forced to abort fetuses against their will if genetic screening exposes a disease or potential risk for a specific disability. To some extent, they temporarily transfer control of their body to the 'intended parents' and/or the agency that hires them. Feminist scholars opposed to commercial surrogacy, such as Kelly Oliver, call attention to the fiction of 'equality' because 'using the jargon of rights, the liberal framework conceals social and class interests behind the illusion of formal equality in contracts' (Oliver, 1989: 96). In other words, women who enter into these commercial pregnancy contracts typically do not possess the power to negotiate terms. This is illustrated by the experiences of Aasia Khan, an Indian gestational surrogate and married mother of three children who was featured in the documentary film *Made in India* (2010). The film provides some insights into the challenges that gestational surrogates encounter when they attempt to negotiate their wages, in this case following medical implications.

Made in India: the case of Aasia Khan Aasia has entered into a commercial surrogacy contract with Planet Hospital.[2] Lisa and Brian Switzer, two White Americans from Texas, have tried without success to conceive a child for seven years. Desperate to form a family with a genetically related child, they have come to Planet Hospital to assist them in finding a surrogate.

The film moves back and forth between the perspective of the Switzers and that of Aasia, the Indian gestational surrogate who ultimately delivers twins for them. Although most of the story is told from the perspective of the American couple, there are moments when Aasia's voice and her analysis are shared with the viewer. Although the Indian government has not required clinics to provide national data, a growing number of studies, including research by national women's organizations such as Sama Resource Group for Women and Health (2012) and the Centre for Social Research (2010, 2012), has revealed the profile of the 'average' or typical Indian surrogate whom in many ways Aasia represents. She is married, an impoverished mother, and she has already delivered healthy children. She also has few desirable alternative job prospects. Thus, as a 'temporary' contract worker and a form of surplus labour, she has little, if any negotiating power with the agency.

After spending twelve days in the hospital and delivering premature twins, Aasia receives only $2,500 in payment, $4,500 less than she had expected. Following a difficult birth and out of desperation, she approaches the Switzers to ask for additional money.

Speaking to the film director, Lisa responds that she sympathizes with Aasia and that she appreciates her labour but she is not willing to offer even an additional $2,000 for the twins. In an interview, Lisa establishes the limits of what she will pay as a 'bonus':

I want to give her a little extra money. I think what she's done is admirable ... I think what she's had to go through with the obstruction and the emergency. And she carried twins ... I don't mind giving a little extra. I just can't give this huge amount of money. ... quite frankly, I think people think we have a lot of money cause we're Americans and we have dollars... . I don't think that they realize that we're not wealthy. We don't have an extra $2000 to just hand out to anyone who is asking.

The Switzers had been told that Aasia would be paid $7,000. When Aasia prematurely delivered twins by caesarean section, she had only received $1,100. She ultimately earned a total of $2,500 for delivering twins – roughly $18,000 to $25,000 less than a US surrogate would earn for a single birth. Moreover, this was significantly less than what the Switzers were told she would be paid. Despite this, at the end of the film, Aasia is seriously considering entering into a second commercial surrogacy contract due to her economic need.

What do we learn from Aasia's experiences as a gestational surrogate? As an uneducated and impoverished mother whose husband is unemployed, she desperately needs this job. She has few, if any transferrable skills and no bargaining power. Aasia was penalized for not moving into the dorm and living with other surrogates at the beginning of her pregnancy because she did not want to be separated from her three children for that long.

While some may argue that Aasia is a 'free agent', exercising her reproductive agency, we also see that she is embedded in a national context in which there is an oversupply of poor mothers – women who are disposable and desperate, and thus can be easily replaced if they refuse to accept the terms of the labour contracts offered to them. They are making decisions within a larger context of scarcity.

The experiences of Aasia suggest that the 'reproductive rights' of women working as gestational surrogates on commercial pregnancy contracts need to be protected and require state intervention. The language of choice conceals the degree to which women like Aasia are subordinated and disempowered due to their poverty, maternity (as mothers they have children whom they wish to raise with dignity) and the absence of state investments in their health and family.

From female contract labourers to 'repropreneurs'

The idea of human capital theory, which is central to neoliberalism, has been critiqued and analysed by transnational feminists studying global capitalism. In a qualitative ethnographic study of Danish citizens engaged in the global surrogacy industry and who travel to India as reproductive tourists, Krølokke and Pant (2012: 234) argue that:

> Neoliberal ideology promotes the idea that (in)fertile individuals should take personal responsibility for their fertility and make behavioral and lifestyle choices that maximize their chances of pregnancy and upward mobility, while simultaneously turning reproductive matter into particular types of commodities. (In)fertility and surrogacy are situated within a rhetoric of choice and draw upon an understanding of the body (and its parts) as individually owned and governed ... In this manner, the ideology of neo-liberalism reconfigures the individual or surrogate into a rational choice-making and responsible individual.

Following and building upon the theoretical arsenal of the UK sociologist Nikolas Rose, they developed the term 'repropreneur' to analyse the 'recoding of infertile Westerns and poor, yet fertile, Indian surrogates into reproductive agents' (Krølokke and Pant, 2012: 239).

Vivid examples of how gestational surrogates strategically employ their bio-capital and assert their agency as female contract labourers are further provided by Pande's groundbreaking work, already extensively cited in relation to post-colonialism and fertility regulation in India. In *Wombs in Labor* (Pande, 2014a), Pande draws upon research that she conducted between 2006 and 2011 with more than 100 surrogates, their husbands, doctors, surrogacy brokers, nurses, hostel matrons and others in the industry. Referring to the surrogates' agency as workers, she describes a wide range of responses and strategies to negotiate power. Although it is not clear how representative the women interviewed are of the surrogacy industry, Pande's rigorous field research suggests that at least a segment of the women working in it perceive surrogacy as a 'career' and enter into these pregnancy contracts multiple times to achieve their economic and familial goals.

Below are two more cases of Indian surrogates, interviewed by Pande, who, in contrast to Aasia, are financially successful 'repropreneurs'. They asserted their agency by insisting upon their right to work as gestational surrogates and refused to obey their husbands or fathers-in-law.

Puja is a 27-year-old woman who is now pregnant for the second time as a surrogate. She intends to enter into commercial surrogacy contracts at least two more times to reach her remaining goals. In her words (Pande, 2014a: 110):

> I built one house and bought another plot of land in the city with the money I got from my first surrogacy. When I become a surrogate again, I will build another house on that plot. I want to do this again and again. He [her husband] did not want me to do this again. But I convinced him that we need money to educate our children. My father-in-law was very against it from [the] start. But I told him it's my life.

Puja discusses gestational surrogacy as a career that will enable her to achieve her financial and familial goals. She is enthusiastic and expresses pride in what she has achieved for her family.

In a second case, we meet Rita, a 29-year-old gestational surrogate and the daughter of a surrogacy broker. Like Puja, she is a veteran in the industry and is carrying a second baby under a commercial pregnancy contract. She expresses amazement at her earnings and pride in her achievements (Pande, 2014a: 109):

> I am the fourth to be a surrogate in my family. Our whole family runs on this [industry]. I've already delivered a baby girl to a couple last year and they asked me to do it again this year. I used the money to pay back some debt and reconstruct the roof of my house. I put the rest of it in the bank in a fixed deposit. ... This is the first time I am working out of the house and am earning so much more than he [her husband] ever has. He was reluctant, but he let me do this the second time. I want to buy a house with the money I earn this time.

Rita, like Puja, appears to feel empowered by the earnings that she is bringing to the family. The balance of power in these marriages may be altered by the ability of these married women to outearn their husbands. In any case, there are unlikely to be any other jobs in which they could earn as much income in such a short time.

Of course Rita and Puja represent the 'success' stories. In striking contrast to Aasia from *Made in India*, their lives have been materially transformed by the wages that they earned. In Aasia's case, she did not receive what she had expected. After enduring medical complications and giving birth prematurely to twins, she was left with very little. In addition, she was penalized financially for not moving into the surrogate dorm at the beginning of her pregnancy.

How do we explain the differences in the financial outcomes for Aasia when compared with Rita and Puja? First, all three women share a desire to work as gestational surrogates again. Aasia desperately needs the money and did not achieve any of her financial goals with her first contract pregnancy. Second, as the daughter of a surrogacy broker Rita may have been able to secure a better financial deal, including not being implanted with multiple embryos therefore avoiding the potential difficulties that can arise from carrying twins. The ability to negotiate the terms of the contract may vary for those women who are part of a 'family' of experienced surrogates. This suggests that, not unlike the US, there are 'premium' surrogates and donors. It is possible that because of their first successful deliveries of singletons, Rita and Puja gained a special status. Being requested a second time by the same couple may confer eligibility for a slightly higher wage.

Towards a reproductive justice agenda

In 1994, a group of US Black feminists coined the term 'reproductive justice' and created a framework for mobilizing women in the US. They shifted the frame from one that focused on 'choice' to a broader agenda that included not only a woman's 'right to have a child' (or not) but also the right to raise her children 'with dignity in safe, healthy and supportive environments. This framework repositioned reproductive rights in a political context of intersecting race, gender and class oppressions' (Roberts, 2015).

Today, SisterSong Women of Color Reproductive Health Collective mobilizes women and plays a central role in the reproductive justice movement. This movement is concerned with the holistic experiences of women as mothers. Defining its objectives, Loretta Ross (n.d.), a founder and national coordinator of SisterSong, writes that the reproductive justice framework

> analyzes how the ability of any woman to determine her own reproductive destiny is linked directly to the conditions in her community and these conditions are not just a matter of individual choice and access... . Moving beyond a demand for privacy and respect for individual decision making to include the social supports necessary for our individual decisions to be optimally realized, this framework also includes obligations from our government for protecting women's human's rights.

Feminist scholars and legal theorists continue to debate the merits and ethics of commercial surrogacy and specifically the power asymmetries among women who sell or rent their reproductive labor in exchange for payment. Are they simply independent contracts selling their 'body' parts? Are they exploited labourers? Are they making a rational choice in the context of capitalist labour markets? Are they the victims of the commodification of women and children?

Amrita Banerjee (2010: 109) discusses the 'problematics of consent' and argues for 'a nuanced ethical paradigm suited to the needs of a complicated and messy globalized world':

> Based on this aspect of commodification, the exploitation paradigm argues that the surrogate is exploited because her labor and her body are judged on the basis of their use-value. This paradigm also highlights the fact that choice does not occur in a socio-cultural vacuum. What appears to be a choice of the individual surrogates is often the outcome of explicit or tacit coercion.

As we have seen in the case of Aasia, Puja and Rita, the three Indian gestational surrogates discussed in this chapter, while two of them achieved their short-term financial goals, they still needed to continue to work in order to provide economic security for their families. The degree of unpredictability and vulnerability that accompanies any pregnancy, combined with a 'surplus' of impoverished married mothers seeking additional income to support their families, suggests that gestational surrogates who enter commercial surrogacy contracts need a guaranteed income. The Indian mothers interviewed by Pande are 'choosing' to enter commercial pregnancy contracts and serve as gestational surrogates in the context of poverty, gender inequality and the desire to provide economic security and upward mobility for their children. Thus, the 'constrained' agency that surrogates describe reflects neoliberal discourses that position them as 'entrepreneurs', or in Krølokke and Pant's term, 'repropreneurs'.

The challenges that gestational surrogates face must be analysed in the context of a larger (in)fertility system that includes access to abortion, contraception, and sterilization. Gestational surrogates need internationally recognized basic human rights and labour protections. Applying the concept of reproductive justice to the situation of commercial surrogates, I argue for a transnational regulatory framework that protects women who, for whatever reasons, may not be able to deliver a healthy baby. The 'unsuccessful' gestational surrogates should be guaranteed a minimum wage as well as lifetime access to reproductive health care.

In an ideal situation India, the European Union, the US and the Asian countries most involved in the commercial surrogacy industry would be obliged to contribute funds to provide an insurance policy for surrogates in cases of illness, death or other incidents that could impact upon their ability to care for their families. At this time there are no legal protections for gestational surrogates. Given the profits to be made in this growing global industry, guidelines are needed that will protect their basic rights. At the minimum, they should be provided with interpreters and advocates who can help them understand the terms of the contracts they sign. The expansion of global capitalism and with it the 'medical tourism' industry, the collapse of state socialism in Eastern Europe and the liberalization of economies in countries such as India have allowed women to perceive jobs in the reproductive tourism industry as desirable options. Regulation and protection may go some way towards addressing some of the concerns discussed, but only by challenging structural inequalities related to poverty, women's reproductive health and women's reproductive rights can true reproductive justice ever be achieved.

Acknowledgements

I am deeply thankful to Miranda Davies for her guidance, patience and editorial support in writing this chapter. I also thank Allan Cronin for his comments on earlier drafts.

Notes

1 In October 2015, ahead of the ratification of the Assisted Reproductive Technology (ART) Bill, the Indian government announced a ban on non-Indian passport holders seeking the services of Indian surrogates (Perappadan, 2015). This is in addition to the clampdown on same-sex couples, unmarried couples and couples who have been married for less than two years imposed in 2012 (Malhotra and Malhotra, 2016). The effects of the ban and how far it will be enforced remain to be seen (see Pande, Chapter 19).

2 Planet Hospital ceased to operate in July 2014 after its owner, Rudy Rupak, was forced into involuntary bankruptcy following investigation by the FBI.

References

Audi T and Chang A (2010) Assembling the global baby. *Wall Street Journal.* Life/Style section. <http://online.wsj.com/articles/SB10001424052748703493504576007774155273928>

Banerjee A (2010) Reinventing the ethics of transnational surrogacy as a feminist pragmatist. *The Pluralist* 5(3): 107–27.

Brunet L, Carruthers J, Davaki K et al. (2013) *A Comparative Study of the Regime of Surrogacy in EU Member States: Report Submitted to European Parliament's Committee* on Legal Affairs. <www.europarl.europa.eu/RegData/etudes/etudes/join/2013/474403/IPOL_JURI_ET(2013)474403_EN.pdf>

Centre for Social Research (2010, 2012) *Surrogacy Motherhood: Ethical or Commercial?* Reports from Delhi and Mumbai and Surat-Gujarat. <www.csrindia.org/surrogate-motherhood>

Colen S (1995) Like a mother to them: stratified reproduction and West Indian childcare workers. In: Ginsburg FD and Rapp R (eds) *Conceiving the New World Order: The Global Politics of Reproduction*. Berkeley/Los Angeles, CA: University of California Press, pp. 78–102.

Das A (2003) Two children, countless wrongs. *India Together*, 1 October. <http://indiatogether.org/twokids-health>

Hansen R and King D (2013) *Sterilized by the State: Eugenics, Race, and the Population Scare in Twentieth-Century America*. New York: Cambridge University Press.

Hardt M and Negri A (2000) *Empire: The New World Order*. Cambridge, MA: Harvard University Press.

Johnson CG (2013) California was sterilizing its female prisoners as late as 2010. *Guardian*, 8 November. <www.theguardian.com/commentisfree/2013/nov/08/california-female-prisoner-sterilization>

Krølokke CH and Pant S (2012) 'I only need her uterus': neoliberal discourses in transnational surrogacy. *NORA: Nordic Journal of Feminist and Gender Studies* 20(4): 233–48.

Lemke T (2011) *Bio-Politics: An Advanced Introduction*. Trans. Eric Frederick Trump. New York and London: New York University Press.

Malhotra A and Malhotra R (2016) *Surrogacy in India: A Law in the Making – Revisited*. Delhi: Universal Law Publishing.

Market Data Enterprises (2013) U.S. fertility clinics & infertility services market worth $3.5 billion: recession is not a factor. Press release, 5 November. <www.marketdataenterprises.com/wp-content/uploads/2014/01/Fertility%20Clinics%20PR%202013.pdf>

Oliver K (1989) Marxism and surrogacy. *Hypatia* 4(3): 95–115.

Pande A (2009) Not an 'angel', not a 'whore': surrogates as 'dirty workers' in India. *Indian Journal of Gender Studies* 16(2): 141–73.

Pande A (2010) Commercial surrogacy in India: manufacturing a perfect mother-worker. *Signs: Journal of Women in Culture and Society* 35(4): 969–92.

Pande A (2014a) *Wombs in Labor: Transnational Commercial Surrogacy in India*. New York: Columbia University Press.

Pande A (2014b) The power of narratives: negotiating commercial surrogacy in India. In: DasGupta S and Dasgupta SD (eds) *Globalization and Transnational Surrogacy in India: Outsourcing Life*. Lanham, MD: Lexington Books, pp. 87–106.

Perappadan BS (2015) ART Bill may close surrogacy door for foreigners, unmarried people. *The Hindu*, 23 October. <www.thehindu.com/news/cities/Delhi/art-bill-may-close-surrogacy-doors-for-foreigners-unmarried-people/article7793884.ece>

Phillips A (2013) *Our Bodies, Whose Property?* Princeton, NJ, and Oxford: Princeton University Press.

Roberts D (1998) *Killing the Black Body: Race, Reproduction and the Meaning of Liberty*. New York: Pantheon.

Roberts D (2009) Race, gender and genetic technologies. *Signs* 34(4): 783–804.

Roberts D (2015) Reproductive justice, not just rights. *Dissent Magazine*, Fall. <www.dissentmagazine.org/article/reproductive-justice-not-just-rights>

Ross LJ (n.d.) What is reproductive justice? The Pro-Choice Public Education Project. <www.protectchoice.org/section.php?id=28>

Sama Resource Group for Women and Health (2012) *Birthing a Market: A Study on Commercial Surrogacy*. New Delhi: Sama.

Smith A (2005) *Conquest: Sexual Violence and American Indian Genocide*. Cambridge, MA: South End Press.

Vora K (2009) Indian surrogacy and commodified vital energy. *Subjectivity* 28(1): 266–78.

7 | NETWORKS OF REPRODUCTION: POLITICS AND PRACTICES SURROUNDING SURROGACY IN ROMANIA

Enikő Demény

Introduction

Policies and laws related to surrogacy in different countries range from permissive legislation through non-regulation to a total ban, making it one of the most contested of all the assisted reproductive technologies (ARTs). The extensive feminist literature on surrogacy offers excellent insights and analysis on the issue from legal, philosophical, ethical, anthropological, sociological or political perspectives. However, it mainly draws on practices in India, the US or other countries where surrogacy has been established for well over a decade. Little has been published from parts of the world that only recently became players in the global reproductive market, such as some of the countries of Eastern Europe (Stoicea-Deram, 2016b).

In discussing surrogacy policies and practices in one of these countries, namely Romania, this chapter aims not to cover the topic but to open it up for further investigation. Romania may not be the centre of the reproductive market in relation to surrogacy in the region, but the various practices some of its citizens are engaged in show that it is clearly connected to the global market of assisted human reproduction.

Various scholarly articles have helped contribute towards our understanding of the wider context in which ART practices are embedded in Romania (e.g. Cutaş, 2008; Demény, 2013; Frunza, 2010; Guţan, 2011; Lundin, 2012), but until recently very few have specifically addressed the topic of surrogacy. Two of these in particular stand out. The first (Hostiuc *et al.*, 2016a) is a philosophical analysis of the ethical issues related to surrogacy arrangements; the other (Hostiuc *et al.*, 2016b) uses four Romanian court cases on contested parenthood to discuss the question of maternal filiation in surrogacy arrangements and the role of genetic information in establishing kinship. In addition, the outcomes of the first feminist debates on surrogacy in Romania were recently published in a special edition of *AnaLize:*

Journal of Gender and Feminist Studies (Stoicea-Deram, 2016a). Contributors point out the scarcity of literature on and lack of preoccupation with the topic of surrogacy among feminist activists in Eastern Europe and Romania (Stoicea-Deram, 2016b) and present valuable theoretical insights (Agacinski, 2016; Gheaus, 2016; Stoicea-Deram, 2016b) including, as a starting point, examples from India (Marinescu, 2016; Saravanan, 2016). One particular contribution tackles the issue of surrogacy from an empirical standpoint by presenting the legislative and policy context of surrogacy in Romania, as well as discussing the motivations of potential surrogates based on phone interviews with these women (Iacob and Stoian, 2016). The authors highlight the difficulties of carrying out empirical work on surrogate motherhood in Romania, partly because these arrangements take place in such an unregulated and legally grey area. They also point out the absence of relevant qualitative and quantitative data (Iacob and Stoian, 2016: 59).

This chapter aims to bring into discussion some publicly available documents and empirical material concerning, on the one hand, legislative and juridical debates on surrogacy in Romania, and on the other hand, publicly expressed opinions from influential actors in these debates such as feminist/women's organizations, churches or NGOs active in the field of human reproduction. It also seeks to capture the attitudes of those directly engaged in surrogacy arrangements, namely intending parents and potential surrogates, by analysing their views as expressed in forums, blogs or comments following articles on surrogacy, as well as using the few publicly available interviews conducted by journalists with would-be surrogate mothers. The forums, blog and articles were identified by searching on the terms *mamă/mame surogat* (surrogate mother), *reproducere asistată* (assisted reproduction), 'IVF' and 'forum/blog'. All this material was written in the Romanian language during the period 2009 to 2015.

The role of the internet has been widely acknowledged in the development and functioning of a transnational surrogacy market (e.g. Morgan, 2003) since this is the forum where the supply and demand sides so often find each other. Consulting forum discussions and blogs is a time-consuming method of investigation, which does not result in a systematic analysis corresponding to scientific exigencies. Moreover, it is no substitute for research based on anthropological fieldwork and in-depth interviews. My aim here is simply to present some insights into how surrogacy is practised in a non-regulated context in an Eastern European country, leaving room for future analysis to test the ideas formulated here using more consolidated methods.

Background

Romania is one of those European Union member countries that has not yet adopted specific legislation on medically assisted reproductive technologies. Despite the abolition of restrictive abortion and contraception policies in the aftermath of the 1989 revolution, their legacy continues to have an impact, making the regulation of medically assisted human reproduction (MAHR) in Romania a very sensitive and complex issue (Kligman, 1998). The abortion and pro-natalist policies of state-socialist Romania represented a specific model of state involvement in the spheres of reproduction and the family. Wishing to increase the birth rate, in 1966, Ceaușescu promulgated Decree No. 770 restricting abortion and contraception. Contraception became illegal and, with the exception of pregnancy through rape or incest, or perceived risks arising from a specific medical condition, only women over the age of 40 (45 in 1985–9) who had at least four children (raised to five in 1985–9) were eligible for abortion. Mandatory gynecological check-ups and penalties against unmarried people and childless couples completed these pro-natalist measures. The consequences were far-reaching: in the period 1966–89 almost 10,000 women died as a result of illegal abortions. At the same time, many children ended up in child care institutions (Morrison, 2004). Documentaries presenting the miserable conditions in many Romanian orphanages made international headline news and in the 1990s the country was the main provider of children for intercountry adoption worldwide (Selman, 2010).

Given the severe restrictions on reproductive rights, it was not surprising that after the collapse of the state-socialist regime one of the first legislative measures concerned the legalization of abortion.[1] This regaining of reproductive freedom resulted in alarming abortion statistics in the first period after liberalization. Since then, the number of abortions has decreased although Romania still has one of the highest rates in Europe (United Nations, 2013). Additionally, in 2010, the country recorded the lowest number of births since 1955. This severe drop in the birth rate, together with the high number of abortions, a rise in the mortality rate (still well above average for the EU) and unprecedented numbers of, mainly young, Romanian citizens leaving to work abroad since the 1990s, has resulted in a negative demographic trend. These factors and the advent of reproductive tourism, as well as the economic crisis, are intrinsic to the social and political circumstances in which the new technologies of reproduction are applied and have to be regulated in Romania.

Up until 2006, Romania had no legislation concerning MAHR and in vitro fertilization (IVF) clinics functioned in an unregulated context (Cutaş, 2008). The only existing regulations during this period were those self-imposed by the medical profession, such as the necessary informed consent process required before embarking on any form of IVF. Specific legislation on MAHR does not exist, even today, as not one of the six legislative proposals concerning this field has been adopted.

Not being expressly prohibited, both altruistic and commercial forms of surrogacy are to some extent practised in Romania. However, rather than taking the risk, many intended parents for whom altruistic surrogacy is not an option, and who have the necessary financial means, prefer to use the surrogacy services offered in Ukraine where commercial surrogacy is legal. At the same time, Romanian attitudes towards surrogacy inevitably vary according to people's individual values, motivations and interests. On the one hand, the major churches, pro-life organizations and some women's associations regard it as an exploitation of women, degradation of motherhood and commodification of the child, and call for an outright ban; on the other hand, those women with a medical condition which means that using a surrogate mother represents their only chance of having 'their own baby' hope for some form of legalization.

These are the two poles between which Romanian authorities are situated when they try to regulate MAHR and surrogacy. In the 1990s, following the abolition of restrictive abortion policies it would have been difficult to introduce any policy that could have been interpreted as intervening in the reproductive rights and freedoms of Romanian citizens. It is therefore not surprising that those years saw a liberal or laissez-faire attitude towards the work of IVF centres, accompanied by some optimism regarding the scientific progress taking place in the field of reproductive technologies. This positive stance was confirmed by the increasing numbers of babies born in Romania with the help of these technologies, including some via surrogacy.[2] However, the exposure of controversial practices (discussed below) eventually led to a more precautionary attitude.

Since 2006 IVF procedures have been regulated by Chapter VI (on the Procurement and Transplant of Human Organs, Tissues and Cells for Therapeutic Purposes) of Law 95/2006 on the reform of the health care system. The aim of the legislator was to provide a legal framework to regulate the activities of IVF centres and also to safeguard the non-commercialization of human biological material and stop the trafficking of these and human organs.³ The law introduced strict sanctions prohibiting and criminalizing any payment for any kind of donation, including ova and sperm.

The New Civil Code (Law No. 287 of 2009, Articles 441–7) entered into force on 1 October 2011 and was the first legal instrument to address the wider implications of third-party MAHR, especially its impact on family relationships and filiation (*Official Gazette*, 2011). The provisions of the Civil Code clearly set out some limits for the proposed new regulation. For example, it restricts the sphere of access to ART procedures to heterosexual couples and single women. It also states that third-party reproduction does not create any kind of lineage between donor and child. No responsibility in this regard can be claimed against the donor and nobody can dispute the lineage of the child for reasons related to third-party reproduction, nor may the child contest her or his lineage for this reason (Guțan, 2011).

As stated above, the New Civil Code on third-party human reproduction does not explicitly address surrogacy so it does not prohibit it. Only one of the many legislative initiatives on MAHR attempted to introduce such regulation. This Draft Law on Medically Assisted Human Reproduction (2011) proposed to allow only altruistic surrogacy and under certain conditions. These included: the age of the surrogate mother is limited to 18–40 years; she should have her own child; all parties involved in the surrogacy arrangement must be evaluated by a commission and offered psychological support; and the adoption of the child by the genetic parents would need to take place before the implantation of the embryo in the surrogate mother. It also proposed the establishment of a register of surrogate mothers. However, like all the other initiatives in the field of MAHR, this draft proposal has not been adopted and there has been no further attempt to regulate surrogacy.

Any controversial cases are individually dealt with by the courts. For instance, in 2014, a genetic mother was recognized as the legal mother of her twins born through an altruistic surrogacy arrangement. This case concerned a married women who had lost her uterus after giving birth to her first child. Later the couple wanted to have another child and decided to achieve this via surrogacy with the genetic mother's sister as gestational surrogate. When she gave birth to twins, in the first instance, the surrogate mother and her husband were registered as the legal parents of the child. The case was about granting legal parentage to the commissioning couple (see Barac, 2014). Despite the fact that the genetic mother was recognized as the legal mother of the twins, this case did not set a legal precedent regarding all genetic mothers having a baby this way because the Romanian judicial system is not based on case law.

The above case was an exception because currently in Romania one can have a child using a surrogate mother only by adopting that child after birth. First, the child is declared as the offspring of the surrogate mother and the biological father. The birth certificate is issued with their names before the surrogate mother gives up the child for adoption. The biological father then 'decides' to adopt the child together with his wife, also the genetic parent, from the competent authorities. Following a successful adoption a new birth certificate is issued to the genetic parents.[4] Surrogacy contracts are non-enforceable. This means that having a valid surrogacy contract will not give parental authority to the genetic (intending) mother over the child. If the surrogate mother changes her mind and wants to keep the child, no one can take the child from her since she is the legal mother in the first instance.

Lack of specific regulations, and therefore law enforcement, meant that for a couple of years Romania became a target country for reproductive tourism for IVF procedures using eggs obtained from Romanian ova 'donors'/sellers, but there is no evidence to suggest that this included surrogacy services. Although a surrogacy industry similar to that in India or Ukraine does not exist in Romania, this does not mean that Romanian citizens do not have a presence in the global surrogacy market.

A growing demand

Surrogacy in Romania, albeit limited, is driven by familiar factors. First of all, widespread use of the internet has made it very easy to find information about reproductive technologies and procedures available at home or abroad. Although mainstream media and portals cover some information on these technologies, the main sources are the IVF centres' own web-pages and social media sites, translated into many languages, as well as the specific sites created to address issues related to infertility, children and family or reproductive health.[5] Forum discussions on these sites, as well as various blogs, add personalized information and offer space in which to share stories and/or express opinions on these topics.

Second, supply and demand exist in the Romania surrogacy market and are most visible on the internet sites mentioned above. Due to the rising percentage of couples facing infertility problems there is an increasing demand for IVF treatment, egg donation and surrogacy. For example, between 2006 and 2011, an estimated 20 per cent of couples were diagnosed as infertile (Sandu, 2011). At the same time, in the context of economic crisis, high rates of unemployment and increasing social inequalities, many women find themselves in situations in which a certain amount of money becomes a powerful incentive to sell their ova and/or become surrogate mothers. Thus, a rising number of women are looking for a surrogate mother or donated ova, and more women are willing to offer such 'services'. They post online ads, but it is also common for comments following articles about surrogacy to contain offers and requests for these arrangements. In terms of their profiles, based on the information shared on the internet, those who offer to be surrogate mothers tend to be aged between 18 and 36 years, have one or more children, are usually married, 'healthy, serious and able to keep privacy', while those who are looking for a surrogate mother are 'serious couples'. Contact details, such as phone number and/or email address are included in the ads as well as some information about the requested or offered price – between 15,000 and 60,000 euros.

Third, this market is part of the global surrogacy business. While in Romania there are women who seek surrogates and can pay for this service and others offering to be surrogates, plus there are IVF centres where the process can be carried out, these types of transactions do not represent the most widely practised form of commercial surrogacy in the country. From reading the blogs and forums it seems that the preferred solution is to employ the services offered by IVF centres in a neighbouring country where commercial surrogacy is legal, specifically Ukraine.

Romanian intending parents who have no financial resources are not in a good position in the global reproductive market. They can enter into a surrogacy arrangement in their home country, with all the risks entailed, but still can find themselves at a disadvantage during the negotiations as there may well be foreign couples seeking women to carry babies for them in Romania who can pay more. In one case reported by Iacob and Stoian (2016: 62), even where the potential surrogate initially wanted 'to help' a family from Romania, she eventually made an agreement with a French family who were likely to be able to offer more money. For many Romanians the only affordable and safe solution to having 'their own baby' would be the legalization of surrogacy in Romania.

Going overseas is also an alternative for those offering to be surrogates. For example, some Romanian internet sites recruit potential surrogates for IVF centres in Greece. Regarding Romanians living abroad, or foreign citizens, while they may use donated genetic material from Romania, for surrogacy they tend to recommend the use of centres such as BioTexCom, which clearly capitalizes on the legal status of surrogacy in Ukraine. While US websites tend to appeal to couples' dreams and longings for a family, the BioTexCom approach, as expressed on the opening page of the company's website, is a lot more pragmatic:

> In the sphere of surrogacy, Ukrainian legislators have proven to be far more progressive than many of their European colleagues. Today, Ukraine is one of the very few surrogacy friendly countries in Europe. Unlike other nations that limit or even ban surrogacy, in Ukraine the intended parents of child are considered to be biological parents from the moment of conception, and they are specifically named as biological parents in the birth certificate without any mentioning of surrogate mother.

Crackdown on the illegal egg trade

Although the crisis in Ukraine in 2013 triggered increased interest in services inside Romania, it has yet to become a target country for commercial surrogacy. This is partly due to recent changes in the attitude of Romanian authorities towards the IVF industry following the exposure of illegal practices, mostly in the form of paid ova donation obtained in conditions of questionable informed consent.

Marcy Darnovsky (2009) publicized the first wave of arrests in 2009 in a BlogPost that also highlights the transnational reach of the clinic's fraudulent activities:

> Last month, authorities in Romania detained 30 people and arrested a number of Israeli physicians at the Sabyc fertility clinic in Bucharest in connection with illegal payments to women for their eggs. Israeli newspapers reported that the eggs were provided by university students and Roma women, some of them as young as 15. Romanian prosecutors confiscated documents, computers and over 130,000 euros (US$185,000) in cash from the clinic, whose mostly Israeli and German clientele reportedly paid 10,000 to 15,000 euros (US$14,000 to $21,000) for fertility treatment. A statement by the country's organized crime department said that the women who provided eggs were paid the equivalent of $270 to $335.

This was the first criminal prosecution concerning the egg trade and eventually resulted in the condemnation of medical doctors and administrative staff, giving a clear signal that the authorities were determined to stop illegal activities related to IVF centres, to enforce non-commercialization principles and to ensure that medically assisted reproduction and related activities are conducted in accordance with the relevant regulations. Law enforcement measures continued with further arrests and closures of IVF centres (Demény, 2013). The most recent such case, in May 2014, concerned a clinic in the city of Timisoara where not only the Greek manager of the centre but also thirteen surrogates were arrested. Since surrogacy is not prohibited in Romania, again, the accusation focused on egg trafficking. (The surrogates came from Romania, Hungary and Slovakia while the beneficiaries were from Romania, Hungary and Norway.)

Attitudes and motives for pursuing surrogacy: views from the internet

Intending parents As stated in my introduction, attitudes towards surrogacy depend on the values, motivation, experiences and interests of those concerned. Most directly involved are the surrogates (and their families) and the commissioning couple/person. From studying the available information, together with online forum discussions featuring those looking for and offering surrogacy services in Romania, it is clear that the voice of intending couples/persons is more represented and elaborated than that of potential surrogates. They form a community to represent their interests and to share their problems, often revealing the whole story of their struggle with infertility. Although it is usually 'serious couples' looking for a surrogate, it is predominantly women who are active on these sites.

These women are well informed about IVF technology and procedures and not only share with each other new information and personal experiences, but also provide mutual support during difficult times. In making their interests public they employ the language of reproductive rights, embrace IVF technology, discuss issues of access and militate for more state-financed support for infertility services. Until 2011, there was no publicly financed IVF in Romania. That year, a programme was introduced that offered state financing for heterosexual couples and single women. Nowadays new information is shared, from the latest developments in uterus implantation to court decisions on surrogacy-related issues and other legislative initiatives. Often women would like their condition (e.g. lack of a uterus or incapacity to carry a baby to term) to be recognized as a disease and to have legal access to surrogacy in Romania. Given the perceived risks in the current legal climate, although we know from court cases on issues related to the establishment of legal parenthood in altruistic surrogacy that some such domestic arrangements take place, these experiences do not appear to be shared in these forums.

Overseas surrogacy is another story. In terms of Romanian salaries, the costs of using the services of IVF centres in Ukraine are high. However, there are middle-class couples or women who manage by making great efforts and seem only too happy to share their experiences online. The issues discussed on the online accounts and websites I looked at vary from the quality of the roads and accommodation to preferred criteria for selecting a surrogate. For example, a number of intending mothers were seeking some kind of resemblance with the surrogate such as brown hair/eyes and same blood type. One woman had chosen a surrogate from Lyviv on the grounds that it is the Ukrainian city located furthest from Chernobyl.

Usually Romanian clients of centres such as BioTexCom were pleasantly surprised by the quality of the services, including administrative and medical support, although they found the state of the roads to be very bad! In the forums I looked at how both success stories and unsuccessful attempts were shared. Those who returned home with a baby had no problems getting into the country since Romania recognizes the birth certificate issued in the intending parent/s' name, on the basis of which the Romanian consulate in Kiev provides the necessary travel documents for the baby. There were no specific warnings about the centres, but intending parents are advised to read the contract very carefully, and decisions to turn to another clinic imply negative experiences.

Of course not all women in need of a surrogate have the financial resources to go to Ukraine or even to pay a woman in their own country. For them the only affordable and safe/non-risky solution to having 'their own baby' would be the legalization of surrogacy in Romania.

Surrogates The reasons for offering to be a surrogate can be deduced from occasional forum discussions but also from interviews with would-be surrogate mothers. Not surprisingly, lack of money, coupled with the desire to provide a proper home or a better future for their family and child, are what motivates most women to offer their services. Renting out their womb represents the ultimate chance to change their miserable financial situation. Altruistic motives are also evident in the views of women who explain that having their own child and realizing what a blessing it is has made them determined to help a woman for whom this is the only chance of becoming a mother. This doesn't mean that they wouldn't request money but financial incentive doesn't appear to be the sole motive behind their decision. These would-be surrogate mothers also might mention altruistic impulses in order to justify their financial motives, by arguing that there is nothing morally wrong in their action since they are doing something that it is good for both of the contracting parties: the surrogate mother and the intending parents. The would-be child rarely features in these discussions as a subject who might be harmed by such an arrangement.

Class and race issues are sometimes raised, for example in a blog discussion about the ethics of surrogate motherhood where it was claimed that many surrogates are poor, uneducated Roma women from villages.[6] However, this is unlikely to be true. Such women may well have been over-represented among the paid ova donors used by unscrupulous clinics in the past, as in the 2009 Sabyc egg-trafficking scandal mentioned above, when the foreign intending parents were not really aware of the source of the eggs they used. However, taking into account public perceptions and discrimination against Roma communities and the high numbers of available offers from Romanians, it is unlikely that poor, uneducated Roma women form the most significant group from which surrogates are recruited. Rather, would-be surrogates tend to live in cities, have some education, are using the internet and know something about IVF and surrogacy procedures.

Very few interviews with surrogates are publicly available and those in existence were recorded under cover. One example is the story of a young woman who, like so many others, offered her services on the internet.[7] At the time, she was 26 years old and living in a Romanian city. She worked in a shop, had a 2-year-old child and resided with her partner in her mother's apartment. Her monthly salary was approximately 220 euros; the price she asked for being a surrogate mother was 25,000 euros. She explained that the couple had been together for a long time and already had a child but they had never had enough money to get married She decided to offer to be a surrogate mother so they could have their own apartment since living with the parents was getting more and more difficult. When asked whether her partner agreed with this, she said that it was her own decision and that when she decides something no one can make her change her mind. From the interview it is evident that she did not see herself as a victim of the surrogacy industry but rather as an active agent who could do something to change her situation. She was not in a position to think about the long-term consequences of her action or about any psychological or philosophical issues raised by surrogacy. For her it was simply an opportunity to improve her living conditions and she probably didn't have many, if any, alternatives.

She was aware that it would be difficult not to form an attachment with the child growing in her womb, so from the start planned to think about the baby as belonging to the intending couple with herself as a temporary carrier. She empathized with the intending couple with whom she was discussing this arrangement: it is clear that, although her primary motivation was financial, she was happy to help them to have a child, telling them how she knew first-hand what a blessing it is. She did not think she was doing anything immoral and explained that she wished to do it only once and didn't want to make a business out of it. We also find out that some time in the future she would like to have another child of her own. This particular interview does not touch upon what she will tell her child about the baby in her belly, clearly a delicate topic, especially when the surrogate mother's child/ children are old enough to ask such questions. However, where this problem is addressed in other interviews and comments, it is seen simply as an issue to be resolved and not something that would lead a potential surrogate to change her mind.

One such example was presented in a 2016 documentary broadcast on a Romanian TV show, *La Maruta*. A 38-year-old married woman with a teenage son posted an announcement that she would like to become a surrogate for 10,000 euros. When contacted by reporters from the TV channel she accepted their offer of an interview and agreed to participate in a live TV show to present her case. The resulting programme reveals that her main motivation was to earn money to buy a bigger home. At the time, she was living with her husband and son in a one-room apartment. She explains that her husband agreed with her plan and her son, with whom she had also discussed it, had no objections. The woman is determined to go ahead despite challenges from the lawyer and psychologist also present in the studio. She appears to have no doubts related to not forming an attachment with the baby, perceiving herself as merely an incubator and not his/ her mother. When asked if the couple have tried alternatives to obtain money to improve their lives – for example, a loan from the bank or taking on other jobs – the woman explains that they have tried many avenues in the past without success. One thing they do not want to do is to go abroad for work, as it is important for them to stay together with their son. She doesn't see anything immoral in her action as her intentions are good: she would like to provide a better life for her son and at the same time help another couple.[8]

The women presented in these interviews do not appear to see themselves as victims of the surrogacy industry but rather as active agents who have an opportunity to do something to change their situation. They are not in a position to think about the long-term consequences of their action or about any of the psychological or philosophical issues raised by surrogacy. For them being a surrogate mother represents a chance to improve their living conditions in the face of few, if any, alternatives. Explaining the socio-economic and cultural context that lies behind their 'choice' is beyond the scope of this discussion.

To summarize the attitude of intending and commercial surrogates, I would say that once they have decided to go ahead, both parties have a highly pragmatic attitude towards the whole arrangement. Each is very much focused on the process and appears to avoid thinking about long-term issues or moral dilemmas. They no doubt face such quandaries, but they don't stop to think and talk about them until they have committed themselves to the arrangement.

Probably the most visible difference in attitude towards surrogacy between those directly involved and those not personally affected is that while the first avoid thinking and talking about the long-term effects, implications, consequences or simply the 'bigger picture', the second take all this into account. Being more detached, they measure someone's desire to have his or her own child against all these issues in accordance with their respective values, motivation and experiences.

The Church and public opinion

Since there has been no public debate on surrogacy in Romania and it is not a common topic in everyday discussion, the attitudes of the general population (i.e. people who are not directly engaged in such arrangements) towards surrogacy are manifested usually around some specific event; for example, the draft legislation of 2011 on MAHR or the landmark court decision granting legal motherhood to the genetic intending mother (referred to earlier), both of which generated opinions from all sectors, from churches to civil society, including women's associations and professionals such as doctors and lawyers. The court's decision in this case sparked controversy, especially among professional lawyers, not so much in relation to the public's reservations about it – namely that this decision could be used as a legal precedent in other similar cases – but because, as one lawyer argued, it was taken on incorrect premises. One of the most interesting aspects of this discussion from a feminist perspective is the arguments on using different standards for the recognition of genetic motherhood and fatherhood (Barac, 2014).

In Romania the Orthodox Church has a big influence on bioethical issues related to reproductive technologies. The draft law intended to legalize surrogacy encountered strong opposition from both the Orthodox and the Catholic Church, according to which it constitutes a serious attack on human dignity, the integrity of the family and the equilibrium of society. In a public letter Mon. Cornel Damian, auxiliary Bishop of Bucharest and Chairman of the Committee for the Family (Magisteriu, 2012: *Donum vitae*, II.2), states that any use of artificial insemination:

> offends the common vocation of the spouses who are called to fatherhood and motherhood: it objectively deprives conjugal fruitfulness of its unity and integrity, brings about and manifests a rupture between blood Conception, blood relation of the task and duty of education. Such damage to the personal relationships within the family has repercussions on civil society: what threatens the unity and stability of the family is a source of dissension, disorder and injustice in the whole social life.

However, some theological or pro-life critiques of surrogacy are based on doctrinal arguments, but also well informed about feminist positions that oppose the exploitation of women and commodification of children. They condemn surrogacy on the premise that it treats women as human laboratories for experimentation using reproductive technologies to separate sexuality and reproduction (Moldovan, 2014). At least one prominent bioethicist takes a similar line – that surrogacy must be treated with caution as it raises so many sensitive ethical questions and could transform the surrogate mother into a living incubator (Cuvantul Ortodox, 2011).

Two Romanian pro-life associations and the Association of Romanian Women signed a petition against surrogacy under the heading, 'No Maternity Traffic', which was initiated by the International Union for the Abolition of Surrogacy (2015) and submitted to the Council of Europe. Their views were also presented in writing to The Hague Conference on Private International law concerning surrogacy (HCCH, 2014a, 2014b). The petition calls for the abolition of surrogacy and non-recognition by national laws of the legal parenthood of intending parents of children born this way. They believe that any regulation regarding the consequences of surrogacy, especially in relation to parenthood, would imply complicity in the surrogacy business, a situation that any state caring about human dignity, children and women's rights should definitely avoid.

Another women's organization with a different ideological platform, the Romanian Women's Lobby (ROWL), the Romanian member of the European Women's Lobby (the largest umbrella organization for women's associations in the European Union), joined the Feminists for the Abolition of Surrogacy platform initiated by the European Women's Lobby, the American Center for Bioethics and Culture, the French NGO CoRP (Collectif pour le Respect de la Personne) and other feminist and human rights organizations, who also submitted a petition to The Hague Conference (CoRP, 2015).

Romanian academic feminists have yet to express a public opinion on issues concerning surrogacy, but their views can be gleaned from their publications on this and related topics. The first feminist debate on the issue of surrogacy in Romania was initiated in 2015 by Laura Grunberg and consisted of workshops convened by the feminist organization 'Ana' and 'The Coalition for Gender Equality'. Some outcomes of the debate were recently published in a special edition of the journal of gender and feminist studies *AnaLize* titled 'What is surrogacy for (East-European) feminism?' and coordinated by Ana-Luana Stoicea-Deram (2016a). One strand of argument on surrogacy she puts forward is based on the feminist ethical theory of a leading Romanian feminist, Mihaela Miroiu, who highlights the importance of valuing women's experiences of giving birth and proposes to include both rational choice and empathy as criteria for morality (Miroiu, 1996; Stoicea-Deram 2016b: 44–6). Besides raising awareness among Romanian feminists, the special edition and ensuing debate offer pertinent analysis of some aspects of surrogacy and propose possible theoretical frameworks for interpretation and policy that pave the way for a more contextualized approach to the issue.

What are the implications of Romania's non-regulated surrogacy for its citizens? Once the state recognizes children born via a surrogate overseas and there is a legal solution for surrogacy arrangements in that foreign country, non-regulation in Romania merely makes the process more costly (with citizens having to travel abroad for commercial surrogacy) and more risky (since the surrogacy contract is non-enforceable). It protects neither the infertile couples in need of a surrogate nor the surrogate nor the child who might never be able to discover the conditions of her or his birth.

In Romania there appears to be a significant consensus that transnational commercial surrogacy should not be an accepted practice. If a country is determined to impose a ban, it must first expressly prohibit it and second, enshrine in law that from a certain date the state will no longer recognize the legal parenthood of the intended parents for children born this way. However, following the recent decisions of the European Court on this issue,[9] this important step may no longer be an option for member states (HCCH, 2015: 4):

> [t]he wide margin of appreciation afforded to States regarding the decision not only whether or not to permit surrogacy, but also whether or not to recognise a legal parent–child relationship between children conceived abroad and intending parents ... has to be reduced in light of the fact that, 'an essential aspect of the identity of an individual is at stake where the legal parent–child relationship is concerned'.

If it is not possible to implement a total prohibition of commercial surrogacy, countries must introduce clear regulations and not force their citizens to engage in reproductive tourism and exclude the possibility of using reproductive technologies for those couples or individuals who cannot afford to travel abroad for this purpose.

Notes

1 Decree No. 1 of December 26, 1989 repealing the Decrees 770/1966 and 441/1985, as well as Articles 185–8 on the abortion of the Penal Code. Later Article 185 on illegal abortions was reintroduced in the Penal Code through Law no. 140/1996.

2 The first known case of a Romanian surrogate mother bearing a child took place in this period, in 1998, at the Bega clinic in Timisoara, western Romania (Nicolova, 2010).

3 This is also because Romania signed (1998) and ratified (2001) the Council of Europe Convention on Human Rights and Biomedicine (1997), known as the Oviedo Convention, which stipulates strong non-commercialization principles (Article 21 – 'The human body and its parts shall not, as such, give raise to financial gain'); also the EU Directive on Human Tissues and Cells (2004/23/EC) had to be implemented in the run-up to Romania's entry into the European Union in 2007.

4 For a precise account of the current legal situation relevant for surrogacy concerning filiation, see the questionnaire submitted by the Romanian authorities to The Hague project on surrogacy in 2013. Available (in French) at: <www.hcch.net/upload/wop/gap2014pd3ro.pdf>.

5 For the first see, for example, the biotex.com web page <http://mother-surrogate.info> and in Romanian <http://www.mamasurogat.net> and Facebook

site <www.facebook.com/pages/Clinica-Biotexcom-Mama-purtatoaresurogat-si-donare-de-ovule/621601117891596?ref=hl>. For the later categories see, for example, the SOS infertility site <http://infertilitate.com> or despre copii nostrii site, topics on surrogacy <http://comunitate.desprecopii.com/forums/topic/69832-fiv-mama-surogat>.

6 See <www.garbo.ro/comunitate/forum/view_topic/16364/vreau-sa-am-un-copil-caut-mama.html>.

7 The link to this story is no longer available.

8 See <www.youtube.com/watch?v=Z7R2okQ8sQs and www.youtube.com/watch?v=oKlUfC2mELo> (original source: *La Maruta*, PRO-TV, 24 July 2016).

9 The decisions of the European Court of Human Rights in *Mennesson v. France* and *Labassee v. France*, 26 June 2014. Application numbers 65192/11 and 65941/11.

References

Agacinski S (2016) La maternité mise sur le marché. In: Stoicea-Deram A-L (ed.) What is surrogacy for feminism? *AnaLize* 6(20): 12–19.

Barac L (2014) *Câteva considerații privind implicațiile juridice ale tehnicilor de reproducere umană asistată medical (RUAM)*, 3 March. <www.juridice.ro/311847/cateva-consideratii-privind-implicatiile-juridice-ale-tehnicilor-de-reproducere-umana-asistata-medical-ruam.html>

BioTexCom (n.d.) Law on surrogacy in Ukraine. <http://biotexcom.com/law-on-surrogacy-in-ukraine>

CoRP (2015) Hague Conference: Feminists for the abolition of surrogacy. <http://collectif-corp.com/2015/03/24/hague-conference-feminists-for-the-abolition-of-surrogacy>

Cutaș D (2008) On a Romanian attempt to legislate on medically assisted human reproduction. *Bioethics* 22(1): 56–63.

Cuvantul Ortodox (2011) *Dr Vasile Astarastoae despre proiectul legislativ ce instituie MAMELE SUROGAT: nu cumva transformam femeia intr-un incubator viu?* <www.cuvantul-ortodox.ro/recomandari/2011/02/24/dr-vasile-astarastoae-despre-proiectul-legislativ-ce-institutie-mamele-surogat-nu-cumva-transformam-femeia-intr-un-incubator-viu>

Darnovsky M (2009) Israeli feminists respond to Romanian egg scandal. *Biopolitical Times*. <www.biopoliticaltimes.org/article.php?id=4843>

Demény E (2013) Medically assisted reproduction: challenges for regulation in Romania. In: Sandor J (ed.) *Studies in Biopolitics*. Budapest: Center for Ethics and Law in Biomedicine, pp. 91–102.

Draft Law on Medically Assisted Human Reproduction (2011) <http://www.senat.ro/legis/PDF%5C2011%5C11b078FG.pdf>

Frunza M (2010) Etică și vulnerabilitate în reproducerea asistată: Studiu de caz. *Studia Universitatis Babes-Bolyai. Bioethica* 2: 15–22.

Gheaus A (2016) The normative importance of pregnancy challenges surrogacy contracts. In: Stoicea-Deram A-L (ed.) What is surrogacy for feminism? *AnaLlize* 6(20): 20–31.

Guțan S (2011) *Reproducerea Umană Asistată Medical și Filiația*. Bucharest: Humangiu.

HCCH (Hague Conference on International Private Law) (2014a) *The Desirability and Feasibility of Further Work on the Parentage/Surrogacy Project*. Preliminary Document No. 3B. The Hague: HCCH.

HCCH (2014b) *A Study of Legal Parentage and the Issues Arising from*

International Surrogacy Arrangements. Preliminary Document No. 3C. The Hague: HCCH.

HCCH (2015) *The Parentage/Surrogacy Project: An Updating Note*. Preliminary Document No. 3. The Hague: HCCH.

Hostiuc S et al. (2016a) Ethical controversies in maternal surrogacy. *Gineco.eu* 12: 99–102. <http://gineco.eu/system/revista/34/99-102.pdf>

Hostiuc S, Iancu CB, Năștășel V, Alua M and Renția I (2016b) Maternal filiation in surrogacy: legal consequences in Romanian context and the role of the genetic report for establishing kinship. *Romanian Journal of Legal Medicine* 24(1): 47–51.

Iacob AA and Stoian SA (2016) A reproductive justice lens towards the reasons to be a surrogate mother in Romania. In: Stoicea-Deram A-L (ed.) What is surrogacy for feminism? *AnaLize* 6(20): 50–65.

International Union for the Abolition of Surrogacy (2015) 'No Maternity Traffic': Surrogate Motherhood and Human Rights. <www.nomaternitytraffic.eu/wordpress/wp-content/uploads/2015/09/2015-Contribution-HCCH-No-Maternity-Traffic-EN.pdf>

Iusmen I (2013) The EU and international adoption from Romania. *International Journal of Law and Policy on Family* 27(1): 1–27.

Kligman G (1998) *The Politics of Duplicity: Controlling Reproduction in Ceaușescu's Romania*. Berkeley, CA: University of California Press.

Lundin S (2012) 'I want a baby; don't stop me from being a mother': an ethnographic study on fertility tourism and the egg trade. *Cultural Politics* 8(2): 327–43.

Magisteriu (2012) Letter of the representatives of the Catholic Church to the Ministry of Health on the issue of Draft Law on Third Party Medically Assisted Reproduction, 8 March. <www.magisteriu.ro/scrisoarea-deschisa-a-cer-despre-reproducerea-umana-asistata-medical-2012>

Marinescu R (2016) Surrogacy: from commodification to empowerment: a literary perspective. In: Stoicea-Deram A-L (ed.) What is surrogacy for feminism? *AnaLize* 6(20): 89–107.

Miroiu M (1996) *Convenio: On Women, Nature and Morals*. Bucharest: Alternative Publishing House.

Miroiu M (2015) On women, feminism and democracy. In: Stan L and Vancea D (eds) *Post-Communist Romania at Twenty-Five: Linking Past, Present, and Future*. Lanham, MD: Lexington Books, pp. 87–106.

Miroiu M and Otilia Dragomir O (eds) (2010) *Nașterea: Istorii trăite*. Bucharest: Polirom.

Moldovan S (2014) *Școala Provita. Probleme fundamentale de bioetică (V). Sănătatea reproducerii și drepturile sexuale* [Provita School. Fundamental problems of bioethics (V). Reproductive health and sexual rights]. <www.culturavietii.ro/2014/01/23/sanatatea-reproducerii>

Morgan D (2003) Enigma Variations: surrogacy, rights and procreative tourism. In: Cook R, Sclater SD and Kaganas F (eds) *Surrogate Motherhood: International Perspectives*. Oxford and Portland, OR: Hart Publishing, pp. 75–92.

Morrison L (2004) Ceausescu's legacy: family struggles and institutionalisation of children in Romania. *Journal of Family History* 29(2): 168–82.

Nicolova D (2010) Women head East for wombs to rent. *Balkan Insight*, 28 October. In English <www.balkaninsight.com/en/article/women-head-east-for-wombs-to-rent>; in Romanian <www.bejeus.com/2010/01/interviu-cu-o-mama-surogatpurtatoare.html>

Official Gazette [the official legal publication of the Romania State] (2011) Part I, No. 505 of 15 July 2011.

Sandu MI, MP (2011) Reasoning submitted for the legislative proposal on medically assisted human reproduction. <www.senat.ro/legis/PDF%5C2011%5C11b078EM.pdf>

Savanandan S (2016) 'Humanitarian' thresholds of the fundamental feminist ideologies: evidence from surrogacy arrangements in India. *AnaLize* 6(20): 66–88.

Selman P (2010) Intercountry adoption as globalized motherhood. In: Chavkin W and Maher J (eds) *The Globalization of Motherhood: Deconstructions and Reconstructions of Biology and Care*. New York: Routledge, pp. 79–104.

Stoicea-Deram A-L (ed.) (2016a) What is surrogacy for feminism? Special issue of *AnaLize* 6(20).

Stoicea-Deram A-L (2016b) Devant une pratique silencieuse, un féminisme muet. La maternité de substitution en Europe de l'Est. In: Stoicea-Deram A-L (ed.) What is surrogacy for feminism? *AnaLize* 6(20): 32–49.

United Nations (2013) *World Abortion Policies 2013*. <www.un.org/en/development/desa/population/publications/policy/world-abortion-policies-2013.shtml>

8 | SURROGACY ARRANGEMENTS IN AUSTERITY GREECE: POLICY CONSIDERATIONS IN A PERMISSIVE REGIME

Konstantina Davaki

Introduction

Global commercial surrogacy is a highly divisive and controversial issue. Legal and ethical aspects, such as citizenship, parentage and the human rights of children, and the protection of life and genetic material have been extensively researched (Anderson, 1993; Ber, 2000; Brunet *et al.*, 2013; Deonandan, 2013). In particular, the intrusion of the market into childbearing opens up the potential for the exploitation of all the main parties concerned: surrogates, egg providers, intended parents and the children born through surrogacy. Political parties, institutions, medical associations, religious groups, social movements and private and public interests all contribute to specific policies and legislation. Culture and kinship structures, attitudes towards new technologies and ethical dilemmas also inform various state responses.

Cross-border reproductive care, often seen as the outcome of limited public services or prohibiting legislation in the home country, has increased challenges around surrogacy. Destination countries lack the regulation and transparency to expose unprofessional, unethical or illegal practices (Crozier, 2010; Deonandan *et al.*, 2012). Globalization and the pervasiveness of information technologies have enhanced cross-border surrogacy, itself facilitated by an escalation of fertility tourism (Gamble and Ghevaert, 2009; Vasilakou, 2010). The proliferation of agencies, clinics and law firms has increased competition (Berend, 2012) and highlighted the profound inequalities between buyers and sellers of surrogate services (Martin, 2009; Pande, 2011).

All the above delineate surrogacy as a unique individual experience, conditioned by ethical dilemmas, socio-economic circumstances, and cultural and regulatory contexts, as well as the relations between the parties involved. Surrogates are not a uniform category. Those living in the more wealthy regions of the global north are generally well-informed, professional, networked and often perfectly capable of negotiating the terms of contracts. By contrast, their counterparts in low-income settings are much more prone to exploitation.

The case of Greece is of particular interest, as it is the first EU member state where altruistic gestational surrogacy is permitted and regulated. The relevant bill was voted unanimously by the Greek Parliament in 2002 and resulted in 2005 in Law 3305/2005 – Enforcement of Medically Assisted Reproduction, while it is also regulated by the combination of Articles 1458 and 1464 of the Greek Civil Code. Since the law came into force, there have been a considerable number of rulings authorizing surrogacy; passing reference will be made to some significant court rulings that went beyond the letter of the law.

This chapter presents the legal and sociological background of surrogacy in Greece. Using specific examples, it goes on to provide a critical analysis of the main challenges, arguments and attitudes of institutions, legal and medical experts, feminists and the media in relation to transnational surrogacy arrangements.

The Greek context

Facts and figures Over the last seven years, Greece, with a population of 11 million, has been experiencing the worst economic crisis of its recent history; tough austerity measures imposed by its European partners have led to soaring unemployment, increasing poverty and a shrinking population.[1] Due to its geographical location, it also constitutes the entry point for refugees and migrant workers who arrive in their thousands every day – a phenomenon that has acquired unprecedented dimensions and requires a solution on a European level.

Some very recent and significant developments took place in 2015. For the first time in Greece's modern history a party of the radical left, Syriza, came to power. One of its electoral pledges included passing a law permitting civil unions for same-sex couples, a matter that had been pending since November 2013, when the European Court of Human Rights found that Greece had violated Articles 8 and 14 of the Convention by denying such access to homosexual couples. The bill was passed by the Greek parliament on 23 December 2015 in a climate of significant resistance and controversy (Reuters, 2015). Now, for the first time, same-sex couples can enter an agreement of cohabitation that gives them the right to civil partnership. Nevertheless, the right for them to adopt children or use surrogacy as a method of creating a family was not granted.

Family in Greece is culturally very important and plays a key role in people's welfare. In the 1970s and 1980s the country had a highly active and ideologically influential autonomous feminist movement. Many of its claims were subsequently adopted by the 'women's movement', an umbrella term encompassing the feminist branches of political parties that were visible on the political scene in the 1980s. This period was marked by the rise to power of Pasok, a social democratic party that introduced a series of reforms related to family law. These incorporated many of the key claims of autonomous feminists, among them legalization of abortion and the overall extension and recognition of women's rights. This piece of legislation was highly advanced and did not correspond to the mentality of most of Greek society at that time (Davaki, 2001).

Against this background, in recent years, Greece has become an increasingly popular destination for 'reproductive tourism'. IVF treatments have multiplied, with couples coming from thirty-four countries. Favourable circumstances include cheaper prices (compared to double prices in the UK and quadruple in the US) and high success rates (Velissaris, 2015). However, there are some significant details: for instance, known donors are used only in fertility treatment for married couples and a marriage certificate is asked for.

Greek law

Description/rationale Even though surrogacy practices existed in Greece prior to 2002, these were not regulated. Legally, children born to surrogate mothers 'belonged' to them. A landmark ruling (31/5803/176/1999) of the multi-member Court of the First Order in Herakleion in Crete in 1999, which approved the application of a couple to adopt twins who had been born by a surrogate mother but using their own genetic material, paved the way for a new law (Agallopoulou, 2004). This case was the first application for parental rights by the woman who was the genetic but not the gestational mother. The court recommended a law reform to address the gap in law concerning legal parenthood, as it felt 'unnatural' for a woman to adopt a child produced by using her own genetic material (Brunet et al., 2013).

In 2002, Law 3089/2002 on 'medical assistance in human reproduction' was passed. It was meant to regulate a number of issues in reproductive medicine following advances in biomedicine and relevant legislation in other countries. The law included specific rules concerning the permissibility of the practice of gestational surrogacy[2] and challenged traditional Greek ideas about family formation.

Three years later, Law 3305/2005 on the 'implementation of medically assisted human reproduction' established that the surrogate and the intended mother had to be permanent residents of Greece. It also provided further details on the permissibility of surrogacy by stipulating the concept and meaning of 'reasonable expenses' paid to a surrogate and introducing criminal and civil sanctions for violations of the legislation (Brunet et al., 2013). 'Reasonable expenses' comprise necessary expenses for IVF, pregnancy and delivery, as well as restitution of damages and lost wages for any unpaid leave of absence during the pregnancy. The amount of compensation is regulated by the National Independent Authority for Medically Assisted Reproduction and is currently set at 10,000 euros, which symbolically includes ten months' salary (nine for gestation and one after birth) for the surrogate. This amount was fixed at a relatively low level in order to stress the altruistic dimension of surrogacy (Fotiadi, 2014; Nikolaou, 2015). A contract is signed without any remuneration other than the above-mentioned expenses (Petroulia, 2012). In the contract all parties involved need to ascertain that the children to be produced will be the children of the commissioning party and not the surrogate.

Requirements for the surrogate mother are:

- that she is younger than 50 and absolutely healthy (this has to be demonstrated through relevant medical examination) and suitable for bearing a child;[3]
- that she is a permanent resident in the country (without necessarily being a Greek national);
- that she is willing to sign the contract between the commissioning parents and herself and that she has the consent of her husband, if married (if she proceeds without this, he is entitled to legal compensation for violation of his human rights);
- that she does not own the eggs used, thus reducing the chance that she might in future claim to be the mother of the child.

Requirements for the intended mother are:

- that she is a permanent resident in the country (without necessarily being a Greek national);
- that she has health problems that prevent her from conceiving or gestating a child or make pregnancy a serious risk (e.g. uterus problems, hormonal imbalance or more serious health issues such as liver failure or heart disease) – these have to be demonstrated

through a doctor's diagnosis and relevant testimonials. It is not enough that a woman might not be able to reproduce through natural means;
- that she is in the reproductive stage of her life and willing to donate her egg or request eggs from a donor (this is to avoid having a child at a very advanced age);
- that she submits an application to her local court of justice to obtain permission to enter the surrogate arrangements; the application should include a copy of the proposed surrogate agreement, including the proposed compensation (Agallopoulou, 2004).

Article 1464 of the Civil Code determines that motherhood rights belong to the intended mother and not the surrogate. The legislator tried to prevent issues that could possibly arise and lead to litigation; for instance, circumstances whereby the surrogate refuses to relinquish the child or the intended mother refuses to accept the child, or in the event that the intended mother or parents die before the child is born[4] (Agallopoulou, 2004). The rights and interests of any resulting child are protected as well as the individuals' rights to personal freedom, family formation and autonomy. Laws 3089/2002 and 3305/2005 are in harmony with the moral principles, rights and obligations of the Greek Constitution and consistent with the European and international laws and inter-country agreements on human rights, and on the protection of and respect for the children's welfare.[5]

By setting strict conditions the law safeguards both the intended parents and the surrogate. Several doctors and lawyers have ascertained that 'it constitutes one of the most pioneering legal frameworks in the world' (Nikolaou, 2015; Paraschos, 2012). In addition, Article 1456 (para. 1) of the Greek Civil Code determines that medical assistance for human reproduction purposes can be requested by (married or unmarried) heterosexual couples, or unmarried women without a partner; such assistance is not available to same-sex couples (gay or lesbian) or single men.

Surrogacy cases are in the first instance examined by civil courts; judges do not look into the reasons why the parties engage in the agreement, they just request proof of inability of the intended mother and residency status. Hatzis (2010) attributes this to the interest of the vast majority of Greek legal professionals who tend to prioritize doctrinal consistency rather than the efficacy of the law.

New surrogacy law Commercial surrogacy or transnational arrangements were banned under Law 3089/2002, which determined that both the intended mother and the surrogate were domiciled in Greece (Article 8). As in other countries, this clause was intended to prevent cross-border reproductive tourism and was produced following discussion in parliament (Agallopoulou, 2004). In terms of interpreting the domicile principle, the judges would request proof that both women had been resident in the country for a certain amount of time and that they would stay for a long period in the future. However, research has shown that this second condition was not given serious consideration and that *de facto* judges did not request proof of future intention on the part of either the surrogate or the intended mother to remain in Greece (Brunet *et al.*, 2013).

In the summer of 2014, during the Greek holiday season and in an extremely tense political climate, Law 4272/2014 was passed. According to Article 17 of this new piece of legislation, one of the two parties, namely the intended mother or the surrogate, needs to be a permanent resident of Greece; the other may have a temporary residence. This has attracted criticism: first, it officially opens the door to reproductive tourism; second, it creates circumstances conducive to the trafficking of women from poorer countries for surrogacy services; third, it can create problematic situations, for instance, when the legal conditions for maternity are different between Greece and the intended mother's country of origin (Stamatoukou, 2015).

In fact, the surrogate and the intended mother do not even need to be EU citizens, which opens the door for further commercialization of surrogacy. As Greece was the first EU country with a regulated and legal surrogacy programme, and due to the limitations of using donated oocytes or sperm in other EU countries, Greece has already become a market for ARTs (www.globalsurrogacy.world.com). For some media, the advantages of Greece as a surrogacy haven include high-quality fertility clinics and a solid legal framework that will help the country 'soon become a new leader in the surrogacy world' (www.fertilitysolutionsinternational.com).

As mentioned, the intended parents can be either a married or unmarried couple or a single woman; there have been cases of single or gay men applying and being approved by the court, but often these have been overturned at the Greek Appeals Court. Whether this is in accordance with the sex equality principle of the Constitution is debatable. At the time of writing, same-sex couples (either gay or lesbian) cannot apply for surrogacy; however, since same-sex unions are now permitted, it is expected that in the future homosexual couples will be allowed to have children with surrogacy as an option.

While the law sets out the requirements for a surrogacy arrangement to take place, these have not been interpreted consistently by judges. For example, in one case the permission granted to an intended father (part of a commissioning couple) was subsequently considered illegal by a higher court (after twins had been born via surrogacy) and parentage was taken away from him on the basis that the application should have been submitted by the mother (Tsimpoukis, 2014). The law does not allow a single man's application for surrogacy arrangements; however, recently this was seen as in breach of equality of the sexes.[6]

Surrogacy in practice

Empirical data are scarce and precise figures on successful cases of surrogacy are hard to estimate. There are two main reasons. First, although gestational surrogacy clearly requires medical intervention, officially reported statistics do not necessarily record the surrogacy arrangement but only the IVF procedure. Second, in many countries there is simply no regulation or licensing regime for fertility treatment and/or surrogacy. The lack of formal reporting mechanisms makes *ad hoc* collection of statistics by individual organizations the only option. Nevertheless, fertility clinics are reluctant to provide data, as we experienced first-hand when working on the empirical part of a recent study (Brunet *et al.*, 2013).

Despite these difficulties, we can point to a number of factors that signal a rise in surrogacy practice. A simple internet search reveals a plethora of agencies and clinics that explicitly seek to facilitate surrogacy arrangements in Greece and boast about their success rate. Some are voluntary organizations that set out to match willing surrogate mothers and hopeful parents on a non-commercial basis; others are for-profit and operate either as part of a fertility clinic or in partnership with fertility clinics. The role of intermediaries is hard to regulate, one of the particularities of Greece being the high number of medical doctors and their immense power as a professional category.

Since 2005, over 120 court decisions have granted permission to couples wishing to become parents through surrogacy, including many from overseas, and it is estimated that there are about ten decisions per year. However, complaints are often expressed regarding delays due to the necessary legal and administrative procedures. According to research by Ravdas (2012) and based on 200 court rulings, 24 per cent of the couples resorting to surrogacy have done so by using a member of their family or a friend paying only 'reasonable expenses'. The rest employ specialized IVF clinics where the remuneration starts at 20,000 euros (Fotiadi, 2014).

Reports have demonstrated that couples from many EU countries now use the services of Greek fertility clinics to have a child (Stamatoukou, 2015). In many ways the conditions are favourable. For example, unlike Australia, by Greek law IVF donors are completely anonymous, meaning that couples do not come into contact with them and do not have to face complications such as the risk of the donor and the child reuniting (Velissaris, 2015).

The socio-economic context also lends itself to commercial surrogacy. The unemployment rate among young people is currently estimated at about 50 per cent. This has led to a rising number of young women offering to act as surrogates in order to generate some income. Doctors also see it as a money-making business with different profit margins: in one case, a doctor asked for 70,000 euros to find a surrogate for a commissioning couple (Nikolaou, 2015).

According to data provided by one of the main Greek newspapers *Ta Nea*, by 2010 over 100 surrogacy arrangements had been authorized by the courts. Out of these, 90 per cent of surrogate mothers were not relatives but 'best friends' of intended mothers (Tsoulea 2010). Another survey of court decisions in Athens, Piraeus and Thessaloniki, showed that out of ninety-two cases only thirteen had involved close relatives, while the remaining seventy-nine involved 'best friends' who were ten to twenty years younger than the intended mothers and mainly from Eastern Europe (Hatzis, 2010). In the same vein, research using legal cases over the period 2003–12 has shown that 91 per cent of the applicant women were Greek and 6 per cent foreign nationals, and all were married and without children. In contrast, over half (54 per cent) of the surrogates were foreign nationals and just over one-third (38 per cent) Greek; they were 33 to 39 years of age, 53 per cent were married and 48 per cent had their own child. Of the foreign surrogates, 35 per cent were from Eastern Europe and the ex-Soviet Union and 21 per cent from the Balkan states. The Greek surrogates were either relatives or friends of the intending mothers. Among the foreign surrogates, 17 per cent had a work relationship (domestic workers) with the intended mother. A significant question raised in the study is whether these data reveal altruistic behaviour or whether they constitute the expression of new forms of the female body being put to work (Ravdas, 2012).

Public attitudes

Surrogacy in Greece is gaining ground with more and more couples using it as a childbearing method. However, many are discouraged when the candidate surrogate mother requests exorbitant fees. For example, in one typical case, a husband and wife had agreed to 20,000 euros, but when the ultrasound showed twins the surrogate requested the amount be doubled to 40,000 (Fotiadi, 2014).

The debate on surrogacy in Greece both reflects the global surrogacy debate and presents its own particularities. On an ethical level, viewpoints on surrogacy, whether traditional or gestational, altruistic or commercial, differ greatly. Most churches and relevant organizations are especially against its commercial form, which is seen as immoral and a threat to the institution of marriage and the dignity of children. According to liberal views, however, the parties entering surrogacy arrangements are the proper judges of their own welfare; thus, a contract that makes all parties better off should be enforced rather than prohibited by law (Hatzis, 2003). It is interesting that the aforementioned case of the father whose parentage was denied because he did not have the right to apply for fatherhood via the court was regarded with sympathy by the public, fuelled by indignation at what was seen as mishandling on the part of the legal system. However, the case also attracted comments on the complications to be expected from such arrangements, with many people seeing gestational surrogacy as being against the law of nature – an impediment to the normal functions of society.

Qualitative research involving a number of women in Greece who have resorted to ARTs has shown that difficulties in producing a child often reinforce the desire for parenthood, enabling women to tolerate long-term and psychologically painful procedures. Attitudes of prejudice and the possible stigmatization of childless couples contribute to this desire as Greek society is seen to exert pressures towards childbearing. The same research found a high number of abortions in the women studied and concluded that the intensity of desire for a child varies during the period of attempts to conceive (Papaligoura *et al.*, 2013).

Greek society seems to be divided by surrogacy. As more infertile couples resort to it as a method of achieving parenthood, attitudes are gradually changing and it is becoming less of a taboo. However, the degree of acceptance and public feelings on the matter are mediated also by changing forms of family, the role of the church and education (Petroulia, 2012). Interestingly, most Greek feminist activists are against (Gasouka 2014) for reasons to do with autonomy and the opposite of views expressed by religious people and proponents of traditional family (see Papathanasopoulos, 2014).

The media also play a considerable role in shaping attitudes as they tend to be dominated by religious and also homophobic opinion. For example, some media outlets have expressed negative views towards the potential approval by the courts of the application of single men for surrogacy on the basis that a child's upbringing should incorporate influences from both sexes. A survey by Kapa Research in April 2015 showed that 39.3 per cent of the Greeks asked were actually in favour of same-sex unions (Chiotis, 2015). Following the recognition of such unions by the Greek Parliament in December 2015, a further survey found that only 14 per cent of the participants endorsed the legalization of family creation for same-sex couples (Public Issue, 2016), as opposed to those who are increasingly in favour of new trends in family raising (Chrysostomou, 2015).

People with fertility problems perceive the legal framework very positively. They consider the chance to use surrogacy under a sound legal framework as a golden opportunity. As surrogacy is often between relatives or friends empathy plays a significant role. Bearing the child of one's best friend carries feelings of responsibility and love. On such occasions surrogacy is underpinned by altruism and solidarity between women towards achieving the 'natural' female goal of reproduction. Many Greek surrogates consider it a vocation (Stamatoukou 2015). For radical feminists though, it has been condemned as a practice that is about satisfying the selfish desire of middle-class intended parents while exploiting surrogate mothers, who are forced to sell 'their children' (Konstantinidi, 2015).

New media such as blogs provide opportunities for the exchange of views and questions regarding the availability and procedures of surrogacy for those in need. Civil society organizations (such as the Association for Fertility Support, Kyveli, active since 1995) are increasingly present and offer support services to couples or individuals who face fertility problems (Nikolaou, 2015).

The progressive law seems to be fitting in with the dominant place of family in Greek social life. Family support plays a vital role in the successful implementation of surrogacy law, in the sense that relatives help the family member who acts as a surrogate to carry out her task by relieving her from other family responsibilities, including in many cases caring for her own children (Fotiadi, 2014). Indeed, quite a few cases have involved grandmothers giving birth to their grandchildren or aunties to their nephew or niece (Kapernarakou 2011).

Feminist critiques

Surrogacy is a very controversial topic for feminists. Liberal feminists (Scott, 2009) take a positive stance, stressing the right of women to determine their reproductive rights, whereas socialist and radical feminists are strongly against, using the commodification argument and expressing fears about disadvantaged women being transformed into an army of surrogate labour often without any legal rights (Anderson, 1993; Kimbrell, 1993). Divisions within women include inequalities between those who can take advantage of new ARTs and those in need of generating an income who offer their body for this purpose. These dichotomies lie at the heart of the surrogacy debate in Greece (Gasouka, 2014). Different attitudes are also linked to broader ethical considerations regarding the concepts of parenthood and childbearing, as well as sociological questions related to the nature of the contemporary family and the parent–child relationship (Karagianni, 2013).

In this debate *autonomy* and *informed consent* are key concepts. It is presumed that a woman who decides to become a surrogate is autonomous, but economic or emotional pressures should not be underestimated (Ber, 2000). In such cases, the western liberal emphasis on the right to choose comes up against the risk that this 'choice' might be 'imposed'. Informed consent may be compromised by coercion (e.g. by family, poverty and unemployment), uncertainty as to the emotional and psychological impact on the surrogate and her surroundings, lack of knowledge about pregnancy complications, complexity of contracts and uncertain ethical implications for the wider community (Storrow, 2005; Tieu, 2009). Furthermore, intended parents and/or physicians can impose invasive procedures, changes in diet or lifestyle or termination of pregnancy in the case of a defective fetus.

What motivates intended mothers and surrogates in Greece is under-researched and extensive qualitative work is required. Sample texts from internet adverts give some idea of this diverse landscape (see Tables 8.1 and 8.2). Intended mothers tend to be driven by health issues and the familiar desire for at least some genetic link with the child. Surrogates posting their services online tend not to mention payment, though this is presumably understood. One exception here is Fotini (Table 8.2), who chooses not to have children of her own due to lack of financial resources but wishes to experience pregnancy and childbirth and appears willing to forego payment – although a contribution to her father's health care clearly would be appreciated.

TABLE 8.1 Profiles of Greek intended mothers as presented in adverts or press articles

Polly: Greek/English, late 40s, professional musician, single, residing in Athens	Polly decided to have a child after she had turned 40 after separating from her long-term partner. Following six years of failed attempts to conceive through donor sperm, she decided to resort to surrogacy. She became a mother of a son whose donor-father has already fathered 30 children across mainly the US. Polly has identified some of them through the online donor registry and is in touch with those families that wish to communicate. She would never adopt. She believes a lot in DNA and wanted her child to have a genetic link with her, which she does not consider a selfish attitude. On the contrary, she considers it more selfish for a mother to work and neglect her children or to have many children in order to get social protection benefits (as in the UK). Her only source of concern is that her son may try to find his biological father when he turns 18 (Papadimitriou, 2012).
Katerina: Greek, 34 years old	'After trying for two years already, due to health problems I will not be able to conceive. Looking for women who would like to help us hold the baby we so desire' (http://forum.eimaimama.gr, October 2010)
Eleni: Greek, living in a provincial town and married	Eleni was unable to conceive due to womb dysplasia and was looking for a surrogate mother. She had made numerous attempts to find one through fertility centres but the minimum cost would be 50,000 to 100,000 euros, which is way above their budget (Athanasiadou, 2012).
Stella: 26 years old from Cyprus	After four years of fertility treatments Stella fell pregnant but the embryo died at 36 weeks, causing septicaemia that almost killed her. Suffering from endometriosis and numerous other problems, she will not be able to conceive. She is desperately looking for a surrogate mother and will do her best, given her limited finances (http://SuperMomRocks.me, January 2015).

Informed consent presupposes access to and availability of information. In the case of Greece, raising awareness is an urgent priority. Surprisingly, Greek feminists have not dealt enough with the topic. A possible explanation may be that feminists (the only ones who

TABLE 8.2 Profiles and attitudes of surrogates

Fotini: Greek, living in Athens, 28 years old, single and childless	Fotini decided to never have children of her own because of austerity and lack of financial means to support them. She volunteers to carry a baby because she wants to experience pregnancy and childbirth but does not wish to be paid. If the intended parents want to help financially, they could contribute towards the expenses for her father's health care (http://SuperMomRocks.me, April 2013).
Mihaela: Non-Greek but does not state nationality	Mihaela stresses that she is a foreigner, 28 years old, single with no children. She is offering to become a surrogate for financial reasons (http://SuperMomRocks.me, February 2015).
Olga: 25 years old, married, healthy and a mother herself	Olga wishes to become a surrogate but does not state why. However, from the use of language in the advert it is obvious she is not Greek (http://SuperMomRocks.me, May 2015)
Voula: Greek, 18 years of age	'I am 18 years old and wish to become a surrogate mother' (http://SuperMomRocks.me, March 2015).

have reacted) adopt the commodification argument fully and dismiss surrogacy altogether.

Policy considerations and the economic crisis

Surrogacy in Greece is still altruistic on paper. In reality, large sums of money are requested from intended parents and Greece, compared to many countries, is a very attractive destination for fertility treatments because prices are comparable to those of Eastern Europe and India, with the additional advantage of the security offered to intended parents by the legislative framework (see Table 8.3).

There have been cases where the altruistic nature of the relationship between the contracting parties is doubtful and the consent of the surrogate uncertain, while the remuneration arrangements can include informal payments to her; in general, there tends to be a lack of transparency with respect to the details of each arrangement, giving rise to concerns about possible exploitation. In reality, as research has shown, on many occasions the arrangement was between Greek women and foreign nationals, who happened to reside in Greece and fulfilled the relevant requirements. Often they were domestic helpers of the intended parents or their extended family (Brunet *et al.*, 2013).

TABLE 8.3 Surrogacy costs

	Greek islands	Cyprus	Eastern Europe	India
Surrogacy with a clinic donor	From €26,000	From €24,000	€26,400	Indian egg donor: From US$26,500
Surrogacy with an agency donor	From €34,000	From €28,000		From US$36,500
EU surrogate with a clinic donor	From €47,000	From €40,000	€32,500	
EU surrogate with an agency donor	From €49,500	From €49,000		

Source: www.reproductive-solutions.com

When fertility clinic gynecologists are asked by representatives of the media about what motivates a woman to become a surrogate, their answer is typically 'altruism'. They argue that they are mothers themselves and they want to help less fortunate women to experience motherhood. However, when one of these well-known doctors was asked about the feelings of the surrogate mother right after giving birth, he said that, 'of course there is a bond that ceases existing because the baby is not genetically related to the surrogate mother' (www.ivf-embryo.gr/exosomatiki-ivf/dorea-oarion-emvryon/parentheti-mitrotita). It may help to re-examine the rhetoric in the light of the high cost of fertility treatments and some facts about the c-section rates in Greece, which keep rising.[7]

Evidence about commercial surrogacy in Greece can be collected from abundant websites. Commodification and exploitation of the female body is manifested in practices such as changing the surrogate during the preparation and replacing her with another for a number of reasons (abnormal thickness of the endometrium, too much blood flow during preparation of the surrogate and non-synchronization of the fertility cycle between the surrogate and the egg donor are the usual medical causes calling for a replacement candidate before impregnation takes place; http://newlifegreece.com). One wonders how changing a surrogate can be so easy when, according to intended mothers' blogs, some have been trying for years to find an altruistic surrogate while for clinics such as New Life it seems so easy.

Such practices show complete lack of respect for the health of surrogates who may have been subjected to treatments without reaching their target. As explained in some detail in Chapter 5 of this collection, their health can be affected by the hormone treatments and risks related to IVF, pregnancy and labour (Chaves, 2011; Montgolfier and Mirkovic, 2009). Neglected dimensions include the biological bonding of the surrogate with the child, relinquishment and the resulting psychological impact. Financial need and lack of regulation expose surrogate mothers to greater health risks.

Conclusions

This chapter has attempted to shed light on different aspects of surrogacy arrangements by looking at legislation, practice and attitudes against the broader socio-economic background of Greece in the midst of a severe economic crisis. It has identified the shortcomings of a 'progressive' legislative framework that seems to be increasingly deployed to facilitate commercial surrogacy arrangements.

Evidence shows rising numbers of foreign and Greek young women offering to act as surrogates, while scandals about huge sums of money involved in deals with clinics and intermediaries come to light. Greece features as a fertility haven all over the internet, yet Greek judges and doctors insist on the rhetoric of altruism.

A better understanding of this complex phenomenon and intertwined interests is urgently required, and considerable efforts at increasing public awareness of the related problems should lead to appreciation of the need for more regulation and for ethical and fair future policies to improve the circumstances of everyone involved.

Without disregarding potential risks and room for the exploitation of intended parents by surrogates, it appears that the latter remain the most vulnerable party. More qualitative research is needed to unravel the motives behind women's decision to act as surrogates and bring to the fore the network of interests that may lead to intricate situations calling for further regulation to safeguard the rights, health and self-determination of surrogate mothers in a European landscape of constant flows of immigration.

Notes

1 According to the latest figures from the Greek Statistical Authority (ELSTAT) on natural population change, there were 111,794 deaths in 2013 compared to only 94,134 births, resulting in an overall population decrease of 17,660. This trend has been picking up steam in the last few years. In 2012, the decline amounted

to 16,297 people, almost four times that of 2011 when the figure was only 4,671. Moreover, the number of abandoned babies in maternity hospitals keeps rising (Vassilopoulou, 2015).

2 The law defines surrogacy as: 'the transfer of fertilized eggs, which do not belong to the surrogate mother herself, into the body of another woman, so as to gestate them. This is allowed when there is a written agreement, without any financial benefit, between the parties involved, meaning the person(s) wishing to have a child and the surrogate mother, and her husband, if she has one. The court authorization is issued before the transfer and following an application by the woman who wants to have a child, provided that evidence is adduced proving that the intentional mother is unable (for medical reasons) to bear a child, and that the woman offering to become the surrogate is, with regards to her (physical and mental) health status, suitable for it.'

3 In certain clinics, at least, the surrogate undergoes extensive psychological and medical screening and is subject to a trial for six months before being presented to a candidate couple as a potential surrogate.

4 In the event of the death of the intended mother or both intended parents before the birth, the child is still considered their child and by law carries the relevant property and other rights.

5 More specifically, Greek laws on assisted reproduction are in line with the provisions of the European Convention of Human Rights (ECHR), the Directive of the EU Parliament and of the Council of 31 March 2004 (2004/23/EC), and the European Convention on the Exercise of Children's Rights CETS No. 160, which are inserted into the national legislation, as well as the UN Convention on the Rights of the Child (Brunet *et al.*, 2013).

6 For example, cases 2827/2008 by the One Member Court of First Instance of Athens and 13707/2009 by the One Member Court of First Instance of Thessaloniki (see Panagos, 2011).

7 C-section is the method used for surrogacy deliveries for the convenience of the surrogate mother and safety of those 'precious' babies. However, it is worth noting that Greece has an extremely high caesarean percentage rate and that accurate statistical data are missing from international tables. According to a recent article in a Greek newspaper (Bouloutza, 2015) it has reached the level of 50–70 per cent (among the highest in the world), with the majority carried out in private hospitals. The EU average is around 25 per cent while the WHO recommends 15–20 per cent. Research on the causes of this phenomenon has shown that the of main factors are doctors' convenience, the fact that there is a booming market in the private sector, mothers' socio-economic status and fear of going through labour. In public hospitals higher informal fees by physicians may play another decisive role (Mossialos *et al.*, 2005).

References

Agallopoulou P (2004) Surrogate motherhood. <http://docplayer.gr/docview/22/1712111>

Anderson E (1993) *Values in Ethics and Economics*. Cambridge, MA: Harvard University Press.

Athanasiadou S (2012) Help me bring my child into the world. <http://supermomrocks.me/2012/01/15/%CE%B2%CE%BF%CE%B7%CE%B8%CE%B7%CF%83>

Ber R (2000) Ethical issues in gestational surrogacy. *Theoretical and Medical Bioethics* 21(2): 153–69.

Berend Z (2012) The romance of surrogacy. *Sociological Forum* 27: 913–36.

Bouloutza P (2015) Greek record in c-sections. *Kathimerini*, 13 December. <http://www.kathimerini.gr/842110/article/epikairothta/ellada/rekor-kaisarikwn-tomwn-sthn-ellada>

Brunet L, Carruthers J, Davaki K et al. (2013) *A Comparative Study of the Regime of Surrogacy in EU Member States: Report Submitted to European Parliament's Committee on Legal Affairs*. <www.europarl.europa.eu/RegData/etudes/etudes/join/2013/474403/IPOL-JURI_ET(2013)474403_EN.pdf>

Chaves M (2011) Homoaffective parentage in relation to medically assisted reproduction: a parallel between Brazil and Portugal. In: Atkin B (ed.) *The International Survey of Family Law: 2011 Edition*. London: Jordan Publishing.

Chiotis V (2015) Kapa Research Survey: Greek Orthodox but just once a year. *To Vima*, 11 April.

Chrysostomou M (2015) Surrogate motherhood: myths and realities. <www.news.gr>

Crozier GKD (2010) Protecting cross-border providers of ova and surrogacy services? *Global Social Policy* 10(3): 299–303.

Davaki K (2001) Women in the labour market and the family: policies in Germany and Greece. Unpublished PhD thesis, University of Kent, Canterbury.

Deonandan R (2013) An introduction to the ethical dimensions of reproductive medical tourism. In: Labonté R, Runnels V, Packer C and Deonandan R (eds) *Travelling Well: Essays in Medical Tourism*. Ottawa: Institute of Population Health, University of Ottawa, Chapter 1.

Deonandan R, Green S and van Beinum A (2012) Ethical concerns for maternal surrogacy and reproductive tourism. *Journal of Medical Ethics* 38(12): 742–5.

Fotiadi I (2014) The Greek 'industry' with surrogate mothers. *Kathimerini*, 13 April. <http://www.kathimerini.gr/762582/article/epikairothta/ellada/ellhnikh-viomhxania-me-paren8etes-mhteres>

Gamble N and Ghevaert L (2009) The chosen middle ground: England, surrogacy law and the international arena. *International Family Law*, November: 223–7. <www.nataliegambleassociates.co.uk/uploads/docs/535faf6133845.pdf>

Gasouka M (2014) New reproductive technologies, new forms of inequality. <fylosykis.gr>

Hatzis A (2003) Just the oven: a law and economics approach to gestational surrogacy contracts. In: Boele-Woelki K (ed.) *Perspectives for the Unification or Harmonisation of Family Law in Europe*. Antwerp: Intersentia.

Hatzis A (2010) *The Regulation of Surrogate Motherhood in Greece*. Working Paper, Social Sciences and Research Network. Athens: University of Athens.

Kapernarakou K (2011) There is only one mum ... or two? <http://efikountouraki.com/2011/12/20>

Karagianni G (2013) New reproductive technologies and parenthood. <http://www.dramini.gr>

Kimbrell A (1993) *The Human Body Shop: The Engineering and Marketing of Life*. New York: Harper.

Konstantinidi M (2015) I am selling my child for 10,000 euros. <http://ravenet.gr>

Martin LJ (2009) Reproductive tourism in the age of globalization. *Globalizations* 6(2): 249–63.

Montgolfier de S and Mirkovic A (2009) Maternité pour autrui: du désir d'enfant à l'enfant à tout prix. *Médecine/Sciences* (Paris) 25(4): 419–22.

Mossialos E, Allin SM, Karras K and Davaki K (2005) An investigation of caesarean sections in three Greek hospitals: the impact of financial incentives and convenience. *European Journal of Public Health* 15(3): 288–95.

Nikolaou V (2015) Wanted: woman to give birth to our child. <www.e-typos.com/gr/ellada/article/124922/ziteitai-gunaika-gia-na-gennisei-to-paidi-mas>

Panagos K (2011) *Surrogate Motherhood: The Greek Regulatory Framework* and the Extension to Criminal Law. Athens and Thessaloniki: Sakkoulas Publications.

Pande A (2011) Transnational commercial surrogacy in India: gifts for global sisters? *Reproductive Medicine Online* 23(5): 618–25.

Papadimitriou L (2012) How I had a baby by a sperm donor. *BHMagazino* <www.tovima.gr/vimagazino/views/article/?aid=460020>

Papaligoura Z, Papadatou D and Bellali T (2013) The formation of the wish for a child. Third scientific one-day conference of Psychology Department, University of Thessaloniki, Greece.

Papathanasopoulos GN (2014) When the birth of a human being is reduced to a consumer good. <aktines.blogspot.gr>

Paraschos T (2012) Surrogacy from the legal and medical perspective. <www.eimastegynaikes.gr>

Petroulia N (2012) Surrogacy from the legal and medical perspective. <www.eimastegynaikes.gr>

Public Issue (2016) Attitudes toward same-sex unions. <www.publicissue.gr/wp-content/uploads/2016/01/34.jpg>

Ravdas P (2012) Surrogate motherhood: legislators' expectations under the challenges of statistical data. In: Papadimitriou AC and Kounougeri-Manoledaki E (eds) *Family Law in the 21st Century: From Incidental to Structural Changes*. Athens and Thessaloniki: Sakkoulas.

Reuters (2015) Greece passes bill allowing civil partnerships for same-sex couples. *Guardian*, 23 December. <www.theguardian.com/world/2015/dec/23/greece-passes-bill-allowing-same-sex-civil-partnerships>

Scott E (2009) Surrogacy and the politics of commodification. *Law & Contemporary Problems* 72(3): 109–45.

Stamatoukou E (2015) My best friend gave birth to my child. <www.athensvoice.gr>

Storrow RF (2005) Quests for conception: fertility tourists, globalisation, and feminist legal theory. *Human Reproduction* 57: 295–330.

Tieu MM (2009) Altruistic surrogacy: the necessary objectification of surrogate mothers. *Journal of Medical Ethics* 35: 171–5.

Triantafyllou D (2015) With two mothers and two fathers. <www.talcmag.gr/sizitondas/rainbow-families>

Tsimpoukis P (2014) The law deprives father from twins acquired through surrogate mother. <www.protothema.gr/greece/article/363934/o-nomos-sterei-apo-patera-ta-diduma-pou-apektise-me-parentheti-mitera>

Tsoulea R (2010) The grandmother who gave birth to her ... granddaughter. <http://ygeia.tanea.gr/default.asp?pid=8&ct=13&articleID=10351&la=1>

Vasilakou K (2010) Bioethics and surrogate mothers. <https://sciencearchives.wordpress.com/2010/09/13/%CE%AE-%CE%AD-%CE%AD>

Vassilopoulou T (2015) New data reveals birth rate decline in crisis-hit Greece. <www.equaltimes.org>

Velissaris H (2015) 2000 Aussie babies born thanks to Greece. <http://neoskosmos.com/news/en/2000-Aussie-babies-born-thanks-to-Greece>

Blogs and relevant websites

<https://anarchypress.wordpress.com/2011/04/29/%CF%84%CE%B5%CF%87%CE%BD%CE%BF>
<http://aktines.blogspot.gr>
<http://www.childrenparenting.com>
<http://www.fertilitysolutionsinternational.com>
<http://forum.eimaimama.gr>
<http://globalsurrogacy.world>
<https://greeksurrogacy.com>
<https://www.ivf-embryo.gr/exosomatiki-ivf/dorea-oarion-emvryon/parentheti-mitrotita>
<http://www.newlifegreece.com>
<http://www.reproductive-solutions.com>
<http://SuperMomRocks.me>
<http://www.talcmag.gr/sizitondas/rainbow-families>

PART THREE

WHAT ABOUT THE CHILDREN?

9 | WHAT ARE CHILDREN'S 'BEST INTERESTS' IN INTERNATIONAL SURROGACY? A SOCIAL WORK PERSPECTIVE FROM THE UK

Marilyn Crawshaw, Patricia Fronek, Eric Blyth and Andy Elvin

Introduction

More than twenty-five years after the United Nations Convention on the Rights of the Child came into force in 1989, social workers are identifying new threats to the rights and interests of children. The growing global market in 'medical tourism' coupled with the development of ever more cutting-edge assisted reproductive technologies (ARTs) have made it increasingly possible to create new family forms resulting from international surrogacy arrangements. Jurisdictions across the world are challenged to respond appropriately – especially where commissioning parents are either unclear about the law or are determined to circumvent it. The burgeoning numbers of commercial brokers and doctors with financial interests, together with pressure from within the consumer lobby and the fertility industry to loosen international and domestic restraints on surrogacy arrangements, mean that these new challenges require new responses to ensure that the best interests of the children are adequately catered for.

Surrogacy is probably the longest established form of family-building using a third party, with several references to it in the Bible (Genesis 16:1–2; 30:1–12), albeit making use of female slaves as surrogates rather than 'free' women. Surrogacy practices today arouse a great deal of controversy, condemned outright by some of the world's major religions, notably Islam and the Roman Catholic Church, but not necessarily opposed by others such as Buddhism (Blyth and Landau, 2009). Many jurisdictions, e.g. France, Portugal, Pakistan, Italy, prohibit all surrogacy – commercial and altruistic – by law (Ory *et al.*, 2013); others, e.g. Israel, the UK and some Australian states, permit certain forms as long as they are subjected to state regulation and legislation; yet others, such as California (Spivack, 2010) and India (DasGupta and Dasgupta, 2014), allow surrogacy arrangements to prosper in a relatively unfettered market.

Surrogacy in the UK

The UK was one of the first jurisdictions to introduce legislation to regulate surrogacy. The Surrogacy Arrangements Act 1985 was focused primarily on deterring commercial surrogacy and was widely seen as a knee-jerk reaction to the storm of outrage generated by the so-called 'Baby Cotton' case, in which a British woman, Kim Cotton, signed up as a surrogate for a US commercial agency.

The Act was aimed specifically at prohibiting a third party (other than the surrogate or commissioning parents) from taking part in negotiations for a commercial surrogacy agreement, the offer or agreement to negotiate such an arrangement or the compilation of information intended to be used for such purpose, including advertising in relation to surrogacy services. Private arrangements between surrogates and commissioning parents and the presence of non-commercial surrogacy agencies were not made illegal and regulation of the latter was not introduced.

Within a few years, the government had a second opportunity to consider suitable regulation with the introduction of what was to become the Human Fertilisation and Embryology (HFE) Act 1990. It essentially drew on the recommendations of the Warnock Committee that had been prompted by the birth in 1978 of Louise Brown, the first baby born of in vitro fertilization (IVF). Chaired by the philosopher Mary Warnock, the Committee was established to inquire into the rapidly developing technologies of IVF and embryology and come up with principles and recommendations regarding some form of national regulation (Department of Health and Social Security, 1984). Largely because the Committee itself had been unable to reach consensus on an appropriate regulatory approach to surrogacy, the proposed legislation was silent on the matter. It was only a serendipitous chain of events during the parliamentary debates that led to the current legislative framework for surrogacy arrangements. When a case of gestational surrogacy came to public attention, the commissioning parents' MP championed their cause and tabled an amendment to the bill (Blyth, 1993a, 2010). The result was a truncated version of the existing provisions for dealing with the adoption of infants, but with fewer safeguards for surrogate children. In practice, it was not until 1994 that the new measures were implemented. In explaining the delay, the then Health Minister was forced to acknowledge that surrogacy situations were 'considerably more complex than they first appeared' (Sackville, 1994: col. 974).

Despite the legislation, problems regarding the regulation of commercial surrogacy were soon evident and led to a government review in 1998 (Brazier et al., 1998). However, no action was taken to implement the resulting recommendations. Minor changes were enacted ten years later through the HFE Act 2008, to sanction the operations of not-for-profit surrogacy agencies so long as they do not engage in any prohibited commercial activities. UK regulation of surrogacy arrangements now deals with two other major areas:

- provision for the transfer of legal parenthood of the child to the commissioning parents (including since 2010 same-sex parents and unmarried couples); and
- access by the child to information about her or his biographical and genetic heritage.

Currently in the UK a woman who gives birth to a child, including all surrogates, is considered the child's legal mother regardless of any genetic connection. Subject to the formal consent of the surrogate (and any other person who is regarded in law as a parent of the child, such as her husband), a commissioning couple who are married, in a civil partnership or 'in an enduring relationship', and where at least one of whom is a genetic parent, may apply for a Parental Order transferring legal parenthood of the child to them. At the time of the application both applicants must be resident in the UK and the child must be living with them. In addition, the application must be made within six months of the birth of the child and no payment must have been made to the surrogate other than 'reasonable expenses'.

A court considering a Parental Order application is obliged to treat the welfare of the child as 'paramount' but this is the first point at which it is given such prominence (since the Parental Orders (Human Fertilisation and Embryology) Regulations 2010). If treatment has been provided by a licensed fertility clinic in the UK, the clinic must have taken account of the welfare of the child in accordance with section 13(5) of the HFE Act 1990 (as amended), although with no particular priority (Blyth, 2007, 2014). What attention to the welfare of the child means in practice, even in Parental Order applications, remains ill defined and inconsistent (Crawshaw et al., 2013; Fronek and Crawshaw, 2015). Given that the surrogate has effectively relinquished care and custody of the child to the commissioning parents by this stage and the child is domiciled with them, courts are faced with few realistic alternatives. Decisions to grant Parental Orders, even where there has been a clear breach of the regulations regarding payment, have thus been justified by reference to the child's welfare (see e.g. *J v. G* [2013] EWHC 1432 (Fam)).

As regards access to information about biographical and genetic heritage, an individual who is subject to a Parental Order may request disclosure of the identity of the surrogate from the relevant General Register Office when they reach the age of 18 in England, Wales and Northern Ireland, and at age 16 in Scotland. Self-evidently, the individual needs to be aware that she or he is subject to a Parental Order in order to make such a request, and even then, there is no statutory requirement for them to be informed of their rights under the HFE Act to information about the donor – where one was used – thus leaving them with potentially incomplete information about their genetic parentage (we return to this below).

Since the operation of commercial agencies is prohibited in the UK, domestic surrogacy arrangements tend to be initiated and executed directly between a surrogate and commissioning parents, sometimes involving a not-for-profit agency, such as Surrogacy UK or Childlessness Overcome Through Surrogacy (COTS). These enable relationships to be built between surrogates, surrogates' families, and commissioning parents and their families that may extend beyond the delivery and handover of the child (Jadva *et al.*, 2015; van den Akker, 2007). An associated characteristic of domestic surrogacy arrangements in the UK is that many commissioning parents appear willing to inform their child of the circumstances of their conception, as is considered important in other non-traditional methods of forming families such as donor conception and adoption (Blyth, 1995; Golombok *et al.*, 2004, 2006a, 2006b, 2011, 2013; Imrie and Jadva, 2014; Jadva and Imrie, 2014; MacCallum *et al.*, 2003; Shelton *et al.*, 2009) – although there is some evidence that this does not necessarily extend to information about whether the surrogate was also their genetic parent (Jadva *et al.*, 2012).

Scant research has been undertaken regarding the outcomes for or experiences of children born of surrogacy, limited further by being carried out with small numbers of participants and focusing on domestic arrangements in the UK. Findings from these indicate that the psychological development and emotional adjustment of children up to the age of 10 years are within the normal range for the samples studied (Golombok *et al.*, 2004, 2006a, 2006b, 2011, 2013; Jadva *et al.*, 2012; MacCallum *et al.*, 2003; Shelton *et al.*, 2009). In a number of instances, surrogates and their own children remained in contact with the surrogate child and commissioning parents, and such contact was generally regarded positively (Jadva *et al.*, 2003, 2012; Imrie and Jadva, 2014; Jadva and Imrie, 2014).

Two studies have investigated the impact on surrogates' children. In the first (Jadva *et al.*, 2003), thirty-four surrogates were interviewed approximately one year after they had given birth to a surrogate child; thirty-two of these had children of their own and all claimed to have discussed the surrogacy arrangement with their offspring at least 'to some extent'. Most of the children were reported to feel positive during the pregnancy, at the time of the handover and a year following the birth of the surrogate baby, and none were reported to feel negative about the process. The second study (Jadva and Imrie, 2014) investigated the experiences of thirty-six children of surrogates aged 12–25 years. Most participants had positive views about the surrogacy arrangement. Nearly half were in contact with the resulting child, all of whom reported positive relationships with her/him. Involvement in surrogacy neither impacted adversely on relationships within their own family nor on their psychological health, with no differences evident between genetic and gestational surrogacy arrangements.

Criticisms of the current UK system

Critics have argued that the failure by successive governments to develop a systematic policy has resulted in a fragmented approach that does not protect the interests of those concerned. Specific problems (in no particular order) include:

- The arbitrary nature of the six months' deadline for applying for a Parental Order does not permit any extension in the event of exceptional circumstances or the realities of demands faced by new parents.[1]
- The requirement that only a couple may apply for Parental Orders does not allow for exceptional and/or unexpected circumstances, such as a separation or the death of one of the commissioning parents before an order is made (see e.g. *A v. P (Surrogacy: Parental Order: Death of Applicant)* [2011] EWHC 1738 (Fam), [2012] 2 FLR 145). It also discriminates against single people, despite their ability to become legal parents through other assisted conception routes or adoption.

- The lengthy period between the child's birth and the granting of a Parental Order carries the potential to hinder bonding with the commissioning parents, as does the uncertainty created by resulting legal and practical difficulties. This includes whether or not commissioning parents can give informed consent for health procedures or travel outside the UK with the child. Some have thus argued for Parental Orders to be made much earlier than at present, for instance through transfer at birth and/or pre-birth binding contracts (Horsey, 2010).
- The cost and complexity of Parental Order proceedings, it is argued, may deter some commissioning parents from applying for an order, thus prejudicing both their own and their child's legal positions.
- Critics argue that the retrospective sanctioning by courts of payments that exceed 'reasonable expenses' makes the ongoing prohibition of commercial arrangements outdated (Martin and Kane, 2014).
- The role of professionals such as social workers in determining the welfare of children coming so late in the process risks this becoming mere rubber stamping (Crawshaw et al., 2013).
- Inadequate recording systems and lack of utilization of DNA testing lead to the possibility that neither commissioning parent is a genetic parent of the child (despite their intentions or expectations), a risk heightened where arrangements are made in unregulated practices overseas.
- Although an individual subject to a Parental Order can only access information about the surrogate at age 18 in England, Wales and Northern Ireland, s/he is entitled to apply for an adult passport at age 16. This becomes problematic if there is no Parental Order in place as the Passport Office would need to investigate the surrogacy arrangement and establish whether the surrogate consented, is who she claims to be and was unmarried/divorced/widowed at the time of the birth.
- Information about biographical and genetic heritage, to which an individual is legally entitled, does not include information about gamete or embryo donors who may have contributed to her/his conception since such details are not recorded on the original birth certificate or Parental Order. Further, safeguards to ensure that children grow up knowing about their origins and have the right as adults to seek out information are not in place. These types of omission carry implications for both medical history and

identity, and conflict with Parliament's intentions under the HFE Act 2008 and adoption legislation.
- Perceptions that the recruitment of surrogates is easier and sometimes cheaper overseas because of domestic restrictions lead to all parties concerned having potentially fewer safeguards for their rights and well-being.

If the current UK law is, as critics argue, not well placed to deal adequately with domestic surrogacy, the ramifications of international surrogacy render it even less fit for purpose.

A growing international surrogacy market

In recent years, increasing attention has been given to international surrogacy. Its prevalence is impossible to determine with any accuracy as most such arrangements are *ad hoc*. As such they may or may not involve an intermediary and tend to bypass any formal recording systems pertaining to assisted reproductive services – where they exist. International travel for surrogacy is premised largely on the more ready availability of surrogates in the destination country, for example because explicit payment is permitted (as in California) or because the services of surrogates may be obtained more cheaply (as in India, Mexico and Ukraine) than at home, or because same-sex couples and single people face fewer restrictions and less discrimination in destination countries, or because surrogacy is illegal in the 'home' country. Research undertaken by Crawshaw *et al.* (2012) and Blyth (2014) indicated both an increase in the annual number of Parental Orders made since 1995 and in the proportion of Parental Orders made in respect of children born as the result of international surrogacy arrangements. The number of Parental Orders granted in the UK rose from 52 in 1995 to 203 in 2012, with marked annual rises since 2008. From 2008, the data collected by the General Register Offices have included the location of the surrogate and reveal an increase from 2 per cent of surrogates located overseas in 2008 to 39 per cent in 2014 (the latest figures available at the time of writing), indicating a significant growth in the use of *commercial* surrogacy arrangements by UK citizens in Asia, Eastern Europe and the US in particular.

Notwithstanding the rise in the number of Parental Orders, there is considerable circumstantial evidence to suggest that these numbers fail to reflect the true increase in the use of international surrogacy. In 2012, the UK newspaper, the *Daily Telegraph*, estimated that during the previous year, Indian surrogates delivered as many as 1,000 births for British commissioning parents (Bhatia, 2012). The credibility of this figure was subsequently endorsed by UK government officials in January 2014, at an international roundtable held in London (Blyth et al., 2014) although there remain no robust data. It appears that not all overseas arrangements lead to applications for a Parental Order, meaning that at least some commissioning parents operate 'under the radar'. Possible reasons include lack of knowledge of the legislation and its process, avoidance of contact with authorities for fear of being found to have acted illegally by entering into a commercial agreement, fear of having the child removed, perceptions that the Parental Order process is time-consuming and expensive (Parental Order applications involving an international surrogacy arrangement are dealt with exclusively by the High Court), belief that it is considered unnecessary if parental status has been recognized by an adoption or other court order made in the destination jurisdiction, or parents feeling tired and overwhelmed with early parenting tasks.

It is the case, however, that further disincentives may result from the absence of processes at border controls to reliably identify children born through surrogacy arrangements, the absence of follow-up (or sanctions) for parents who identify themselves and declare their intention to apply for a Parental Order to obtain entry clearance and then fail to apply, and the lack of any visa process specific to surrogate children.

Currently no follow-up research has been undertaken involving children born as a result of an international surrogacy arrangement, regardless of whether an application for a Parental Order has been made. Neither is there any information about whether such parents encounter any difficulties when registering them with the National Health Service (NHS), applying for school places, passports, and so on. However, it has been reported anecdotally that there appear to be growing numbers of cases dealt with by family courts when couples separate and parents find they have no legal status in relation to the child; robust data collection is needed.

Current law in the UK seems ill-prepared to deal with the *additional* challenges posed by international surrogacy including those where arrangements take place in destination jurisdictions that:

- Do not provide access to adequate medical care for the child or surrogate (deaths of surrogates and donors have been reported), especially delivery and postnatal care, and do not give adequate consideration to matters of informed consent by the surrogate (Tanderup et al., 2015).

(There are health risks to children, surrogates and donors associated with ovarian hyperstimulation, embryo transfers and multiple implantations, multiple and premature births, disability and caesarean sections in surrogacy (Martin and Kane, 2014). Health issues for the newborn can also delay plans to leave the country and return to the UK and mean unforeseen costs that commissioning parents may not have taken into account. Evidence is also emerging of the potential significance for the child's health of the 'uterine environment' and the overall health of the pregnant woman (in this case the surrogate) regardless of whether she is the biological mother (Knoche, 2014; van den Akker, 2012).)

- Do not provide access to relevant biographical and genetic heritage information for the individual born following a surrogacy arrangement.
- Apply a different system to that in the UK for determining parental status, e.g. where commissioning parents are regarded as the legal parents or where adoption of the child is permitted, but are not subsequently recognized in the UK, with implications for legal parentage, nationality and citizenship status.

In addition, there are now numerous cases reported internationally where commissioning parents have been unable to effect the transfer of legal parentage of the child, establish the child's citizenship status or return to their home country with the child, sometimes because of their own disregard of advice about the legality of their intentions prior to travel (Trimmings and Beaumont, 2013). Also the lack of robust data on both domestic and international surrogacy hinders inter-agency and inter-departmental collaboration on policy and practice development.

Recent cases highlight the serious risks to human rights and child welfare, in the absence of adequate regulation, including child selling and child trafficking (Yaxley, 2014). An Australian man and his partner claimed to have become parents through international commercial surrogacy, sexually abused the child and made him available to an international paedophile network (Marr, 2012). A convicted Israeli paedophile lives with his daughter produced through overseas commercial surrogacy and the authorities have been unable to remove her (Kumar and Chopra, 2013). Children have also been abandoned due to illness, disability or being an unwanted twin, as in the case of Baby Gammy mentioned elsewhere in this volume. Most recently, reports are emerging of underground baby-selling rackets that trade the 'extra' children from multiple births, a not uncommon occurrence in risky surrogacy practices (Ronan, 2015). The existence of these children may or may not be known to commissioning parents or surrogates.

The severity of problems has been recognized by the European Parliament (Brunet et al., 2013), International Social Service (ISS) (2013) and The Hague Conference on Private International Law (HCCH). The latter has for some time been deliberating whether to develop a convention on international surrogacy, drawing on the experiences of intercountry adoption and related conventions (Baker, 2013; Fronek et al., 2014; HCCH, 2012) and has currently deferred a decision on whether and how to pursue this project (HCCH, 2014a, 2004b).

A social work response to the challenges posed by international surrogacy

Social work has increasingly contributed to surrogacy-related and assisted conception research and policy development from its unique perspective (Blyth, 1993a, 1993b, 1995; Cheney, 2014; Cuthbert and Fronek, 2014; Fronek and Crawshaw, 2015; Gagin et al., 2004; Karandikar et al., 2014; Rotabi et al., 2015). Given internationally recognized human rights conventions for both children and adults that set out the right to be free of exploitation, and social work's long concern with the potential for exploitation of vulnerable children and adults, social work is well placed to make a strong contribution.

Social work's mandate to bring a critical perspective to bear on international surrogacy is derived from its expertise in child and family welfare and safeguarding and the definition of social work by the International Federation of Social Workers (IFSW) and International Association of Schools of Social Work (2014 and its predecessor) that includes the values of social justice and human rights and 'promotes social change and development, social cohesion, and the empowerment and liberation of people'. This informed the adoption by the IFSW in 2008 of a policy statement on 'cross-border reproductive care' that included reference to international surrogacy arrangements (Blyth and Auffrey, 2008). It clearly articulated the risks of exploitation for all parties, particularly in relation to: the commodification of life, sperm, eggs, embryos; the exploitation of women, especially the poor and Indigenous; a commitment to empowerment and self-determination; the exercise of rights only when it does not impair the interests of others; the right to competent, safe and affordable reproductive and sexual health care free from government, institutional, professional, familial or other interpersonal coercion and that such services should be provided free of charge to gamete and embryo 'donors' and surrogates; and the rights of individuals to full information about their biographical and genetic heritage.

The longstanding activities of the Project Group on Assisted Reproduction (PROGAR), a multi-agency group operating under the auspices of the British Association of Social Workers (BASW) (Wincott and Crawshaw, 2006), have been strengthened by its multi-agency and multi-disciplinary membership (though centrally informed by social work), which includes leading child and family welfare organizations as well as those directly involved in the fertility field. PROGAR has made written contributions to all major consultations on third-party assisted reproduction since its inception in 1984 and has regularly been invited to present oral evidence. In doing so, it has given particular prominence to the importance of lifespan perspectives as well as giving voice to the children affected. One notable UK policy achievement, in which PROGAR took a leading role, was the success of the campaign to enable individuals conceived following gamete or embryo donation in the UK to access information about their biographical and genetic heritage. It is reasonable to suggest that campaign pressure also contributed to Parliament's decision to make the child's welfare paramount in Parental Order applications by adapting the Welfare of the Child Checklist from the Adoption and Children Act 2002, and to recent decisions by the regulator of licensed treatments, the Human Fertilisation and Embryology Authority (HFEA), to adopt a Lifecycle Strategy for donor conception and to pilot a support and intermediary service for those seeking information post donor conception.

In addition, PROGAR's most recent success has been in bringing together relevant government departments, consumer groups and a range of academic and practitioner disciplines to the above-mentioned roundtable in 2014 focusing on the best interests of children in international surrogacy (Blyth *et al.*, 2014). This not only led directly to the establishment of an ongoing cross-departmental working group but also to PROGAR being further consulted during a mini-review of surrogacy legislation. Internationally, both ISS and the IFSW have declared international surrogacy as a particular focus of interest and contributed to the HCCH deliberations on whether to develop an international convention on surrogacy. An International Forum on Intercountry Adoption and Global Surrogacy in August 2014 brought together probably the largest numbers of social workers ever gathered to consider such matters, alongside other advocates of women's health, children's rights and human rights together with legal and policy analysts, many of whom have contributed to this collection.

The importance of biographical and genetic heritage information Social workers have long understood the importance to children of knowing about and having access to information about their biological/genetic relatives and their biographical and cultural story, primarily as a result of their experience in domestic and intercountry adoption (Blyth *et al.*, 2001, 2011; Daniels, 2004; Riley, 2013; Triseliotis *et al.*, 2005). This is acknowledged in the 1989 UN Convention on the Rights of the Child and is a central principle of UK family law.

Access to information can meet a variety of needs, some of which may not manifest for many years. For example, where parents have used a third party for family-building they need sufficient and accurate information about the donor and surrogate from the beginning in order to share this with their child in age-appropriate ways throughout the child's life. Parents also need sufficient understanding of the importance of this information for a child's healthy sense of identity and may need preparatory education and support to achieve this. An individual born following an international surrogacy arrangement may also wish to know about the country and culture of the surrogate (and donor where applicable) and that of her family, since this information is all part of *their* story.

Although some research has begun to emerge of the experiences of overseas surrogates engaged in surrogacy, none has yet investigated the outcomes of these arrangements for commissioning parents or children, whether in the UK or elsewhere. Commissioning parents do not have direct experience of a pregnancy through which to start the bonding process with the child and report frustration and anxiety at the physical distance from the child during pregnancy (Ziv and Freund-Eschar, 2015). It is by no means certain that similar levels of transparency, ongoing relationships between children, commissioning parents and surrogates and their families, and the generally positive outcomes reported in UK domestic arrangements apply to international surrogacy. Indeed, future contact between commissioning parents, children and surrogates (and donors where applicable) are likely to be compromised by barriers relating to language, culture, geographical distance, socio-economic, educational and literacy disparities, norms and expectations. They may not be possible at all where practices are unregulated, clinic records are inadequate and where anonymity between the commissioning parents and surrogate/donor is required. In addition, the impact on children of knowing that a financial transaction brought about their birth remains unknown.

International surrogacy and intercountry adoption: the same or different? For some social work scholars, a concern with international surrogacy has emerged from their previous interest in assisted reproduction; for others it stems from an earlier focus on intercountry adoption (Cheney, 2014; Cuthbert and Fronek, 2014; Rotabi, 2014; Scherman *et al.*, 2016). While there are similarities between the two, there are also differences. Generally speaking, the first involves creating a child with a genetic connection, usually, to at least one intended parent; despite the involvement of multiple actors (donors and surrogates), some view the practice as simply a fertility treatment free from social, legal and medical consequences. Although involuntary childlessness also motivates most of those seeking parenthood through intercountry adoption, there is, usually, no genetic link and quite often an existing family to consider.

The observable parallels between intercountry adoption and international surrogacy lie in the similar ways the practices have gained international popularity. Both have been characterized by: (1) their market-driven approach; (2) the movement of children from poorer to wealthier countries; (3) the belief among prospective parents that their governments would be forced to ratify their actions even if they broke the law or worked around it; and (4) their promotion by interested organizations, influential lobbyists and support from some politicians and celebrities (Fronek, 2009; Cuthbert and Fronek, 2014). Transferable lessons from intercountry adoption include the role of money in enabling corruption and abuses, including the provision of false or misleading information. Further, without robust systems for accessing information and tracing surrogates or donors, and without access to support across the lifespan, issues of identity and in some cases cultural heritage will emerge and/or be troubling. Abuses in intercountry adoption, for many reasons, took years to be fully identified: with surrogacy there is an early opportunity for research and sharing of practice on which knowledge-based policy can be developed.

Unlike in intercountry adoption, there is no requirement for assessing the parties involved in surrogacy prior to commissioning parents leaving the UK, providing education on risks or pre-approving arrangements including financial and citizenship and legal parental obligations. No parenting preparation is required on how best to meet the particular needs of children created through surrogacy, for example in relation to birth identity and heritage or talking to them about how they were born, and there is no follow-up or longer-term support provided. Nor is there any education with regard to expectations and sensitivity towards surrogates or even rudimentary police checks to eliminate those convicted of crimes against children. This is despite accepted good practice with prospective parents of donor conceived children receiving UK licensed treatment of the need for such preparation, endorsed by a Nuffield Council of BioEthics report (2013) to which PROGAR gave both written and verbal evidence. In light of what we currently know about international surrogacy, including the potential for poorer outcomes for the resulting families given that ongoing relationships between surrogates and commissioning parents are harder to achieve, it seems that additional checks and balances and preparation are needed, regardless of whether the surrogate uses her own egg or not. The history of both international and domestic adoptions has demonstrated that parenting desires alone are not always sufficient for raising well-adjusted, healthy children and neither practice necessarily offers 'win-win' outcomes.

Information and money as sources of power and exploitation

Making good-quality information available to commissioning parents and to surrogates and their families and instigating assessment processes independent of those with commercial or other interests carry some potential to redress power imbalances and conflicts of interest. This is of course difficult in unregulated overseas environments. Although the Foreign and Commonwealth Office and Home Office (2014) recently reissued a statement warning parents to seek legal advice prior to entering arrangements, much more is needed. Even in the UK, surrogacy information is disjointed and difficult to access. Government departments, agencies and regulators have tended to compartmentalize processes related to surrogacy, reinforced by the requirements of the relatively newly formed Government Digital Service, which pushes for standardization across portals and does not allow for unique coverage where this is warranted. This is especially worrying given that many information seekers would look to government sites as being trustworthy and reliable and find it difficult when faced with such a complex and incomplete jigsaw puzzle. Until developments following the 2014 PROGAR-run roundtable, there has been little cross-departmental collaboration and planning, and hence no concerted efforts to push for consistency.

There is also no clear definition of commercial surrogacy. It is commonly held to mean arrangements that involve third-party brokers (who may or may not be the clinic owners) who profit financially from the arrangements. Typically, commissioning parents pay a fee to brokers who then apportion payments to the parties involved. Surrogates in impoverished countries receive significantly less than the other players involved (i.e. even when the surrogate is 'allowed' to be recompensed for her labour) and often receive less remuneration than promised or only get paid after the handover of the child. Darnovsky and Beeson (2014) point to the lack of information about what happens when a pregnancy fails or when the surrogate fails to conceive. While commercial surrogacy agencies are banned from operating in the UK, 'not-for-profit' organizations are permitted. Since they are unregulated and the pay rates of staff and the fees for commissioning parents are therefore self-determined, the distinction between the two types may not always be evident to users and onlookers.

One major step in the legal process of applying for Parental Orders comes when commissioning parents are required to show (and Parental Order Reporters to check) that only 'reasonable expenses' have been paid to the surrogate in international as in domestic arrangements. Research has reported that Parental Order Reporters do not interpret the 'reasonable expenses' requirement in a standard way so do not consistently look for exploitation driven by monetary reward, and that the Child and Family Court Advisory and Support Service through which most Parental Order Reporters are appointed does not provide guidance (Crawshaw *et al.*, 2013; Purewal *et al.*, 2012). In addition, the courts have in a number of cases retrospectively authorized substantial payments to surrogates, especially in overseas arrangements (as referred to earlier), leading to calls for domestic commercialism to be allowed. However, it has been argued that such a 'solution' is neither problem-free nor would commissioning parents necessarily regard it as a preferred option to going overseas (Riggs, 2015). It also minimizes the role that money can play in fuelling conflicts of interest and in compromising acceptable standards of practice.

Pulling it all together to find a way forward

The roundtable held in London in 2014 was the first event to bring together government departments, consumer groups, academics and practitioners to engage in dialogue about the complexities and concerns relating to international surrogacy, specifically around the interests of children. Participants identified the following key points requiring early attention and follow-up (not in order of priority):

1. What measures can be put in place to reduce the numbers of UK commissioning parents who do not apply for Parental Orders after bringing children born of surrogacy arrangements into the country?
2. How can the support for qualified extensions to the six months rule be taken forward?
3. How can attention to child welfare be assured/improved? What sorts of checks, assessments and preparation of the parties are needed and when?
4. How can improvements be made to the collection of family and medical history of surrogates and its provision to parents and (later) to the child?
5. What other measures are needed to ensure that the surrogate child's identity needs (including cultural needs) are adequately met, including where a donor egg is used, where the country of birth does not have legislation/systems allowing for identity release and where the opportunities for a personal relationship to build between surrogate and commissioning parents are restricted?
6. How can the information needs of (1) surrogates and (2) commissioning parents be better met? Who will take the lead on addressing the lack of standardized information for commissioning parents, surrogates and surrogate offspring currently available across government departments?
7. Which agencies should be tasked with keeping data to improve understanding of the profiles of surrogates, commissioning parents and children? And how should such data be used to inform policy and practice?
8. How can the debate on the role and impact of commercialization in surrogacy be taken forward?
9. How can the debate on appropriate improvements to regulation of surrogacy activity be taken forward?
10. Is there potential for the development of minimum standards by relevant multi-disciplinary professional organizations such as the IFSW, ISS, PROGAR, the European Society for Human Reproduction and Embryology, the International Federation of Fertility Societies and country-specific organizations?

11. How can it be ensured that organizations concerned with child trafficking are alerted to the potential for surrogate arrangements to be used within such activities?

The roundtable provided an opportunity for at least tentative proposals towards a way forward, including provisional support for an International Convention on Surrogacy, to be explored through the lens of the best interests of the children affected. At the same time, it was recognized that this was a longer-term response and that bilateral agreements between individual countries willing to address the issues may be more feasible in the shorter term.

In the UK, the lack of safeguards afforded by legal parenthood that result from the apparently low numbers of Parental Orders being granted following international surrogacy arrangements prompt very real concerns about the well-being of children born this way. The need to better understand and address the disincentives for making Parental Order applications is urgent. Options might include making prominent and clearer the importance of Parental Orders and legal parentage, providing consistent and clear information for all parties across government departments, extending the timeframe allowed for applications and allowing retrospective orders to be made, and improving the ability of border control staff to identify potential surrogate infants, especially where the destination country has issued a birth certificate or Adoption Order. There may also be merit in introducing a dedicated travel visa for children to enter the UK and then making it compulsory to secure a Parental Order to obtain a UK passport and citizenship. Encouragement of the international multi-disciplinary community to develop and adopt codes of practice and minimum standards for health care professionals involved in surrogacy arrangements would be an important step forward. Lessons from international adoption could also be applied, such as enhancing staffing in UK embassies/consulates in countries that are known to be particularly problematic.

Finally, more research, including large-scale studies with representative samples, is needed into the physical, social and psychological development of children born via surrogacy *and* the children of surrogates as well as studies of the impact on surrogates and commissioning parents.

In this chapter, we have explored international surrogacy through a social work lens, drawing on its widespread professional and academic expertise and commitment to the values of social justice and human rights in child and family welfare, in particular where there is third-party involvement. Using that expertise and its contribution from research to inform the development of policy, legislation and practice can ensure a broader understanding and management of the risks and benefits of surrogacy as they relate to the interests of children and families, providing a crucial counterbalance to the powerful voices from the medical, legal, commercial and 'right to parent' lobbies.

Note

1 However it should be noted that in a recent reported case (*Re X (A child)(Surrogacy: Time limit)* [2014] EWHC 3135 (Fam)) Mr Justice Munby *did* grant a Parental Order after the deadline, saying that Parliament could not have intended the six months rule to be wholly fixed, describing its enforcement as 'almost nonsensical'. This ruling may well lead to other such decisions though the law remains unchanged.

References

Associated Press Canberra (2014) Australian father charged with sexually abusing surrogate twin daughters. *South China Morning Post*, 3 September. <www.scmp.com/news/asia/article/1584032/australian-father-charged-sexually-abusing-surrogate-twin-daughters>

Baker H (2013) A possible future instrument on international surrogacy arrangements: are there 'lessons' to be learnt from the 1993 Hague Intercountry Adoption Convention? In: Trimmings K and Beaumont P (eds) *International Surrogacy Arrangements: Legal Regulation at the International Level*. Oxford: Hart Publishing, pp. 411–26.

Bhatia S (2012) Revealed: how more and more Britons are paying Indian women to become surrogate mothers. *Daily Telegraph*, 26 May. <http://www.telegraph.co.uk/health/healthnews/9292343/Revealed-how-more-and-more-Britons-are-paying-Indian-women-tobecome-surrogate-mothers.html>

Blyth E (1993a) Section 30: the acceptable face of surrogacy? *Journal of Social Welfare and Family Law* 15(4): 248–60.

Blyth E (1993b) Children's welfare, surrogacy and social work. *British Journal of Social Work* 23(3): 259–75.

Blyth E (1995) 'Not a primrose path': commissioning parents' experiences of surrogacy arrangements in Britain. *Journal of Reproductive and Infant Psychology* 13(3/4): 185–96.

Blyth E (2007) Conceptions of welfare. In: Horsey K and Biggs H (eds) *Human Fertilisation and Embryology: Reproducing Regulation*. London: Routledge-Cavendish, pp. 17–45.

Blyth E (2010) Parental Orders and identity registration: one country three systems. *Journal of Social Welfare and Family Law* 32(4): 345–52.

Blyth E (2014) The changing profile of international surrogacy. Opening presentation at PROGAR/SRIP Workshop on International Surrogacy: What are the child's 'best interests' in international surrogacy? National Council for Voluntary Organisations, London, 10 January.

Blyth E and Auffrey M (2008) *International policy on cross border reproductive services*. Policy statement. Geneva: International Federation of Social Workers. <http://

ifsw.org/policies/cross-border-reproductive-services>
Blyth E and Landau R (2009) *Faith and Fertility: Attitudes towards Reproductive Practices in Different Religions from Ancient to Modern Times*. London: Jessica Kingsley Publishers.
Blyth E, Crawshaw M, Haase J and Speirs J (2001) The implications of adoption for donor offspring following donor-assisted conception. *Child & Family Social Work* 6(4): 295–304.
Blyth E, Thorn P and Wischmann T (2011) CBRC and psychosocial counselling: assessing needs and developing an ethical framework for practice. *Reproductive BioMedicine Online* 23(5): 642–51.
Blyth E, Crawshaw M and van den Akker O (2014) What are the best interests of the child in international surrogacy? *Bionews* 742, 17 February. <http://www.Bionews.org.uk/page_397263.asp>
Brazier M, Campbell A and Golombok S (1998) *Surrogacy: Review for Health Ministers of Current Arrangements for Payments and Regulation. Report of the Review Team*. Cm 4068. London: HMSO.
Brunet L, Carruthers J, Davaki K et al. (2013) *A Comparative Study of the Regime of Surrogacy in EU Member States: Report Submitted to European Parliament's Committee on Legal Affairs*. <www.europarl.europa.eu/RegData/etudes/etudes/join/2013/474403/IPOL JURI_ET(2013)474403_EN.pdf>
Cheney KE (2014) Executive summary of the International Forum on Intercountry Adoption and Global Surrogacy. In: Cheney KE (ed.) *International Forum on Intercountry Adoption and Global Surrogacy*. The Hague: Institute of Social Studies (ISS), Erasmus University, 595: 1–40.
Crawshaw M, Blyth E and van den Akker O (2012) The changing profile of surrogacy in the UK: implications for national and international policy and practice. *Journal of Social Welfare and Family Law* 34(3): 265–75.
Crawshaw M, Purewal S and van den Akker O (2013) Working at the margins: the views and experiences of court social workers on Parental Orders' work in surrogacy arrangements. *British Journal of Social Work* 43(6): 1225–43.
Crawshaw M, Fronek P, Blyth E and Elvin A (2014) *What Are Children's 'Best Interests' in International Surrogacy*. Birmingham: British Association of Social Workers. <http://www.basw.co.uk/resource/?id=3176>
Cuthbert D and Fronek P (2014) Perfecting adoption? Reflections on the rise of commercial offshore surrogacy and family formation in Australia. In: Hayes A and Higgins D (eds) *Families, Policy and the Law: Selected Essays on Contemporary Issues for Australia*. Melbourne: Australian Institute of Family Studies, pp. 55–66.
Daniels K (2004) *Building a Family with the Assistance of Donor Insemination*. Palmerston North: Dunmore Press Ltd.
Darnovsky M and Beeson D (2014) *Global Surrogacy Practices*. ISS Working Paper Series/General Series 601: 1–54. <http://hdl.handle.net/1765/77402>
DasGupta S and Dasgupta SD (2014) *Globalization and Transnational Surrogacy in India: Outsourcing Life*. Lanham, MD: Lexington Books.
Department of Health and Social Security (1984) *Report of the Committee of Inquiry into Human Fertilisation and Embryology* (The Warnock Report) (Cm. 9314). London: HMSO.
Foreign and Commonwealth Office and Home Office (2014) *Information for British Nationals Who Are Considering Entering into Surrogacy Arrangements in Foreign Countries*. London: Foreign & Commonwealth Office and Home

Office. <https://www.gov.uk/government/publications/surrogacy-overseas>

Fronek P (2009) Intercountry adoption in Australia: a natural evolution or purposeful actions. In: Sparkes C and Cuthbert D (eds) *Other People's Children: Adoption in Australia*. Melbourne: Australian Scholarly Publishing Pty Ltd, pp. 37–54.

Fronek P and Crawshaw M (2015) The 'new family' as an emerging norm: a commentary on the position of social work in assisted reproduction. *British Journal of Social Work* 45(2): 737–46.

Fronek P, Crawshaw M and Blyth E (2013) Written submission to The Hague Conference on Private International Law consultation on the private international law issues surrounding the status of children, including issues arising from international surrogacy arrangements.

Fronek P, Crawshaw M, Blyth E and Elvin A (2014) International surrogacy: a report from the roundtable. *The Bulletin* (Australian Association of Social Workers) Winter: 30–1.

Gagin R, Cohen M, Greenblatt L, Solomon H and Itskowitz-Eldor J (2004) Developing the role of the social worker as coordinator of services at the Surrogate Parenting Center. *Social Work in Health Care* 40(1): 1–14.

Golombok S, Murray C, Jadva V, MacCallum F and Lycett E (2004) Families created through surrogacy arrangements: parent–child relationships in the 1st year of life. *Developmental Psychology* 40(3): 400–11.

Golombok S, MacCallum F, Murray C, Lycett E and Jadva V (2006a) Surrogacy families: parental functioning, parent–child relationships and children's psychological development at age 2. *Journal of Child Psychology and Psychiatry* 47(2): 213–22.

Golombok S, Murray C, Jadva V, Lycett E, MacCallum F and Rust J (2006b) Non-genetic and non-gestational parenting: consequences for parent–child relationships and the psychological well-being of mothers, fathers and children at age 3. *Human Reproduction* 21(7): 1918–24.

Golombok S, Readings J, Blake L, Casey P, Marks A and Jadva V (2011) Families created through surrogacy: mother–child relationships and children's psychological adjustment at age 7. *Developmental Psychology* 47(6): 1579–88.

Golombok S, Blake L, Casey P, Roman G and Jadva V (2013) Children born through reproductive donation: a longitudinal study of psychological adjustment. *Journal of Child Psychology and Psychiatry* 54(6): 653–60.

HCCH (Hague Conference on International Private Law) (2012) *A Preliminary Report on the Issues Arising from International Surrogacy Arrangements*. Preliminary Document No. 10. The Hague: Hague Conference on Private International Law. <http://www.hcch.net/upload/wop/gap2012pd10en.pdf>

HCCH (2014a) *The Desirability and Feasibility of Further Work on the Parentage/Surrogacy Project*. Preliminary Document No. 3B. The Hague: Hague Conference on Private International Law. <http://www.hcch.net/upload/wop/gap2014pd03b_en.pdf>

HCCH (2014b) *Study of Legal Parentage and the Issues Arising from International Surrogacy Arrangements*. Preliminary Document No. 3C. The Hague: Hague Conference on Private International Law. <http://www.hcch.net/upload/wop/gap2014pd03c_en.pdf>

Horsey K (2010) Challenging presumptions: legal parenthood and surrogacy arrangements. *Child and Family Law Quarterly* 22(4): 449–74.

Imrie S and Javda V (2014) The long-term experiences of surrogates: relationships and contact with surrogacy families in genetic and gestational surrogacy arrangements. *Reproductive BioMedicine Online* 29(4): 424–35.

International Social Service (2013) *International Surrogacy: Preserving the Best Interests of Children: A Call for Action by the International Social Service Network.* <http://www.iss-ssi.org/index.php/en/what-we-do-en/surrogacy>

Jadva V and Imrie S (2014) Children of surrogate mothers: psychological well-being, family relationships and experiences of surrogacy. *Human Reproduction* 29(1): 90–6.

Jadva V, Murray C, Lycett E, MacCallum F and Golombok S (2003) Surrogacy: the experiences of surrogate mothers. *Human Reproduction* 18(10): 2196–204.

Jadva V, Blake L, Casey P and Golombok S (2012) Surrogacy families 10 years on: relationship with the surrogate, decisions over disclosure and children's understanding of their surrogacy origins. *Human Reproduction* 27(10): 3008–14.

Jadva V, Imrie S and Golombok S (2015) Surrogate mothers 10 years on: a longitudinal study of psychological well-being and relationships with the parents and child. *Human Reproduction* 30(2): 373–9.

Karandikar S, Gezinski LB, Carter JR and Kaloga M (2014) Economic necessity or noble cause? A qualitative study exploring motivations for gestational surrogacy in Gujarat, India. *Affilia* 29(2): 224–36.

Knoche JW (2014) Health concerns and ethical considerations regarding international surrogacy. *International Journal of Gynecology and Obstetrics* 126(2): 183–6.

Kumar M and Chopra R (2013) India's shame story: Israeli paedophile adopts girl through surrogate mother. *dna*, 8 June. <www.dnaindia.com/india/report-india-s-shame-story-israeli-paedophile-adopts-girl-through-surrogate-mother-1845195>

MacCallum F, Lycett E, Murray C, Jadva V and Golombok S (2003) Surrogacy: the experience of commissioning couples. *Human Reproduction* 18(6): 1334–42.

Marr D (2012) Boy, 6, taken from gay pair. *Brisbane Times*, 9 February. <www.brisbanetimes.com.au/national/boy-6-taken-from-gay-pair-20120208-1rf17.html>

Martin D and Kane S (2014) National self-sufficiency in reproductive resources: an innovative response to transnational reproductive travel. *International Journal of Feminist Approaches to Bioethics* 7(2): 10–44.

Nuffield Council on Bioethics (2013) *Donor Conception: Ethical Aspects of Information Sharing.* London: Nuffield Council on Bioethics.

Ory SJ, Devroey P, Banker M, Brinsden P, Buster J, Fiadjoe M, Horton M, Nygren K, Pai H, Le Roux P and Sullivan E (2013) *IFFS Surveillance 2013.* <http://www.iffs-reproduction.org/?page=SurveillanceHidden>

Purewal S, Crawshaw M and van den Akker O (2012) Completing the surrogate motherhood process: the experiences of Parental Order Reporters. *Human Fertility* 15(2): 94–9.

Riggs DW (2015) '25 degrees of separation' versus the 'ease of doing it closer to home': motivations to offshore surrogacy arrangements amongst Australian citizens. *Somatechnics* 5(1): 52–68.

Riley H (2013) Exploring the ethical implications of the late discovery of adoptive and donor-insemination offspring status. *Adoption & Fostering* 37(2): 171–87.

Ronan A (2015) Inside the dark realities of the international surrogacy industry.

The Cut, 30 March. <http://nymag.com/thecut/2015/03/dark-side-of-international-surrogacy.html>

Rotabi KS (2014) *Bridging from Knowledge in Intercountry Adoption to Global Surrogacy: Report for Thematic Area 4 of the International Forum on Intercountry Adoption and Global Surrogacy*. The Hague. <www.academia.edu/10165753/Force_fraud_and_coercion>

Rotabi KS, Bromfield NF and Fronek P (2015) International private law to regulate commercial global surrogacy practices: just what are social work's practical policy recommendations? *International Social Work*. doi: <10.1177/0020872814564706>

Sackville T (1994) *House of Commons Official Report*. 26 October, vol. 248, col. 974.

Scherman R, Rotabi KS, Misca G and Selman P (2016) Global surrogacy and international adoption: parallels and differences. *Adoption & Fostering* 40(1): 20–36.

Shelton KH, Boivin J, Hay D, van den Bree MBM, Rice FJ, Harold GT and Thapar A (2009) Examining differences in psychological adjustment problems among children conceived by assisted reproductive technologies. *International Journal of Behavioural Development* 33(5): 385–92.

Spivack C (2010) The law of surrogate motherhood in the United States. *American Journal of Comparative Law* 58: 97–114.

Tanderup M, Reddy S, Patel T and Nielsen BB (2015) Informed consent in medical decision-making in commercial gestational surrogacy: a mixed methods study in New Delhi, India. *Acta Obstetricia et Gynecologica Scandinavica* 94(5): 465–72.

Trimmings K and Beaumont P (eds) (2013) *International Surrogacy Arrangements: Legal Regulation at the International Level*. Oxford: Hart Publishing.

Triseliotis J, Feast J and Kyle F (2005) *A Study of Adoption, Search and Reunion Experiences*. London: BAAF.

van den Akker OBA (2007) Psychosocial aspects of surrogate motherhood. *Human Reproduction Update* 13(1): 53–62.

van den Akker OBA (2012) *Reproductive Health Psychology*. Chichester: Wiley-Blackwell.

Wincott E and Crawshaw MA (2006) From a social issue to policy: social work's advocacy for the rights of donor conceived people to genetic origins information in the UK. *Social Work in Health Care* 43(2/3): 53–72.

Yaxley L (2014) International surrogacy is 'new frontline in human trafficking', says Judge John Pascoe; Indian case sparks renewed calls for inquiry. *ABC News*, 9 October. <http://www.abc.net.au/news/2014-10-09/surrogacy-claims-strengthen-calls-for-inquiry/5800258>

Ziv I and Freund-Eschar Y (2015) The pregnancy experience of gay couples expecting a child through overseas surrogacy. *Family Journal* 23(2): 158–66.

10 | WHAT ABOUT THE CHILDREN? CITIZENSHIP, NATIONALITY AND THE PERILS OF STATELESSNESS

Marsha Tyson Darling

> When is it in the best interests of the child to be stateless? Never!
> (Renate Winter, Member of the United Nations Committee on the Rights of the Child)

As we focus a lens on transnational gestational surrogacy agreements much of our attention rests on assessing adult agency and identifying their stakeholder interests in relation to their desire to arrange for methodically organized conception: the choices, decisions and actions of mostly white commissioning parents and the many people who are involved in providing surrogacy services to the fertility industry; the experiences of the impoverished, mostly brown women who work as gestational surrogates in low-resource countries; the family court judges, legislators and state regulators who enforce laws but also create exceptions to national social policies regarding surrogacy agreements; and the immigration officials who apply criteria and guidelines for determining a child's citizenship status. But what about the children who are the fertility industry's main enterprise, given that producing *them* is the reason the surrogacy industry exists? This article positions a lens on the child's stakeholder interests and explores a number of questions related to several key quality of life issues – legal citizenship, nationality and identity, and statelessness – that denote important challenges for some newborns as well as older children born through transnational gestational surrogacy arrangements. Another important element of a child's stakeholder interests – the right to knowledge – is discussed elsewhere in this volume.

Stateless babies and children: the fundamental dilemmas

The main focus of this chapter is on the children who have faced potentially perilous situations because they were denied citizenship status, both in the countries of their gestational birth and in the countries where their intended parents hold citizenship; these are 'stateless children'. They are important not because in the main their experience constitutes the experiences of the majority of newborns born through transnational surrogacy agreements (though their numbers are increasing), but because their experience, even in its singularity, is important from a human rights perspective (Graham, 2014; Henaghan, 2013; Kanics, 2014; Trimmings and Beaumont, 2013). Stateless children are created when there is a difficulty in a nation state of establishing or recognizing whom it considers the legal parentage of a child to be. The challenge, stated plainly, is that some children fail to acquire the nationality of their nation of birth or the country in which their intended parents legally reside, leaving the child with no legal parents and no state. This dilemma, now several years old, poses very real problems for children and of course for their intended parents, even as it seems to go without mention by those whose focus is on the successes of the emerging biotechnology's ability to provide parenthood for so many adults. Stateless children merit our concern because the challenges they confront are entirely remediable and warrant the close scrutiny and active engagement of international and nation state judicial, immigration and legislative authorities (European Network on Statelessness, 2015a; Trimmings and Beaumont, 2013).

The importance of the child's perspective regarding transnational surrogacy comes into clearer focus when one considers that it does not serve the child's interest to be excluded from the state nationality of their parents who are already citizens. Without a registered nationality a child in some countries is ineligible to access free health care and public education, and as the years pass, the child having become an adult will be unable to vote, work legally (especially in occupations that require that one is bonded) or possibly even live in the country of their parents. Many domestic state regulators are intent upon enforcing existing social policy regarding commercial surrogacy; often state courts send a punitive message towards intended parents and any others considering transnational gestational surrogacy options. From the point of view of a child, such state policies and decisions often impact the children who will bear the adverse *consequences* of adult agency that they had no part in creating.

In representing the child's stakeholder interests the most important question bearing on matters of citizenship, nationality, identity and, as time passes, the right to knowledge concerning one's gestational, biological or genetic ancestry, is who is looking after the interests of the child born through transnational gestational surrogacy arrangements?

What are the circumstances by which newborns are denied citizenship in the countries of their commissioning parents, and how are those circumstances already affecting these babies' 'quality of life'? What complications are newborns and even young children forced to confront if they are rendered 'stateless'? Whose responsibility is it to look after infants born to surrogacy agreements who because of home country regulations are required to remain in orphanages in low-resource countries? What happens if there is no genetic or DNA match that confirms their genetic parentage? What happens to infants who are abandoned because commissioning parents either are unprepared to accept twins or triplets, or because the baby has a visible disability, or because something happens to one or both intended parents? What about a child's right to know information about all of the participants in its gestational process, including the poor brown woman s/he will not likely meet? Who will be responsible for maintaining and providing that information to the adult children who are curious and as the years pass, may have important health and genetic marker transmission concerns regarding their lineage?

As we should hold a child's concern for personal security paramount, we begin with the first question: who is looking out for the interests of the newborn in transnational gestational surrogacy arrangements? In addition to the commissioning adult(s) who have committed time, energy, resources, and likely their gametes, the existence of international law, nation state laws and public policy directed towards insuring the exercise of agreed upon human rights for the child are important contributions to the stakeholder interests of all children. With the *welfare principle of the paramountcy of the best interests of the child* as a normative justice standard, many of the signatories to the Convention on the Rights of the Child (CRC), the most widely endorsed convention ever, have worked to institutionalize a benefits standard for the world's children that stipulates that each child shall have a citizenship (Article 15), an identity (Article 8) and a right to knowledge of their origins (Article 7).[1]

The limitations of international law

Over the course of the past several decades there has been a concerted international effort to use the CRC and The Hague Convention as the legally binding standards for assessing the *best interests of the child*, even as regulatory agencies and officials now engage the challenges of boundary-making regarding transnational gestational surrogacy agreements.[2] In our contemporary engagements with the thorny issues that have arisen in the course of navigating a way through the complexities of how to embrace personal reproductive liberty for adults wanting to create families, while at the same time using state institutions to regulate the boundaries of permissible adult agency as it impacts parentage, countries differ in the criteria and regulations they apply to parentage. Much of Europe, including France, Italy, Germany and Slovenia, as well as Japan and China, bans all forms of surrogacy. The UK, Australia, Israel, Holland and New Zealand allow only altruistic surrogacy, and India, Ukraine, Russia and certain states within the United States, especially California, Florida and Illinois, allow commercial surrogacy (Boyce, 2013).

While domestic regulations in much of the industrialized world restrain most of their citizenry from utilizing commercial surrogacy services in surrogacy-friendly countries, there are increasing numbers of domestic nationals arranging such contracts and then applying to bring their new family members home. It is the home country judiciary that is on the frontline of engaging citizen litigation that seeks relief from restrictive regulations that void surrogacy agreements that violate domestic law. An increasing number of judges adjudicating such litigation are confronted with international law that clearly obligates states that are signatories to the CRC and The Hague Convention to consider issues impacting the child through the available lens provided by both adoption law (a focus on the paramountcy of the *best interests of the child*) and family law (rooted in tradition that every child has paternity as well as a claim to a mother's womb). Hence, because there is little doubt that being rendered 'stateless' is a very untenable and possibly dangerous status for an infant child, a number of state courts and the European Courts of Human Rights and of Justice are vitally important to the child's stakeholder interests.

At the same time, many judges are acutely aware that state-imposed prohibitive measures that deny the intended parents their child serve to punish them for transgressing domestic law and also, very often, customary notions and traditions shaping the rules about how families are to be created. Nonetheless, facing the concrete reality that children born from commercial surrogacy arrangements now exist and require a name, legal citizenship in the nation of their intended parents, and participation in the social categories and relationships that comprise nationality, a home and adults to take care of them, a number of judges have begun to render decisions that secure newborns and children with their intended parents, regardless of the legal violation the adults have committed. In keeping with this chapter's focus on the stakeholder interests of the child, clearly, from the child's perspective s/he has not transgressed any laws and therefore should not be punished for adult agency (especially since the intended parents are for all intents and purposes the child's best lifeline).

A determination of legal parentage is at the centre of the challenges that impede the recognition of who should be responsible for children. As a matter of social policy within many nations, traditional notions of parenthood collide with surrogacy's ability to provide significant reproductive options as it produces two or three mothers and up to two fathers. It is in a child's interest that international law asserts that the right of every child to state citizenship is a fundamental right that should not be withheld based on the method of reproduction by which a child was born. In the US the right of a child to legal citizenship is secured immediately at birth through *jus soli* or after confirmation of *jus sanguinis*, meaning that a child is a citizen of the nation if s/he is born on American soil or is born through the bloodline or biological ancestry (genetic DNA) of an American citizen. While Article 7 of the UNCRC expressly provides 'the right to acquire a nationality', in much of Europe access to home country nationality is through descent from an adult parent to a child (*jus sanguinis*). It is important to note that twenty-seven countries worldwide, including some in Western Europe, prohibit single women who undergo IVF treatment using an anonymous sperm donor within their borders from exercising the right to pass nationality to their children at birth, rendering the infant stateless; in the Netherlands an infant born into such a circumstance will have to wait three years to be eligible to claim Dutch nationality (European Network on Statelessness, 2015a).

Alongside gender bias, discrimination towards LGBT persons is a very real challenge to the enforcement of gender-blind and sexuality-neutral law, even as growing numbers of adults representing non-traditional families come forward to access transnational gestational surrogacy services.[3]

Recent litigation has revealed that there are sometimes *disparate and unequal* additional conditions applied as LGBT intended parents seek nationality for their newborns. For instance, the Helsinki Foundation for Human Rights is arguing a case in Poland where a Polish man who is a citizen seeks to have his paternal ties to four children born through surrogacy in the US recognized so as to provide them with Polish nationality. The man and his male partner are registered on the US birth certificates, but have encountered a problem in that Polish authorities have insisted that he provide details about the identity of the children's biological mother. While these children are not stateless, they have not been allowed by Polish authorities to access their father's nationality (European Network on Statelessness, 2015b).

In Slovenia, a same-sex couple who married in California took custody of a baby girl born through a gestational surrogacy agreement. Returning to Slovenia, they were challenged in that the state does not allow for LGBT adoption nor did it allow surrogacy or adoption outside of heterosexual marriage. In recent litigation the Slovenian District Court issued a ruling 'that the foreign judicial decision must be recognised – and with it the parental link and the rights deriving from that, including acquisition of Slovenian nationality' (European Network on Statelessness, 2015c).

In yet another recent case regarding the challenges that same-sex couples continue to confront in their efforts to secure legal recognition of their familial ties with the children they have commissioned through gestational surrogacy arrangements, in July 2015, in *Oliari and Others v. Italy*, the European Court of Human Rights in Strasbourg (ECtHR) ruled that Article 8 protections of the European Convention of Human Rights (ECHR) (formerly the Convention on the Protection of Human Rights and Fundamental Freedoms) applies to same-sex couples, thereby making it easier for LGBT couples to obtain legal recognition of their parentage rights, which also enables their ability to provide physical security for children.[4]

Can the law keep up?

Continuing with who is looking after the child's stakeholder interests, particularly concerning citizenship and nationality, are the challenges for children born through transnational gestational surrogacy arrangements. A major issue across much of Europe is the inability of national laws to allow transnational gestational surrogacy contracts to be legally binding on state citizenship and nationality requirements. Against the backdrop of patriarchy and with a focus on parentage and kinship, many regulators in Europe are challenged to accept the parentage choices that some of their citizens are utilizing given the rapidly expanded use of reproductive biotechnologies available via transnational gestational surrogacy arrangements. For instance, a new development in reproductive medicine, Mitochondrial Replacement Therapy (MRT) in oocytes or zygotes promises to add yet another technology-enabled dimension to motherhood, namely the ability to prevent the second-generation transference of mitochondrial DNA defects to children. Are we approaching a tipping point where the absence of international regulation of commercial surrogacy allows the technology to be so far out in front of governance making that it renders rule making and enforcement untenable (Darnovsky and Cussins, 2015; Davis, 2010; Gallagher, 2015)?

In a widely quoted speech on 'Children and International Human Rights Law', the thirteenth Secretary-General of the Council of Europe, Thorbjorn Jagland, noted that 'developments in technology have created major challenges for the law'.[5] Indeed, dating back to 2009 the Council of Europe issued a recommendation to its Member States regarding the nationality of children born to surrogacy arrangements, noting that they should 'apply to children their provisions on acquisition of nationality by right of blood if, as a result of a birth conceived through medically assisted reproductive techniques, a child–parent family relationship is established or recognized by law'.[6] The Council's recommendation appeared to refer the issue back to domestic laws, which were already challenged to adapt to changing parenting realities in Europe and abroad.

In those nations that ban commercial surrogacy, the non-enforceability of transnational surrogacy agreements thwarts measures designed to protect a child's stakeholder interests, namely state protection of their human rights. The denial of citizenship and nationality to either newborn infants or older children who accompany intended parents who have commissioned them through transnational gestational surrogacy arrangements is, while being a punitive measure directed at the choices, decisions and actions of adult nationals, arguably not in *the best interests of the child*. If lawmakers in most of Western Europe continue to aim to dissuade their citizens from engaging in transnational gestational surrogacy agreements even as some citizens continue to avail themselves of surrogacy opportunities, especially in low-resource countries, it is the judiciary in European countries that is creating case law that finds the *welfare of the child* to be more important than the legal regimes designed to discourage cross-border commercial surrogacy. The ECtHR and some European judges have decided to confront the issue head on.

The role of the European courts

European Union (EU) law seeks to create and sustain uniformity and a nuanced approach to nation state compliance as its decisions transfer to its Member States. While EU law shares competence with its Member States' laws in areas of social policy, it can exert supremacy over a state's refusal to recognize a citizenship obligation.

Regarding the European Court of Justice (ECJ) in Luxembourg, the decisions made by the Court are intended to establish a 'legal norm', are binding and require Member States to amend their national law. The ECtHR in Strasbourg provides jurisprudence that requires Member States to recognize international legal norms that the *rights of the child should be paramount* (Graham, 2014). With that in mind, we look to several important decisions in which an ECtHR ruling has provided a concern to prioritize the welfare of the child born abroad whose well-being hangs on their access to citizenship and nationality. In *Genovese v. Malta* the ECtHR ruled that the policy of requiring evidence of paternity for the conferring of nationality in cases where a child is born out of wedlock and requiring registration as necessary for the acquisition of nationality by a child born abroad violated Articles 8 and 14 of the ECHR.[7] In 2014 and 2015, Denmark and Sweden amended their laws and researchers at the European Network on Statelessness (2015a: 20) noted that:

> in both Denmark and Sweden, a child born to a citizen father after the entry into force of the new law automatically acquires nationality, regardless of the place of birth or whether the parents are married ... [but] the lack of retroactive effect of these amendments means that the situation of any child rendered stateless due to previously problematic law is not addressed through this reform.

In a landmark case, *Mennesson v. France* decided in June 2014, the ECtHR issued a decision that reversed the decisions of France's highest courts regarding the recognition of the familial status of children born abroad to French parents through gestational surrogacy arrangements. Dominique and Sylvie Mennesson commissioned a surrogate in California to carry twins produced from Mr Mennesson's sperm and a friend's egg. The surrogate was paid US$10,000 and the twin girls, Valentina and Fiorella, were issued US birth certificates naming the Mennessons as their parents. While the children were allowed to accompany the Mennessons back to France they were denied French citizenship because surrogacy is illegal in France.

Over the course of ten years the Mennessons fought unsuccessfully to be recognized as the children's parents and to register them in the National Register. Then, in 2010, the French Court of Appeal allowed recognition of the Mennessons as the children's parents but declined to add the children to the French National Register, thereby refusing them as French citizens despite the Mennessons' position that the interests of the children should be *paramount*. On further appeal, the French Supreme Court upheld the ruling of the Appeal Court, which left the children ineligible for free health care, education, and later the right to vote, reside legally or work in France.

With all avenues of appeal in France closed, the Mennessons took their case to the ECtHR in Strasbourg, which focused on the *best interests of the child* in noting that 'everyone must be able to establish the substance of his or her identity' and further, that the lack of French nationality 'is liable to have negative repercussions on the definition of their personal identity'. The ECtHR found Article 8 of the European Charter of Human Rights instructive and ruled that France had violated the children's right to respect for private life.[8] Also, in June 2014, the ECtHR extended the Article 8 based ruling to *Labbassee v. France*, a case in which another French couple arranged a gestational surrogacy contract in the US in 2001 and after returning to France encountered the same challenges as the Mennessons.[9]

In *D and Others v. Belgium*, a case that also went before the ECtHR in 2014, the Court issued a unanimous ruling that Belgian authorities had been in their rightful authority to insist on 'carrying out checks before allowing a child who had been born in the Ukraine to a surrogate mother to enter Belgium'. The Court rejected the applicants' claim that Belgian authorities interfered with 'their right to respect for their family life', stating that 'Belgium had acted within its broad discretion (a wide margin of appreciation)'. The ECtHR denied any further application for a claim in this case. This case brings to light the most serious consequence of differing standards for assigning parentage, a situation that most intended parents seldom anticipate, namely that their infant will be unable to secure any citizenship and is at risk of being left in an orphanage. The child was commissioned by a married couple listed in the Court's petition as Mr D and Ms R. The couple travelled to Ukraine and arranged a birth with a Ukraine surrogate who delivered a boy in 2013.

Unlike the French couples mentioned above, who paid surrogates in the US for infants who assumed US citizenship at birth even though the couples' names were on the birth certificates, consistent with social policy in Ukraine children born to surrogates are not citizens of Ukraine at birth. Belgian officials refused to issue a travel document to the child who was born in Ukraine to a gestational surrogate mother. The surrogate surrendered any responsibility for the child at his birth (consistent with the terms of the surrogacy contract and with

Ukraine law), and at the same time the child could not accompany his intended parents to Belgium. While the child had no *right* to residence or citizenship in Ukraine he was allowed to remain there having now become stateless – he was neither a citizen of Ukraine nor Belgium. The intended parents travelled to Ukraine several times to visit the infant boy, as they were apart from him for three-and-a-half months.[10]

The risks and realities of separation

Most often, commissioning parents look after some of the interests of the child, but may unintentionally become a party to circumstances that adversely impact the quality of life for newborns. From the perspective of a child's stakeholder interests, being unable to accompany one's commissioning parents to their home country and domicile is a serious threat to personal security as it puts a child who is denied citizenship at risk for neglect, injury, illness and possibly death. The issue of infants rendered 'stateless' or caught up in a quagmire of legal manoeuvres has shadowed the commercial surrogacy industry for some time, primarily because commercial gestational surrogacy contracts are either unenforceable or outlawed in much of the world. Several examples highlight the danger this presents for newborns.

Laurent Ghilain and Peter Meurrens, gay men living in a committed relationship in Belgium where adoption by same-sex couples is legal, sought to start a family having grown weary of the adoption process. A surrogate in the Ukraine gave birth to a boy from Ghilain's sperm and an anonymous donor's egg in 2008. The Belgian Embassy in Kiev refused to recognize Samuel as a citizen of Belgium, even as DNA showed a genetic match with his father, Ghilain. The infant was denied Ukrainian citizenship because Ukrainian law recognizes the commissioning intended parents as the child's legal parentage; the surrogate and her husband do not have a legal responsibility to the child.[11] Samuel was rendered stateless and was forced to remain in the Ukraine while his intended family sought legal solutions. The couple initially placed the infant with a foster family in the Ukraine, but as a year passed and financial resources withered away, the infant was placed in a Ukrainian orphanage. Another year passed with no progress on a legal solution. Finally, a Belgian court ruled in favour of the intended parents' attempts to confer Belgian citizenship status on the child and the Belgian Foreign Ministry issued baby Samuel a passport, two years and three months after his birth. At that time the nation's Foreign Ministry put out a press release cautioning its citizens against commissioning surrogates in a foreign nation (Lin, 2013).

Infants can also be rendered stateless if there is an error committed by the fertility clinic. In 2005 a married couple living in Canada contracted with a fertility clinic in India for a gestational surrogate. Using the husband's sperm and a donated egg the surrogate gave birth to twins, a girl and a boy, in 2006. Consulting the Canadian High Commission in New Delhi for permission to secure Canadian citizenship for both children, a DNA test revealed that the baby girl was indeed the daughter of the commissioning father but the boy was not. With no policy in place to cover the consequence of the clinic's error the Canadian authorities declined to issue travel papers to the infant boy. The family remained in India for five years, until 2011, when a citizen card was issued to their daughter and travel documents were issued to their non-biological son. Once in Canada the couple filed an application on *humanitarian grounds* for citizenship for their non-biological son (Aulakh, 2011).

Some examples from the UK

The UK led the way in creating surrogacy legislation in 1985, and it banned and assigned criminal penalties for commercial surrogacy. The Human Fertilisation and Embryology (HFE) Act forbade payment for surrogacy services greater than 'reasonable expenses', and stipulated a traditional norm for assessing motherhood, namely that the woman who gives birth to a child is its mother. While UK law allowed domestic 'altruistic surrogacy', there were UK citizens who sought to expand their parenting options by engaging the transnational fertility industry.

Three cases in particular highlight the complexities of the unexpected and disquieting situations that confronted three sets of intended parents and young infants who were rendered stateless by the incompatibility of national laws one with another.

A married British couple commissioned a US surrogate who delivered Baby L in Illinois, having paid more expenses than UK law allowed. The agreement was legal in the US – conferring US citizenship and a passport on the child. Baby L entered the UK on a temporary visa, but the UK refused to honour the surrogacy agreement as it violated section 54 of the HFE Act (Ross, 2010).[12] In terms of the stakeholder interests of the child, the judiciary was a key authority as UK Justice Hedley J issued a Parental Order asserting that the welfare of the child was important and therefore *outweighed* social policy invalidating commercial surrogacy arrangements: the interests of the intended parents prevailed.[13]

In 2008, a British couple engaged a commercial surrogacy arrangement with a Ukrainian woman using the sperm of the intended father and a donated egg. Proceeding with a birth certificate from Ukraine identifying the British couple as the parents of the two children, the intended parents applied for a Parental Order in the UK. British authorities asserted that the surrogacy contract violated section 27 of the HFE Act that requires that a birth mother is an infant's mother within and outside the UK. Further, even after a genetic test confirming a match with the twins, the British parents were not considered the children's parents under UK law. Still further, the amount of the payment to the surrogate violated section 54 of the HFE Act. 'Differing legal parentage views between the two systems left the children with no right to entry to the UK and the intended parents had no *right* to remain with the children in Ukraine; the children were *parentless/ orphaned and stateless*.'[14] In waiving the rule, the High Court decided that, despite the arrangement's violation of UK law, where a DNA test confirms the paternity of a UK man with a child, the child could not be denied entry into the UK; and the High Court authorized the £23,000 payment to the surrogate – all in the interests of the *welfare of the children* (Ghevaert, 2009).

In 2011, twin boys were born to a male UK couple by an anonymous Indian gestational surrogate who also provided the egg; a fertility clinic oversaw the arrangement and contract that was legal in India. After birth, the infants were discharged from the hospital to the care of their intended parents, who in the weeks that followed were unable to secure the consent of the surrogate mother to accompany their attempt to secure a Parental Order. Despite repeated requests to the clinic, they were ignored and even rebuked. Failing to secure the consent of the surrogate the intended parents appealed to British authorities for a Parental Order minus the mother's consent (Henaghan, 2013: 6). The UK court, 'emphasising that consent is a very important element to granting parental order as the surrogate is the "natural mother" with a "very special relationship" to the child, the court nevertheless found that in this case her consent would not be required'. However, the court cautioned that its first-time allowance of this provision should not replace due diligence in seeking the approval of a child's birth mother.[15]

In an attempt to stem the incidence of citizens contracting with fertility clinics in India without first consulting with their home country embassy, in 2010 the Consul Generals of Belgium, France, Germany, Italy and Spain, the Netherlands, Poland and the Czech Republic wrote to a number of Indian fertility clinics pressuring them to refer intended parents to their home country embassies before proceeding with surrogacy arrangements (Smerdon, 2013: 188). In response to the disquieting scenarios that have left some newborn infants unable to enter the home countries of intended parents, officials in India provided a 'Draft Bill' (since superseded by the Surrogacy (Regulation) Bill, 2016) that addressed a number of issues in gestational surrogacy arrangements, including the requirement that surrogacy contracts must appoint a local guardian who is legally responsible for a newborn between birth and delivery to its intended parents (up to thirty days).

The situation in the US

Fixing a gaze on the US, which is both a gestational surrogacy provider destination as well as a sending location from which citizens travel abroad to participate in transnational gestational surrogacy arrangements, the *guarantee* of US citizenship for children is attained if the infant is born on US soil (*jus soli*) or if the child is born abroad with a bloodline link to a US citizen (*jus sanguinis*).[16] The Child Citizenship Act of 2000 (CCA) created changes for the acquisition of citizenship for children, setting out criteria for citizenship at birth, citizenship through naturalization after birth and citizenship for children adopted or born through surrogacy arrangements. With mounting concerns that fertility centres and medical personnel abroad have been falsifying medical records of children born of gestational surrogates in order to identify a US citizen as the biological parent, US Consulates often request DNA tests to verify a bloodline link between a US citizen and the infant or child on whose behalf a claim for citizenship is being presented. Regarding the citizenship status of an infant born to an unmarried or married woman who is a US citizen who has undergone IVF utilizing donated sperm, the infant is considered to have been born out of wedlock regardless of the citizenship status of the sperm donor. It is the fact that the woman is not married to the sperm donor that is controlling; the infant in such a situation acquires the nationality of its mother (Law *et al.*, 2010). Because children can be conceived in a variety of ways, US State Department (USSD) regulations can mean that an ART child is not only denied US citizenship, but depending on the law of the country in which the child is born, s/he becomes stateless (Knaplund, 2013: 25–6).

The USSD has cautioned Americans to be aware that careful scrutiny will be applied by US Consulates when they are approached with a request to grant US citizenship to newborn infants. The

Consulate will likely require a DNA test that seeks a genetic tissue link between the US citizen and the infant for whom US citizenship is being sought. There have been instances where intended parents have supplied their own gametes to fertility clinics outside the US, only to later learn at the point of consulate DNA testing of the newborn that the infant lacks any of their DNA materials. It was likely that a mix-up occurred in the fertility clinic laboratory, or that the gametes supplied by the commissioning parent were not viable; either way, the fertility facility implanted an embryo into a gestational surrogate that lacked the commissioning parent's genetic materials. Unfortunately, they only learn of the problem when they approach the consulate for citizenship credentials for their newborn.

Despite *jus sanguinis*, there are instances of infants being rendered *stateless* by US officials. The USSD considers the infant birthed through the use of donated gametes to have been *born out of wedlock* regardless of the marital status of the US citizen(s) who petitions the US Consulate. Recently, the USSD denied US citizenship to the children of three American women, leaving each child *stateless*. Two of the women received anonymously donated gametes and birthed a child, one in Israel and one in Switzerland. The third used donated eggs and gave birth in India; subsequently, the US Embassy refused to accept the birth mother as the child's mother. In all three of these cases the women had a biological but not a genetic link with the infants they birthed, and the USSD refused citizenship to the children, thereby rendering the infants stateless (Knaplund, 2012).

Should intended parents be screened?

In addition to challenges concerning citizenship and nationality, infants born through transnational gestational surrogacy agreements sometimes confront other threatening scenarios, such as abuse or molestation by an intended parent. Domestic and international adoption involves rigorous screening and opportunities to identify intended parents that may not be persons who will act in the best interests of a child. Arguably adults who engage in coital sex that produces a child are often under the gaze of state-sponsored child protective services in much of the industrialized world. But it is clear from the commercial nature of the services provided by fertility clinics, especially in low-resource countries, that they do not undertake to screen commissioning parents. While there are those who would argue that children who cost so much money are valuable and will be taken care of, and while in the main that is from what we know an accurate assertion, it is nonetheless crucial to note the absence of vetting of intended parents and the known instances of sex offenders commissioning infants in India and Thailand (Overdorf, 2013; Pearlman, 2014). Arguably, from a child's stakeholder position there is work to be done on states crafting responsible governance that puts in place an effective screening process or registration procedure for intended parents accessing the fertility industry.

Baby Gammy, a little boy born through a transnational gestational surrogacy arrangement in Thailand, made international headlines in August 2014 when he was abandoned by the married Australian couple who returned home with his twin sister after leaving him with the Thai surrogate who gave birth to him. Gammy, who has Down's syndrome and a congenital heart condition, was conceived using the husband's sperm, and because he did not come out as desired his intended parents abandoned him to the Thai surrogate who was under no contractual obligation to take responsibility for him (*BBC News Asia*, 2014; Topping and Foster, 2014). Reporters grew interested in the intended parents only to learn 'that the husband was revealed to have been convicted of multiple child sex offences that took place between the early 1980s and early 1990s against girls as young as five years old' (Pearlman, 2014). As we consider Gammy's stakeholder interests, if he had been born in Australia, the US or Western Europe would state law have allowed his intended parents to take his twin sister and walk away from him and the legal obligations that accompany giving birth to or commissioning children in the industrialized world (van Wichelen, 2014)?

In addition to a child being rejected because of a visible disability, other equally perplexing situations weigh on the stakeholder interests of children born through commercial gestational surrogacy arrangements. Space limitations prevent this chapter from exploring several more salient questions that bear directly on quality of life issues for the child born this way. What if the intended parents will not pay for twin children when they requested and expected a single child and the surrogate refuses to undergo an abortion? What if an unforeseen legal complication befalls one or both intended parents prior to their taking custody of a newborn surrogacy baby in a low-resource country like India or Ukraine? What if a fertility clinic mix-up results in the birth of a child that is racially different from the expected child?

Conclusion

In conclusion, this chapter has taken the stakeholder position of the child born through transnational gestational surrogacy arrangements who has a right to begin life with the citizenship and nationality of the adults most responsible for the child's survival and well-being. Nowhere are the human rights of infants born through gestational surrogacy arrangements more challenged than when they move across the legal and public policy terrain of nation states regarding parentage. At no point are children born to transnational gestational surrogacy arrangements more vulnerable and at risk for injury, abandonment and death than when they are rendered *stateless* and therefore not entitled to the rights, immunities and protections of any nation. While the judiciary in a number of nations and at the regional governance level in Europe has provided some meaningful relief for the intended parents of infants and children caught between legal systems, being orphaned or without citizenship and nationality in either the country of one's birth or the country of one's intended parents is a perilous situation for a child's well-being. This mounting case law suggests that lawmakers and governance bodies are aware of the necessity to craft a legally enforceable mechanism for recognizing a child's fundamental right of citizenship, as it is simply unacceptable to allow a discriminatory and potentially dangerous circumstance of *statelessness* to obstruct *the best interests of the child*.

Notes

1 Efforts on behalf of the *best interests of the child* have accumulated over time: the Universal Declaration of Human Rights (1948); the United Nations Declaration on Social and Legal Principles Relating to the Protection and Welfare of Children (1986); the World Summit Declaration on the Survival, Protection and Development of Children (1990); the United Nations Convention on the Rights of the Child (1990); and still later the Hague Convention on Protection of Children and Cooperation in Respect to Intercountry Adoption (1993); the Convention on the Reduction of Statelessness; the European Convention on Human Rights; and the European Convention on Nationality.

2 The Permanent Bureau of The Hague Conference has released two reports that focus on surrogacy: *Issues Surrounding the Status of Children, Including Issues Arising from International Surrogacy Arrangements* (HCCH, 2011) and *Issues Arising from International Surrogacy Arrangements* (HCCH, 2012). Both reports note an exponential expansion of transnational international surrogacy and the challenges of crafting responsible governance of adult utilization of commercial surrogacy services while simultaneously advancing a welfare interest on behalf of children. The reports conclude that The Hague Convention, as it exists, is inadequate to deal with the new challenges created by surrogacy arrangements. Nonetheless, in a number of nations that are signatories to international conventions on the rights of the child, judges and lawmakers routinely embrace The Hague Convention's *welfare of the child standard* as a factor alongside *the intent to parent standard* in rendering litigation decisions.

3 The exercise of greater reproductive liberty for women, gays

and lesbians, and single women and men has followed civil rights advances for those political constituents in democratic societies. What was once assumed to be the traditional family now exists alongside new ways in which recently empowered citizens are defining personal identity and family creation. Family issues, specifically noted in this chapter, include: changes in who can be a parent; options for how children are created; issues related to how legal parentage is secured for the well-being of the most vulnerable (who are the children); and requirements for how adults communicate their choices and behaviours to institutions of the state charged with overseeing family, adoption and immigration law are central stakeholder issues for the child.

4 European Court of Human Rights, *Oliari and Others v. Italy*, Application No. 18766/11 and 36030/11, 21 July 2015.

5 Secretary-General Jagland's comments at the 46th Annual Study Session of the International Institute of Human Rights (IIHR), July 2015.

6 Council of Europe Recommendation CM/Rec (2009) 13 of the Committee on Ministers to Member States on the Nationality of Children, 9 December 2009, Principle 12.

7 European Court of Human Rights, *Genovese v. Malta*, Application No. 53124/09, 11 October 2011.

8 European Court of Human Rights, *Mennesson v. France*, Application No. 65192/11, 26 June 2014, and *No Child Should Be Stateless*. London: European Network on Statelessness (ENS), 17 September 2015.

9 European Court of Human Rights, *Labassee v. France*, Application No. 65941/11, 26 June 2014.

10 European Court of Human Rights, *D and Others v. Belgium*, Application No. 29176/13, 9 November 2014.

11 Family Code of Ukraine, Article 123(2).

12 *Re: L (A Minor)* [2010] EWHC 3146 (Fam.).

13 *Re: S (Parental Order)* [2009] EWHC 2977 (Fam.), [2010] 1 FLR 1156.

14 *Re: X & Y (Foreign Surrogacy)* [2008] EWHC 3030 (Fam.); see also *Re: IJ (A Child)* [2011] EWHC 291 (Fam.), a later case involving a UK law and Ukraine and an orphaned and stateless infant child.

15 *Re: D, L (Minors) (Surrogacy) and in the Matter of Human Fertilization and Embryology Act 2008* [2012] EWHC 2631 (Fam.).

16 In the US the right to privacy and the right to procreate – including an immunity from state intrusion when utilizing reproductive services is grounded in ethics and constitutional law: *Skinner v. Oklahoma* (1942), *Griswold v. Connecticut* (1965), *Eisenstadt vs. Connecticut* (1972), *Roe v. Wade* (1973), *Doe v. Bolton* (1973), *Thornburgh v. American College of Obstetricians and Gynecologists* (1986), *Planned Parenthood of S.E. Pa. v. Carey* (1992), *Stenberg v. Carhart* (2000), *Lawrence v. Texas* (2003) and *Gonzalez v. Carhart* (2007).

References

Aulakh R (2011) After six years and fertility mix-up, surrogate twin can come home. *The Star*, 5 May. <www.thestar.com/news/gta/2011/05/05/after_6_years_and_fertility_mixup_surrogate_twin_can_come_home.html>

BBC News Asia (2014) Conflicting claims over Thai surrogate baby case. *BBC News Asia*, 4 August. <www.bbc.co.uk/news/world-asia-28636126>

Boyce AK (2013) Protecting the voiceless: rights of the child in transnational surrogacy agreements. 36 *Suffolk Transnational Law Review* 36: 649.

Daily Telegraph, 11 December. <www.telegraph.co.uk/news/uknews/8194099/Surrogacy-couple-paying-American-woman-was-our-last-chance-for-a-child.html>

Darnovsky M and Beeson D (2014) *Global Surrogacy Practices*. ISS Working Paper Series/General Series 601: 1–54. <http://hdl.handle.net/1765/77402>

Darnovsky M and Cussins J (2015) Britain is on the brink of a perilous vote for 'three person in vitro fertilisation'. *Los Angeles Times*, 8 February. <http://www.latimes.com/opinion/op-ed/la-oe-0209-darnovsky-children-dna-from-3-people-20150209-story.html>

Davis E (2010) The rise of gestational surrogacy and the pressing need for international regulation. *Minnesota Journal of International Law* 21(1). <http://minnjil.org/wp-content/uploads/2015/07/The-Rise-of-Gestational-Surrogacy-and-the-Erica-Davis.pdf>

European Network on Statelessness (2015a) *No Child Should Be Stateless*. <www.statelessness.eu/sites/www.statelessness.eu/files/ENS_NoChildStateless_final.pdf>

European Network on Statelessness (2015b) *Ending Childhood Statelessness: A Study on Poland*. <www.statelessness.eu/resources/ending-childhood-statelessness-study-poland>

European Network on Statelessness (2015c) *Ending Childhood Statelessness: A Study on Slovenia*. <www.statelessness.eu/resources/ending-childhood-statelessness-study-slovenia>

Gallagher J (2015) MPs say yes to three person babies. *BBC News*, 3 February. <www.bbc.co.uk/news/health-31069173>

Ghevaert L (2009) Surrogacy law must be reviewed to stop more British couples ending up in a legal nightmare. *BioNews*, Progress Educational Trust, 12 January. <www.bionews.org.uk/page_38044.asp>

Graham RJ (2014) Citizenship and the stateless child: obligations of the European Union. Unpublished Master of Law in Human Rights Law thesis, Chapters 3 and 4. University of Ulster, UK.

HCCH (Hague Conference on International Private Law) (2011) *Private International Issues Surrounding the Status of Children, Including Issues Arising from International Surrogacy Arrangements*. Preliminary Document No. 11. The Hague: Hague Conference on Private International Law.

HCCH (2012) *A Preliminary Report on the Issues Arising from International Surrogacy Arrangements*. Preliminary Document No. 10. March. The Hague: Hague Conference on Private International Law.

Henaghan M (2013) Children's rights: international surrogacy trends: how family law is coping. Presented at the 6th World Congress on Family Law and Children's Rights. March, Sydney, Australia.

Hutchinson AM (2012) The Hague convention on surrogacy: should we agree to disagree? ABA Section of Family Law. Fall CLE Conference, October.

Kanics J (2014) Preventing and addressing statelessness: in the context of international surrogacy arrangements. *Tilburg Law Review* 19: 117–26.

Knaplund KS (2012) Immigration article of the day: what's blood got to do with it? Determining parentage for ART children born overseas. Immigration Prof Blog. <http://lawprofessors.typepad.com/immigration/2012/12/immigration-article-of-the-day-.html>

Knaplund KS (2013) *Jus Sanguinis*: determining citizenship for assisted reproduction children born overseas. <http://dx.doi.org/10.2139/ssrn.2181026>

Law KS, Steffas I and Strain D (2010) A child's claim to citizenship: birth, surrogacy, and adoption. American Immigration Lawyers Association Immigration Practice Pointers.

<www.ailawebcle.org/resources/Resources%20for%2010-13-11%20Seminar.pdf>

Lin T (2013) Born lost: stateless children in international surrogacy arrangements. *Cardozo Journal of International & Comparative Law* 21(2): 545.

Overdorf J (2013) Israeli sex offender taps India's booming surrogacy trade for baby girl. *Global Post*, 10 June. <www.globalpost.com/dispatch/news/regions/asia-pacific/india/130610/india-israeli-sex-offender-taps-indias-booming-surro>

Pearlman J (2014) Surrogacy case: the history of sex offenses of the Australian accused of leaving surrogate boy in Thailand. *Daily Telegraph*, 6 August. <www.telegraph.co.uk/news/worldnews/australiaandthepacific/australia/11015898/Surrogacy-case-the-history-of-sex-offences-of-the-Australian-accused-of-leaving-surrogate-baby-in-Thailand.html>

Ross T (2010) Surrogacy couple: paying American woman was our last chance for a child.

Smerdon UR (2013) India. In: Trimmings K and Beaumont P (eds) *International Surrogacy Arrangements: Legal Regulation at the International Level*. Oxford: Hart Publishing, pp. 187–218.

Topping A and Foster B (2014) International surrogacy laws in the spotlight amid row over baby Gammy. *Guardian*, 4 August. <http://www.theguardian.com/world/2014/aug/global-surrogacy-laws-deate-baby-gammy-thailand>

Trimmings K and Beaumont P (eds) (2013) *International Surrogacy Arrangements: Legal Regulation at the International Level*. Oxford: Hart Publishing.

van Wichelen S (2014) What chance for international surrogacy laws? *The Drum TV ABC*, 20 August. <www.abc.net.au/news/2014-08-21/van-whichelen-what-chance-forinternational-surrogacy-laws>

11 | TRANSNATIONAL THIRD-PARTY ASSISTED CONCEPTION: PURSUING THE DESIRE FOR 'ORIGINS' INFORMATION IN THE INTERNET ERA

Deborah Dempsey and Fiona Kelly

Much of the growing transnational market in third-party assisted conception (including gestational surrogacy, donor sperm and ova) occurs under conditions in which gamete donors and surrogates are anonymous. Countries allowing payment for clinical assisted reproductive technology (ART) also tend to either mandate or allow donor and surrogate anonymity without identity registration (e.g. the US, Greece, Spain and the Czech Republic). Counter to these trends, it is likely that some children born of transnational ART and their parents will be very interested in knowledge of the gamete donors and surrogates who contributed to their conception and birth, and will be motivated to go to considerable lengths to find out who they are (e.g. Beeson *et al.*, 2011; Rodino *et al.*, 2011). In this chapter, we argue that donor offspring and their parents increasingly have available to them informal, web-based avenues of communication in the quest to obtain knowledge about the third parties who have assisted their conception. It is also feasible to expect that interest in knowledge of genetic and gestational origins will remain high given recent developments in the marketing and uptake of genetic and communication technologies. This makes it imperative for reproductive medicine clinics worldwide to reconsider their policies about privacy and identity registration for third parties involved in assisted conception, and for legislators globally to consider how informal mechanisms interact with formal legislative regimes governing identity registration.

Introduction

In *Distant Love*, Ulrich Beck and Elisabeth Beck-Gernsheim (2014: 165) pose this compelling question about families created through transnational ART:

Can we conceive of a society in which people stop inquiring into the identity of their biological father, their biological mother, and the place and country in which they were born, so that the quest for identity and the sense of belonging can be pursued along quite different paths?

In light of rapid advances in genetic technologies, as well as web-based means for identifying and making contact with 'anonymous' gamete donors, the answer to their question is more than likely to be 'no'.

As large numbers of couples or singles travel to form families through ART, a transnational market in gametes and gestational services flourishes. Many children are now conceived with the cooperation of egg or sperm donors and/or gestational surrogates who are anonymous and geographically dispersed. At the same time as this transnational ART market gains momentum, genetic connections are increasingly understood by many to be constitutive of familial identities. In no arena of social life is this trend demonstrated more starkly than in changing attitudes towards donor conception.

Donor conception was historically shrouded in secrecy and heterosexual couples were encouraged to forget about it and not tell their children. However, it is increasingly accepted in the international literature that, while not all donor-conceived people would find information about their sperm or egg donor necessary, meaningful or useful, 'the state, in its stewardship role, has a duty to ensure that information is available for those who might feel an interest in or need for it' (Nuffield Council on Bioethics, 2013: 123). Furthermore, the internet offers today's recipients and offspring of donor gametes and gestational services many ways to seek and find information, as well as organize themselves into communities of connection and support.

In this chapter, we argue that we can expect interest in knowledge of genetic and gestational origins to remain strong among children born of transnational ART, given developments in various internet-based genetic and communication technologies. These include the marketing of DNA paternity testing and genetic genealogy, the creation of donor sibling registers and the opportunities afforded by photographic 'detective work', software and social media. These means of donor tracing raise questions about the extent to which permanent privacy or anonymity can feasibly be promised to sperm and egg donors, at the same time as use of anonymous third-party assisted conception remains the norm in most parts of the world. It is imperative to encourage reproductive medicine clinics in countries where anonymity remains legal to reconsider their promises of privacy along with their identity registration processes.

First, we outline the various ways in which anonymous third-party assisted conception is used globally. Then we consider how this runs counter to trends in some countries that have, in recent years, introduced legislation mandating identity registration for gamete donors and gestational surrogates. We then situate this increasing emphasis on biogenetic origins information for donor-conceived young people and adults in the context of other developments in genetic and information technologies. Finally, we consider some of ways in which donor-conceived adults and their parents are using the internet to form communities of support, along with the privacy and identity registration issues likely to confront clinics and policy-makers globally in the near future.

The internet now provides a highly successful means for prospective gay and heterosexual parents to research family formation through ART without necessary recourse to medical practitioners at home. Brokerage agencies with global reach provide 'one stop shop' web portals to reproductive travel. Services tailored to the gay communities are a lucrative niche market. Many couples and single adults of diverse sexualities and fertility needs travel to use ART services abroad because these offer them a way to have children not available in their home countries.

For instance, in Australia, clinical compensated surrogacy is forbidden, there are legal restrictions on advertising for surrogates, egg or sperm donors, and women giving birth to children cannot easily contract away their parental rights. For these reasons, and also due to the lower costs associated with fertility treatment in some countries, heterosexual and gay prospective parents are known to travel to countries such as Greece, Mexico and Nepal (previously India and Thailand until legislative change in those countries restricted access) in order to have children. Although it is not a low-cost option, travelling to the US to use commercial surrogacy and donor gametes remains popular because of the favourable legislative regime for commissioning parents and clinical infrastructure in states such as California.

Transnational third-party assisted conception includes gestational surrogacy, ova and sperm donation. Some prospective parents travel for both gestational surrogacy and gamete donation, whereas others only require gametes, particularly donor eggs. During the years 2010 to 2011, there were 394 babies born to Australian gay and heterosexual parents in India alone (most likely to have been born through commercial surrogacy)[1] whereas only sixty were born within Australia through altruistic surrogacy (Millbank 2015). Increasingly, Australian women who cannot conceive using their own eggs are travelling to source donor eggs. According to Australian newspaper the *Sydney Morning Herald*, one fertility specialist in Sydney in 2014 advised more than ninety couples and single women requiring egg donors to travel overseas (Smith, 2014).

Rules and regulations

In most countries that allow compensated surrogacy and gamete donation, laws and policies also support anonymity for donors and a lack of requirements about identity registration. For instance, women from Australia and the UK, where anonymity has now been banned, travel to Greece and Spain for egg donation, where anonymity is permitted. Websites advertising clinical ART services in Thailand, and more recently Mexico, Greece and Spain, have at various times actively promoted the fact that gamete donors can remain permanently anonymous, as an attractive feature of using ART in their countries (see Whittaker and Speier, 2010). Websites advertising fertility treatment in Europe promote donor anonymity as a benefit linked to greater choice of donors and no waiting times. Choice of donors is highly valued so prospective parents can match their own traits to those of the donor, in the event that they want children to 'pass' as their genetic offspring. Time is often a consideration for prospective parents who have been trying to have children for many years unsuccessfully or are struggling with age-related infertility. Some prospective parents are also known to prefer the idea of anonymous gamete donors and no identity-registration for gamete donors or surrogates due to less likelihood of future 'intrusion' into their nuclear or single-parent family unit (see Whittaker and Speier, 2010).

Counter to this anonymity trend, in an increasing number of jurisdictions legislators and policy-makers are arguing for compulsory identity registration of surrogates and egg and sperm donors, along with mechanisms that would enable children born of third-party assisted conception or their donors to have contact in the future. Many donor-conceived adults and young people indicate that they should have a right to knowledge about their genetic and biographical history (e.g. Rodino *et al.*, 2011) and some scholars go as far as to insist that the practice of anonymous gamete donation should be banned (e.g. Allan, 2011). Such is the persuasiveness now of the idea that knowledge of biogenetic origins is a human right and formative of identity, the recording of identifying information about gamete donors is mandatory in a number of countries. These include Australia, Sweden, Norway, Austria, Switzerland, the Netherlands and the UK.

Parents of donor-conceived children in countries that mandate 'identity-release' are very much encouraged to tell their children they are donor conceived, and numerous resources for the parents of donor-conceived children are available to help with providing this information in an age and family-type appropriate way. For instance, in Victoria, Australia, the Victorian Assisted Reproductive Treatment Authority (VARTA) has produced videos and downloadable publications, and runs regular 'Time to tell' public events for parents of children who are donor-conceived. Among lesbians and gay men using sperm donation, egg donation or gestational surrogacy to form families, the absence of a social father or mother in the immediate family encourages openness with children from an early age. Disclosure rates to children among heterosexual parents are known to be increasing and this is true of those who have used donor sperm and/or donor eggs (see Blake *et al.*, 2010; Blyth *et al.*, 2013).

A key policy response to concerns about the well-being of donor-conceived children and adults has also been the emergence of donor linking. This is the process whereby donor-conceived people, donors and/or recipient parents gain access to identifying and non-identifying information, including health information, about each other. Support for donor linking in Australia is facilitated by the decision of three state governments to introduce legislation that permits access to a donor's identity for those conceived after the date of legislative commencement.

In our home state, Victoria, Australia, the right to access identifying information about gamete donors, until recently, depended on the year in which you were born. If you were a donor-conceived person born after 1998, you could get identifying information about your sperm or egg donor because they had been required to consent to identity release when they donated. If you were born between 1988 and 1997 you could also access information provided your donor agreed. However, all donations made pre-1988 were made on the condition of anonymity. The best you could do was to put your name on a voluntary register and hope that your donor did the same (Hammarberg *et al.*, 2014). However, in 2014, Victoria amended its legislation so that donor-conceived people conceived prior to 1988 could access their previously anonymous donor's identity if the donor consented. On the day this legislation came into force, the Victoria government announced further proposed amendments, stating that it intended to retrospectively open all of Victoria's sperm donor records so that donor-conceived people could obtain the name and date of birth of their donor, *regardless* of the donor's consent. Contact vetoes, which can be used to indicate that contact is not wanted or to specify the type of contact the party is comfortable with, have been proposed as a way of ensuring that knowledge does not result in unwanted intrusions into the lives of donors or donor-conceived people (Kelly and Dempsey, 2015). Debate about this controversial issue continues at the time of writing.

These more recent legal and policy developments in Victoria were in part influenced by the tragic story of Narelle Grech, a young woman who campaigned for many years for the rights of donor-conceived people in Australia. Narelle was born in Victoria prior to 1988 and therefore subject to a law preventing her from gaining access to information about her sperm donor. She spent fifteen years searching for her donor, a quest that became more urgent when she was diagnosed several years ago with terminal cancer. It was reported in the media that her cancer was a rare genetic form and that, had she known about the family history, more could have been done about early diagnosis and preventive treatment. Narelle's situation influenced the former Premier of Victoria, Ted Baillieu, to intervene and enable release of information that enabled her to identify, contact and meet her donor before she died at the age of 30. However, for the vast majority of pre-1988 donor-conceived Australians legal impediments to accessing this information remain.

Narelle's story exemplifies the health and identity issues that can be at stake for some donor-conceived young people and adults. Since the mapping of the human genome and growing sophistication of genetic testing, beliefs have intensified about the importance of knowledge of one's genetic inheritance. As biomedical science continues to propose and provide the public with evidence that genetic histories hold the key to predicting an individual's future health and well-being, it becomes harder to ignore that knowing as much as possible about a child's biogenetic make-up is a responsible decision made in the interests of that child's future health. That said, many sociologists and anthropologists of health and illness have also pointed out that the genetic basis for many cancers and other serious illnesses beyond known single gene disorders is rare and complex, and knowledge of family history cannot always facilitate a straightforward preventive solution. However, what

Narelle's situation highlighted was the persuasiveness of the idea for many people that our genetic make-up intrinsically connects us to those who share our substantive constitution.

Harnessing the power of the internet

Although some may criticize the dissemination and uptake of genetic technologies for increasingly medicalizing familial identities, according to Carlos Novas and Nikolas Rose (2000), they also facilitate new means of engaged identity-seeking and citizenship, particularly in the internet era. In the words of these authors, consumers of genetic technologies have available to them ever-increasing 'life strategies' and the obligation to 'calculate choices in a complex interpersonal field' (2000: 488). The creative 'detective work' that donor-conceived young people and adults can engage in as a result of the existence of the internet marketing of genetic technologies and the rise of parent-initiated web-based registers for donor-conceived people are good examples of these tendencies. Many recipients and offspring of donor conception are not proving passively resigned to their fate. As communication and genetic technologies become more sophisticated, they demonstrate ingenuity and creativity in subverting the clinical policies of the past. Donor offspring and their parents increasingly have available to them a range of informal channels in the quest to obtain knowledge about the third parties who have assisted their conception. Here, we use 'informal' to mean avenues beyond identity registration mandated by legislation or required by fertility clinic accreditation policies.

For instance, various companies now promote the use of direct-to-consumer genetic testing via the internet. For relatively small fees, it is possible to send DNA samples through the mail to anywhere in the world and receive in return a comprehensive analysis of maternal or paternal DNA. Some donor-conceived adults are taking steps to utilize these technologies in order to find out information about their donors or even meet them.

As long ago as 2005, the *Guardian* newspaper reported that a 15-year-old boy had tracked down his anonymous sperm donor by sending a swab taken from the inside of his cheek for genetic testing (Sample, 2005). The boy sent his sample to an online genealogy DNA-testing service called Family Tree DNA.com. For the US$289 (£163) testing and registration fee, he was able to make his genetic code available to other site members. Although the boy's genetic father was not registered, the boy was later contacted by two men on the database whose Y-chromosome was a match. These two men were strangers but had the same surname and the genetic similarity of their Y-chromosomes suggested there was a 50 per cent chance that the two men and the boy had the same father, grandfather or great-grandfather. Using this surname, together with information supplied by his mother about the sperm donor's date and place of birth, the boy then turned to another website, Omnitrace.com, which exists to this day and now explicitly markets its services as follows: 'Find Your Birth Parents, Siblings or Adopted Child Fast. We will amaze you!' From this site, he bought information on everyone born in the same place and on the same date as his father. Within ten days he had found a surname match and made contact with his genetic father. Since this time, FamilyTreeDNA and other popular genetic genealogy sites such as 23 and Me have begun actively marketing their services to adopted people and children conceived using donated gametes, featuring videotaped stories of customers searching and finding each other on their websites.

Photographs have also proved to be useful in identifying donors. When donor gametes are sourced from a clinic, there is often a photograph of the donor accompanying his or her profile to assist prospective parents with their choice. It is well known that some prospective parents like to match their own physical characteristics to those of the donor, in order that any children born may more easily 'pass' as their genetic children. Furthermore, some clients are very interested in getting a sense of what the donor is like as a person and the photograph, together with a biographical profile, can provide clues to personality, values and personal style. Extensive profiles and photographs are indeed an attractive web-based marketing tool in countries such as the US and Israel where they are allowed.

In our 'in progress' interview study with single mothers by choice who conceived through use of donor sperm, we have been struck by some women's curiosity about their children's donors and desire to contact them, usually 'just in case' their children happen to express interest. One woman told of how she and another mother who had used the same donor found out the identity of their children's donor through the photograph and donor profile supplied by the sperm bank. In the photo, he was wearing the distinctive uniform of his college sports team. Using the information gleaned from the photograph and other information contained in the donor's profile, the two mothers were easily able to identify the donor through web searches. Though the women have decided not to contact the donor, they were able to access his Facebook profile and print information, including additional photographs, for their children.

As Rosanna Hertz and Jane Mattes (2011) have observed, sperm banks could not have foreseen the possibility that children conceived through sperm from the same donor would find each other through use of the internet. In lieu of access to information about anonymous donors, so-called 'donor siblings', or children who are genetically related through an egg or sperm donor, are becoming linked through websites set up for this purpose. The largest of these is the Donor Sibling Registry (DSR) based in the US. The DSR was created in 2000 by Wendy Kramer and her son Ryan. To quote from the website's home page:

> Certain that other donor offspring would have the same curiosity as Ryan about his genetic origins – yet also knowing that sadly, no public outlet existed for mutual consent contact between people born from anonymous sperm donation – this site was started as the logical next step to making those connections.

In addition to the 47,000 registered members of the DSR, thousands of people check the site, which claims to have 12,000 unique visitors each month.

The DSR enables people to register themselves as recipients or offspring conceived from clinics around the world based on the unique identifier the donor was known by at the clinic. For example, a single mother by choice can look up her child's donor number and find out whether there are any genetic siblings born through use of the same donor's sperm. It is well known that many clinics around the world do not keep accurate records about the number of live births attributed to individual donors, making the DSR one of the few reasonably reliable resources for information about donor siblings. The Register has linked more than 12,600 individuals with donor relatives in more than thirty countries. In some instances, previously anonymous donors have also begun to join these registers and make contact with recipients and offspring.

To date, the research on donor sibling relationships formed through these web-based registries is sparse, but it is beginning to be published. In 2009, Freeman and colleagues surveyed 791 parents who had joined the DSR and asked them about their motivations for searching, the kind of contact they sought and their experiences of contacting donor siblings. One hundred-and-thirty-six of these parents had met their children's donor siblings and introduced the children to each other. Although Freeman *et al.* did not interview the children, their parents reported that the interactions were largely positive and that they often referred to each other as brothers and sisters. The relationship status and gender of the parents also seems to be relevant, in that single mothers and lesbian couples appeared more likely to initiate donor sibling searches than heterosexual couples. Jadva and colleagues (2010) surveyed 165 donor-conceived young people, also contacted through the DSR. They found that about a third of these young people had found donor siblings on the Registry and that 95 per cent of those who had found siblings had also contacted them. Of those who found siblings 50 per cent were in contact with them at least once a month and most found the experience 'very positive'.

In 2011, Hertz and Mattes published exploratory research with parents registering on the DSR site and Hertz *et al.* (2016) followed up with a study of how parents and donor-conceived young people form relationships with donor siblings. In the earlier study, Hertz and Mattes found that for a growing number of unrelated parents who have biogenetically related children, the site offers a range of meaningful ways for them to connect and interact. Of the parents who had searched for donor siblings 84 per cent had found at least one other family who shared the same donor. For some of the parents registering on their children's behalf, the information they obtained served as a kind of 'insurance policy' in the event of future questioning about the donor by their children. Parents who found other parents with children from the same donor were organizing into what the authors called 'clans', in the sense that they kept in touch, monitored each other and shared photographs and health information, without necessarily forming emotional attachments or close social ties. There was particular interest in tracing family resemblances through photographs. For other parents who found each other through the site, the connections were taken 'offline' and became meaningful social relationships. Whereas 74 per cent of parents had made contact with their children's donor siblings in the earlier study, this increased to 91 per cent in the Hertz *et al.* study.

The authors of both studies found compelling evidence that parents and donor-conceived young people who trace donor siblings through these sites are highly motivated to communicate with them. Exchange of emails, photographs and telephone calls remain the most popular ways to keep in touch, with social media connections through Facebook becoming more important since the earlier study. Parents and donor-conceived young people who form relationships with donor siblings often view them as equivalent to 'extended family' with all the nuances of meaning that that term entails when applied to family of origin (Hertz et al., 2016: 28):

> Less than a fifth say that they are equally involved with all families, and although proximity and size of group are clearly factors limiting involvement, so too are shared likenesses and simple compatibility. As is the case for relationships with one's blood/legal family, intimacy and ongoing contact emerge unequally within the [donor sibling] group ... But everyone might keep track of the entire kinship group on Facebook, noting important events as they occur, and maintaining latent ties that can be called on if and when needed.

Concluding thoughts

At the same time as increasing numbers of prospective parents internationally are availing themselves of transnational ART using anonymous gamete donors or gestational surrogates, large numbers of people born through third-party assisted conception are using DNA-based detective work, online donor registries and social media to find their donors and connect with donor siblings. In years to come, developments in internet-disseminated technologies such as face recognition software and programmes that predict what a young person will look like as they age may also be harnessed to the cause of assisting young people in finding out information about the gamete donors and gestational surrogates who contributed to their conception and birth.

The affordances of genetic and communication technologies, coupled with the resourcefulness of those who use them, serve to raise questions about the extent to which clinics will be able to fulfil promises of privacy to gamete donors and surrogates in the future. According to Rene Almeling in *Sex Cells* (2011), an ethnographic study of egg and sperm donation in the US, most egg and sperm donors are not opposed to the idea of having their identity known when asked, but taking steps to ensure this can occur is not the emphasis or focus of the clinical counsellors. More recently, Julia Woodward (2015) points out that many donors to clinics in the US assume that the information they give in an anonymous donor programme is actually shared with the recipients of their gametes. She speculates that the younger donors of today, due to their participation in social media, may have a different understanding of privacy and feel more comfortable with the idea that there are limits to anonymity. Nonetheless, it seems imperative that pre-education for donors and surrogates should include information about the limits to their privacy in the internet era.

Almeling (2011: 172) makes the point that much more needs to be known about the interactional dynamics in gamete markets: 'of how subtle and not so subtle differences of framing the exchange influence how each party relates to the transaction'. The insight of this work is that transactions involve complex choreographies of market and social relations, of exchanges between clients, clinicians and donors that are malleable and open to change. We clearly need more ethnographic work globally, in jurisdictions that mandate or encourage anonymity, in order to uncover the challenges and opportunities for doing this kind of work, particularly in the newer markets in less developed countries. This may generate new and inventive ways to promote identity registration to all involved in third-party assisted conception transactions.

Fertility clinics in countries that currently permit or mandate anonymity could clearly do more to ensure that their records were maintained in such a way so as to support future interest in health and identity information about donors and surrogates. Even in the absence of 'identity-release' laws and policies, they could ensure they keep the kinds of records that assume information-seeking could occur at any time in the life course of a person born of third-party assisted conception. Such record-keeping would enable recipient parents and their children to identify themselves in the future as donor or surrogate linked, e.g. by ensuring that a unique identifier is provided for every donor or surrogate. This identifier should also be known by the gamete donor or surrogate to ensure they also have a means of connecting with offspring through online registers or similar in the future.

In the case of children born from commercial surrogacy in countries such as India that do not support identity registration for egg donors or surrogates, we know very little about the relative importance children may attribute to the 'biogenetic relationship' with the egg donor as opposed to the 'gestational relationship' with the surrogate. It is highly likely that some children will desire information about egg donors and surrogates. Deborah Dempsey, in her research with Australian gay men forming families through commercial surrogacy, has found that the men often downplay the significance to children of the anonymous egg donor in favour of putting their energies into maintaining an ongoing connection with the surrogate and her family

(Dempsey, 2013, 2015). The assumption here is that it is pregnancy and birth that constitutes the more important 'origins information' for children. It remains to be seen if the children will feel the same way. In the future, we may see clients of commercial surrogacy agencies in countries such as India, Thailand and Mexico joining the DSR and similar registers. They may also lobby the clinics that assisted them to set up their own registers and help the children they created to find the information they seek.

In making our case in this chapter, and to again pick up the question posed by Beck and Beck-Gernsheim (2014) in the introduction, we are certainly not arguing that it is intrinsically harmful to children to find out that, in addition to the love and will of their parents, their creation involved a sperm donor from the Ukraine, an egg donor from Spain and the reproductive labour of an Indian surrogate. What is hard to imagine, given the evidence, is that many children won't at least be curious about the people who contributed to their creation and view the circumstances of their conception and gestation as an important part of their heritage. We owe it to these future generations to make it as easy as possible to trace this heritage through the manner in which we encourage this global market to develop, and also pre-empt the privacy issues that may arise for those who donate anonymously, in good faith. To emphasize this is not to fetishize the genetic or gestational connection above and beyond the social ties of parenthood. Rather, it serves to acknowledge that these connections are meaningful and resonant to many people born of third-party assisted conception and likely to continue to be so in the future.

Note

1 These numbers were calculated based on applications for citizenship and passports rather than confirmed births from surrogacy arrangements.

References

Allan S (2011) Psycho-social, ethical and legal arguments for and against the retrospective release of information about donors to donor-conceived individuals in Australia. *Journal of Law & Medicine* 19(2): 354–76.

Almeling R (2011) *Sex Cells: The Medical Market for Eggs and Sperm*. Berkeley, CA: University of California Press.

Beck U and Beck-Gernsheim E (2014) *Distant Love*. Cambridge: Polity Press.

Beeson D, Jennings P and Kramer W (2011) Offspring searching for their sperm donors: how family type shapes the process. *Human Reproduction* 26(9): 2415–24.

Blake L, Casey P, Readings J, Jadva V and Golombok S (2010) 'Daddy ran out of tadpoles': how parents tell their children that they are donor conceived, and what their 7-year-olds understand. *Human Reproduction* 25(10): 2527–34.

Blyth E, Kramer W and Schneider J (2013) Perspectives, experiences and choices of parents of children conceived following oocyte donation. *Reproductive BioMedicine Online* 26(2): 179–88.

Dempsey D (2013) Surrogacy, gay male couples and the significance of biogenetic paternity. *New Genetics and Society* 32(1): 37–53.

Dempsey D (2015) Relating across international borders: gay men forming families through overseas surrogacy. In: Inhorn M, Chavkin W and Navarro J (eds) *Globalized Fatherhoods*. New York and Oxford: Berghahn Books, Chapter 11.

Freeman T, Jadva V, Kramer W and Golombok S (2009) Gamete donation: parents' experiences of searching for their child's donor siblings and donor. *Human Reproduction* 24(3): 505–16.

Hammarberg K, Johnson L, Bourne K, Fisher J and Kirkman M (2014) Proposed legislative change mandating retrospective release of identifying information consultation with donors and government response. *Human Reproduction* 29(2): 286–92.

Hertz R and Mattes J (2011) Donor-shared siblings or genetic strangers: new families, clans, and the internet. *Journal of Family Issues* 32(9): 1129–55.

Hertz R, Nelson MK and Kramer W (2016) Donor sibling networks as a vehicle of expanding kinship: a replication and extension. *Journal of Family Issues*. doi: <10.1177/0192513X16631018>

Jadva V, Freeman T, Kramer W and Golombok S (2010) Experiences of offspring searching for and contacting their donor siblings and donor. *Reproductive BioMedicine Online* 20(4): 523–32.

Kelly F and Dempsey D (2015) The retrospective opening of Victoria's sperm donor records: do contact vetoes work? *The Conversation*, 9 December. <http://theconversation.com/as-victoria-opens-sperm-donor-records-the-key-question-is-do-contact-vetoes-work-51906>

Millbank J (2015) Rethinking 'commercial' surrogacy in Australia. *Journal of Bioethical Inquiry* 12(3): 477–90.

Novas C and Rose N (2000) Genetic risk and the birth of the somatic individual. *Economy and Society* 29(4): 485–513.

Nuffield Council on Bioethics (2013) *Donor Conception: Ethical Aspects of Information Sharing*. London: Nuffield Council. <http://nuffieldbioethics.org/wp-content/uploads/2014/06/Donor_conception_report_2013.pdf>

Rodino IP, Burton J and Sanders KA (2011) Donor information considered important to donors, recipients and offspring: an Australian perspective. *Reproductive BioMedicine Online* 22(3): 303–11.

Sample I (2005) Teenager finds sperm donor dad on internet. *Guardian*, 3 November. <http://www.theguardian.com/science/2005/nov/03/genetics.news>

Smith A (2014) Older women turning to Europe for affordable IVF. *Sydney Morning Herald*, 23 March. <http://www.smh.com.au/national/older-women-turning-to-europe-for-affordable-ivf-20140322-35adx.html>

Whittaker A and Speier A (2010) 'Cycling overseas': care, commodification, and stratification in cross-border reproductive travel. *Medical Anthropology* 29(4): 363–83.

Woodward JT (2015) Third-party reproduction in the internet age: the new patient-centred landscape. *Fertility and Sterility* 104(3): 525–30.

PART FOUR

FEMINIST RESPONSES AROUND THE WORLD

12 | FREQUENTLY *UNASKED* QUESTIONS: UNDERSTANDING AND RESPONDING TO GAPS IN PUBLIC KNOWLEDGE OF INTERNATIONAL SURROGACY PRACTICES WORLDWIDE

Ayesha Chatterjee and Sally Whelan
(Our Bodies Ourselves)

Assisted reproduction in an unregulated global market

A revolution in human reproduction is now here, and it presents unprecedented opportunities in family formation for many, including people with infertility, those in the LGBTQ community and individuals who are single by choice or circumstance. For others, particularly women who provide services in contractual third-party reproduction – as surrogates (or gestational mothers) and egg providers – this far-reaching and innovative era poses historically unparalleled risks and new global inequities.

Commercial surrogacy uses a range of assisted reproductive technologies (ARTs) and is a fast-growing transnational practice, with mediated contracts between people considering commercial surrogacy (intended parents) in one country who hire gestational mothers in another. For some intended parents, these arrangements represent a singular pathway to genetic parenthood; for others, they are reasonably priced alternatives to more expensive options in their home countries. For all, however, gestational mothers represent a lifeline – as women they can pay to gestate, birth and relinquish babies.

Transnational commercial surrogacy agreements tend to neglect the needs of gestational mothers beyond those which directly affect her ability to carry and birth a healthy baby. Instead, they favour intended parents and the different intermediaries that facilitate or broker the practice. These intermediaries include fertility clinics and recruiting agents and, increasingly, businesses related to travel, tourism, law and immigration, all of which prioritize the convenience and experience of intended parents who seek out and pay for their services.

The swell in transnational commercial surrogacy in hubs such as India and Nepal has been encouraged by a set of attractive factors.[1] These countries have open economies that welcome the influx of consumers and capital. Until recently, they offered unfettered access to an abundant pool of women who have few other ways to earn money. They seemed to lack the political will to regulate a prized source of national revenue, perhaps relying on the stigmatization of gestational mothers to drive women and their families to silence and the practice itself off public radar.

India is one example. Medical tourism drives a significant part of the economy and commercial surrogacy has been legal since 2002. By some estimates, surrogacy services in the country account for 25 per cent of a roughly US$2 billion industry in medical tourism (Goodwin, 2015). The Indian Society for Assisted Reproduction has claimed that more than 600 IVF clinics in the country provide an estimated 60,000 assisted reproductive treatments a year (Lal, 2012). Others declare there are no official figures on how large the fertility industry is in India, but they cite a 2012 UN-backed study that estimates the surrogacy business at more than US$400 million a year (Bhalla and Thapliyal, 2013), with a speculated growth of 17 to 20 per cent annually (*Economic Times*, 2015). Regardless of which estimate is cited, it is important to note that much of the demand originates in North America, Australia and Europe. The reason for this is straightforward. According to researchers and women's organizations on the ground, India's advanced – but inexpensive – medical facilities and fertility services, weak regulatory oversight, along with poor social and economic mobility among women who serve as 'surrogates', make the country an attractive hub and, for the global community, a cautionary tale. Yet, regulation has been fraught, with a 2010 ART bill stuck in a 'legislative log jam' and amendments – such as a proposal to ban *only* non-resident Indians and foreigners from hiring Indian gestational mothers – that largely failed to address social inequalities and human rights violations within the practice. In 2016, India banned all commercial surrogacy and now allows only altruistic arrangements with caveats.

As global demand rises, these poorly regulated hubs are venues of aggressive recruitment to ensure a steady stream of cost-effective 'supply'. However, as we note earlier, while transnational commercial surrogacy is a financial opportunity for most gestational mothers, these contractual arrangements are seldom transparent in either intent or implications; and, due to language barriers, many gestational mothers are often unable to consent in an informed manner to the conditions of their participation. As a result, they face a number of health risks and restrictions, which most fertility clinics and agents routinely downplay or disregard while, at the same time, denying gestational mothers health, legal and financial protections. Organizations such as Sama, an Indian health resource group at the forefront of research and activism on surrogacy, as well as other groups and individual researchers, have documented many risky practices and violations. For example:

- contracts that many cannot read and that undermine 'informed' consent
- coercive and other unethical recruitment tactics
- minimal compensation and unfair payment schedules
- dearth of information on health risks associated with gestational surrogacy
- dormitory-style living arrangements with constant monitoring
- restricted movement outside the surrogacy 'residence'
- forced seclusion from family, including children
- high doses of hormones for embryo transfer
- mandated and medically unnecessary caesarean sections
- no independent ability to terminate or continue a pregnancy
- increased risks of pregnancy and birth with multiples
- forced 'reductions' (abortion of one or more fetuses) in cases of multiple pregnancy
- minimal postpartum follow-up, even in cases of unexpected birth outcomes and trauma
- restricted access to independent medical care and/or legal aid
- no independent legal representation, life or disability insurance.

While gestational mothers are uniquely harmed by the unsound practices listed above, and have limited safety nets and avenues of recourse, they are not alone in facing risks. At the other end, there are accounts of intended parents being duped by fertility clinics and recruiting agents; and, in the absence of long-term safety data, growing anecdotal evidence of harm to egg providers, a group in growing demand due to a preference for gestational (over traditional) surrogacy. This includes known side-effects of hormones and procedures used to increase and retrieve eggs – a painful condition called ovarian hyperstimulation syndrome (OHSS) that makes the ovaries swell up and the body retain massive amounts of fluid, as well as cramping, bleeding and infection from surgical extraction.

Beyond individual egg providers, as the demand for specific types of babies increases so has aggressive marketing and compensation to women with specific types of human gametes (eggs) thought to carry desired genetic characteristics. This competitive playing field has opened doors for, and tacit acceptance of, eugenically driven options reflected, for example, in the recruitment of blonde and blue-eyed egg providers in Eastern Europe and young women at prestigious US universities for their 'Ivy league' eggs.

Finally, there is also growing concern for the welfare of the children born within these arrangements. These relate to their health (the most obvious due to multiple births and preterm delivery), legal status (due to a global patchwork of laws on parentage and citizenship) and fears around abandonment and abuse. As related cases come under scrutiny, transnational commercial surrogacy has become a major concern of international bodies such as The Hague Conference's Permanent Bureau. In fact, safeguarding the rights of children was one of the original impetuses for the body's consideration of a Hague Convention on global surrogacy (HCCH, 2014a, 2014b).

Despite the risks, the implications of the practice and the revolution in human reproduction unfolding before us are largely under the public's radar and absent from civil society discourse. There are various reasons for this: issues surrounding ARTs, clinical practices in fertility and new contractual arrangements in childbearing receive inadequate coverage in the news media; they occur largely in the private sector, where there is insufficient conflict-free oversight from public and peer-based institutions; and they travel fluidly across geographic borders to find receptive hubs in lucrative and minimally regulated markets.

Given this scenario, it is not surprising that increasing numbers of women are becoming involved in contractual third-party reproduction, from gestational mothers in resource-poor communities across South Asia and Central America to educated young women in the US recruited for their 'superior' genes/eggs. The market for their services is global, largely unregulated and growing. It is failing them in its disregard of documented risks, evidence-based health information and human rights guarantees. Intended parents are not spared either; they are emotionally, financially and legally vulnerable as they scour the internet for information and negotiate a complex web of fertility clinics, recruiting agents, immigration offices and tourism touts. This leaves all of them – and us – in a dangerous vacuum, asking what we *know* and *need to know* about transnational third-party reproduction. Filling this vacuum is an imperative, with transparent information on risks, meaningful mechanisms of redress and increased participation and pressure from civil society for universally implemented best practices.

Digging deeper: transnational commercial surrogacy on the ground, in the media and online

Researchers, health advocates and concerned citizens around the world are beginning to respond to multi-dimensional questions raised by transnational commercial surrogacy. Our Bodies Ourselves (OBOS) and the Center for Genetics and Society (CGS) are members of this growing network. We have been looking at the 'big picture': the spectrum of information available to the public on transnational commercial surrogacy and the nature of this information, so we can identify the gaps and responsive strategies. With our domestic and global allies, we are making every effort to bring our observations and analysis to a broader civic community.

This exploration started unexpectedly in 2012 with OBOS's partners in Nepal and India. While they were focused on advocating on behalf of gestational mothers and raising awareness of health and human rights risks on the ground, we realized – and they confirmed – that a large segment of demand for gestational mothers seemed to originate in highly developed nations such as the US. This made us curious about three things: the information available to people considering or engaged in transnational commercial surrogacy (intended parents) about the gestational mothers they hire overseas; the sources of this information; and the level of awareness and action on the issue among our broader network of global partners.

In 2014, with support from the MacArthur and Appleton Foundations, OBOS and CGS launched a project to document and increase awareness about practices associated with transnational commercial surrogacy. A first priority was to understand the nature of current information and action on the practice. To do this, we conducted a two-pronged informal survey: the first included a group of women's organizations around the world, to assess awareness and action related to commercial surrogacy in their country; the second focused on a random selection of two types of information sources – news media outlets and websites of surrogacy agents that often serve as public gateways to information.

Our methodology of random selection on the second survey was intentional. We believe it reflected a process similar to that of a lay user interested in learning more about the issue and/or considering a transnational commercial surrogacy arrangement. Our findings have helped clarify the gaps in information available to users and provided guideposts and strategies for increasing awareness, dialogue and collaboration in this area. One such strategy is called Surrogacy360 discussed at the end of this chapter. This refers to a digital platform developed by OBOS and CGS that serves as an information clearinghouse, gathering in one place the information and analysis generated by researchers and advocates who have dug deeper still, so that intended parents and the wider public can easily find and grasp the complexity and current status of transnational commercial surrogacy.

On the ground: a survey of grassroots knowledge and response

We start with findings from a survey of global partners on local awareness and action related to commercial surrogacy. As background, OBOS facilitates an informal global network of women's organizations working on reproductive health and rights and partnering with us on culturally adapting the organization's signature book, *Our Bodies Ourselves* (Boston Women's Health Book Collective, 2011), for women and girls in their countries. One of our partners, the Women's Rehabilitation Centre (the Centre) in Nepal, published six booklets in Nepali based on *Our Bodies Ourselves* in 2008. The series focuses on sexuality and violence against women, as well as the politics of women's health and human rights, and serves as a vital educational and training tool throughout the country. While the Centre was already positioned as a national and international leader in sexual and reproductive health, collaborating with OBOS on this project was pivotal to bringing the emerging issue of transnational commercial surrogacy onto its radar.

In 2012, Sama Resource Group for Women and Health, OBOS and the Centre in Nepal organized a workshop on transnational commercial surrogacy for Nepal's countrywide network of Women Human Rights Defenders and sexual/reproductive health advocates. The goal was to understand and articulate the impact of the practice regionally and internally, for a country abutting the biggest hub in the global supply chain. With the Indian Parliament tightening regulation, the Centre and other women's and human rights advocates anticipated (rightly) cross-border movement of the industry and Nepal's lack of preparedness with a suitable response.

After the workshop, the Centre launched a timely initiative to bring transnational commercial surrogacy into public view. In 2013, the organization completed a situational analysis in the capital, Kathmandu, and along three border areas with India, feeding their findings into an outreach strategy that now spans rural communities and institutional providers. The fulcrum of this strategy is a series of thirty-six radio shows called *My Body, My Rights* on a popular radio station – a smart move in a country where the majority relies on radio for information and news, especially in rural areas where more than 80 per cent of the population resides.[2] Each show includes an interactive session with physicians who have rarely or never talked about assisted reproduction on a public forum, and the series has forced leading newspapers and media outlets in the country to pay attention to transnational commercial surrogacy.

In 2014, OBOS built on this public awareness initiative in South Asia with a survey of the entire global network of OBOS partners. Our goal this time was to gather their perceptions of ARTs, commercial surrogacy and egg retrieval for pay, as well as to identify any action initiatives that they may have undertaken and that could be built upon with network-wide involvement.

The dozen or so OBOS partners who responded to the survey represented Turkey, Senegal, Israel, Nepal, Serbia, Vietnam, Bulgaria, Armenia, Iran and Japan, in addition to a coalition in Latin America. Nearly all the respondents were aware of commercial surrogacy (in-country and transnational) and paid egg donation. They identified the internet and the news media as primary sources of information in their communities, followed by medical providers, and shared many of the health and human rights concerns articulated by OBOS, CGS and our allies. This ranged from the gap between evidence and public awareness to the different health risks, such as OHSS for egg providers, and the implications of premature and multiple births and lack of postpartum care for gestational mothers. Lack of legal oversight and protections was another common concern, together with broader human rights and ethical considerations, such as the commercialization of eggs and babies, the commodification of women's bodies, the economic inequalities between intended parents and gestational mothers, balancing access to fertility treatment with protecting women's human rights, and the exclusion of some – the gay community and single women – from access to new forms of family formation.

Some respondents pointed to the downside of access to reproductive technologies and had particular concerns, for example, pro-natalist government policies and social pressure to use ARTs in Bulgaria and Israel. In one instance, Senegal, there was dissonance between perception and evidence. The Senegalese respondent reported that transnational commercial surrogacy was not a concern in Africa, despite countries like Kenya and South Africa growing into international hubs and gestational mothers being paid as high as US$18,000, although the practice is 'shrouded in secrecy' (Okwemba, 2012). However, since the survey, this partner has planned steps to raise awareness among regional women's rights activists. A key driver in this push is Sama's (2013) film, *Can We See the Baby Bump Please?*, which is serving as an important conversation starter on the issue.

The survey also confirmed that local responses are already underway. OBOS partners in Vietnam and Canada, for example, are incorporating evidence-based content on ARTs and transnational commercial surrogacy into their Vietnamese and French cultural adaptations of *Our Bodies Ourselves*. Others are co-editing anthologies and contributing new research (India and Japan), documenting women's experiences (India and Bulgaria), guiding government legislative responses (India and Bulgaria) and building broad-based knowledge and women's advocacy networks (Vietnam, Canada and Israel).

In South Asia, the work of OBOS's partner in Nepal complements the work of Indian organizations like Sama (2012) and the Centre for Social Research (2010, 2012). Their investigations and related outreach provide helpful insight into the lives and motivations of gestational mothers. They confirm the role of poverty, lack of economic mobility and global market inequalities in the growth of transnational commercial surrogacy. They form indisputable links between these factors and a gestational mother's inability to negotiate transparency, competitive payment and fair work conditions, afford independent legal counsel and medical care, and neutralize social isolation and stigmatization. They unpack the defence of altruism – the oft-touted idea that gestational mothers are providing a selfless and compassionate service – along with the women-helping-women paradigm and the win-win slogan. They lay bare the medical process, treatment side-effects, lack of postpartum care and the emotional conundrum of relinquishing a baby (e.g. Pandey, 2016). They confirm a gestational mother's complete dependence on fertility clinics and agents, as well as on the money as her only viable option out of poverty.

Beyond South Asia, in Mexico, GIRE (Grupo de Información en Reproducción Elegida) is focused on gathering basic information about the conditions and extent of transnational commercial surrogacy in Tabasco, building awareness of the health and human rights risks to gestational mothers and advocating for federal and local policies that secure sustainable protections.

These organizations represent a growing body of evidence and activism, led by women's, human rights and social justice organizations positioned to document human rights violations associated with surrogacy. They are joined by other field researchers, including contributors to this book, who are building knowledge around the full range of the practice and people most affected by it; with ears to the ground, their collective perspectives are critical to framing the conversation and related outcomes.

Despite this growing body of knowledge, the public's ability to access evidence-based information seems limited. We believe this is partly due to the few and restricted spaces where reliable information can be found by lay communities, and partly to the biased and unbalanced information that inundates the vast majority of open community spaces off and online. This brings us to our second survey.

In the news media: a survey of trends in coverage

In the media: from news flashes to sustained coverage The first portion of our second survey comprised a random selection of news media reports on transnational commercial surrogacy. Thus far, the news media have played a major role in guiding individual and collective thinking on this issue via different pulpits: print, broadcast, digital and mobile. For organizations working on the ground, these media would ideally be a reliable channel that brings the documented violations to the public domain. Given this watchdog role, it seems worthwhile to take a look at their past and current engagement with transnational commercial surrogacy.

Some of the earliest news reports date back to 1985, when the 'Baby M' case in the US catapulted commercial surrogacy to centre stage, with eye-opening analysis on the role of social class in assisted reproduction. The furor seemed to abate in mainstream news media until 2006, despite the fact that the business of surrogacy had been growing steadily behind the scenes. That year, in an episode titled 'Journey to Parenthood', Oprah Winfrey blazed her spotlight on a US couple who travelled to a fertility clinic in the Indian city of Anand to commission a baby.[3] In minutes and in front of millions (the Oprah show is reportedly broadcast in 145 countries) America's favourite talk show host portrayed the arrangement as a 'win-win for everyone'. On an aside, Dr Nayna Patel, who runs the Akanksha Fertility Clinic in Anand and appeared on the Oprah Winfrey show in 2007, acknowledges charging intended parents an average of US$25,000 to US$30,000 but paying gestational mothers around US$6,500 (Vogt, 2014). According to this article, Patel plans to open a clinic to house hundreds of Indian women, delivery rooms, an IVF department, restaurants and a gift shop.

For years after Oprah's 'unveiling' of transnational commercial surrogacy, other US news outlets seemed to follow suit. From Fox News in 2007 to CNN and Huffington Post in 2013, these channels mostly emphasized the 'women helping women' paradigm and the experiences of (frequently celebrity) intended parents, along with images of gestational mothers living in close and comfortable camaraderie, and soundbites on the altruism embedded in transnational commercial surrogacy arrangements. References to the treatment of gestational mothers, if made, were in passing and with little analysis. Along with Oprah, they lost many early opportunities to broaden social discourse and help the public to understand the realities and risks faced by gestational mothers, children and intended parents. What they did do, and did well, was repackage the practice to make it palatable, hailing 'the new phenomenon of Americans going to India to hire surrogates on the cheap' as cultural ambassadorship and a 'warm and fuzzy example' of 'women helping women' (Brooks, 2007).

In our exploration of news media coverage, we asked whether there has been progress. Based on our sample of news reports, a provisional answer is 'yes' with a looming 'but'.

Inclusion of gestational mothers and children Human interest stories about intended parents in the news media have given long overdue visibility to issues traditionally associated with stigma and silence, focusing on those who have walked the slow and painful journey of infertility, or have faced legal barriers to parenting. However, in the attempt to provide this focus, the longing of childless people to have children seems to take centre stage to the exclusion of other stakeholders (Sloan and Lahl, 2014). Recently, some news outlets have delivered fuller coverage by focusing on all participants in surrogacy arrangements. They have finally also turned their attention to the question of where gestational mothers and children fit into the 'human interest' equation. This expanded perspective, though sporadic and largely triggered by specific events, suggests a readiness to stretch the conversation beyond celebrities and the 'women helping women' trope. It also underscores the news media's role as a watchdog that can corroborate the findings of researchers and advocates on the ground and bring these into mainstream conversation.

The BBC is a heartening example. Picking up from 2013, a *Hard Talk* interview with Nayna Patel dug relentlessly into the less ethical practices that have come to exemplify the transnational business in commercial surrogacy, including many of the violations cited in this chapter. Other articles have also examined, for example, the risks in multiple embryo transfers to gestational mothers and the living conditions and restrictions placed on them in countries like India. At the time of writing, there are countless more on the BBC website, most recently a feature on India's proposed legislation to ban commercial surrogacy for all foreigners (*BBC News*, 2015).

Another example of responsible coverage comes from the *New York Times*, which, in 2014, published a series of articles on transnational commercial surrogacy. While a few focused on the US as a destination for intended parents from countries with restrictive legislation, one (Haberman, 2014) provided useful historical insight into the practice, starting with the case of Baby M. This item was part of a series of documentary videos re-examining major news stories in the country from years past. Another featured Planet Hospital in Mexico, at one time a leading facilitator of transnational commercial surrogacy and now bankrupt and under investigation by the US Federal Bureau of Investigation, 'as a cautionary tale about the proliferation of unregulated surrogacy agencies, their lack of accountability and their ability to prey on vulnerable clients who want a baby so badly that they do not notice all the red flags' (Lewin, 2014). It included interviews with ex-employees who admitted agency-wide unsavoury practices such as non-payment of bills, unauthorized egg splitting and inappropriate or careless selection of gestational mothers. Other sources have since revealed that Planet Hospital paid bonuses to gestational mothers who agreed to be impregnated with sperm from HIV positive donors, and routinely subjected them to medically unnecessary caesarean section deliveries to accommodate convenient travel for intended parents.

Standards set by news media outlets like the BBC and the *New York Times* seem to have resonated with others including, for example, the *Guardian* (Tuckman, 2014) and National Public Radio in the US in 2014, and spilled over into 2015. Articles appeared in *Foreign Policy* (Drennan, 2015), *Huffington Post* (Goodwin, 2015) and Al Jazeera (Kumar, 2015), as well as follow-up pieces on the BBC[4] in response to recent developments in Thailand to address legislative gaps; others were precipitated by new crises, such as Israel's evacuation in quake-hit Nepal of babies commissioned by Israeli intended parents (Ilic, 2015; Kamin, 2015; also see Chapter 3).

The most groundbreaking, perhaps, has been the Home Box Office (HBO) series *VICE* (2015) in which the network's exposé of transnational commercial surrogacy in India tackles the issue head on (without fear of reprisal from advertisers or censors) and, given its capacity to reach a large audience, has opened new doors for non-mainstream news voices. In minutes, journalist Gianna Toboni delves deep into the underbelly of baby making and baby selling in the country, unearthing many of the risks described here. A recruiter is filmed searching, on commission, for potential gestational mothers while her employer, a physician, insists women are never pressed into participating. Toboni, undercover as a potential client, is offered – for a price – an 'extra' baby on the spot over dinner in a public café (see Ronan, 2015).[5]

Together with a growing attention on gestational mothers, the human rights of children born within transnational arrangements have also garnered focus. Driven perhaps by intended parents who have met cross-border legal obstacles, the news media now have impetus to understand how the unique circumstances of these babies' births can affect their citizenship, parentage and safety; and, in comparisons with adoption, their need in later life for a coherent birth narrative and open access to official records.

In 2014, in the wake of the Baby Gammy case,[6] Al Jazeera published articles on the legislative minefield around transnational commercial surrogacy (e.g. Ahmed, 2014). One piece carried interviews with Our Bodies Ourselves staff and allies. Another focused on families scammed by Planet Hospital and grew out of conversations between intended parents on parent and surrogacy blogs that had paid the agency vast sums of money and never seen their babies. In the same year, a popular TV news magazine in Australia, *60 Minutes*, published an eye-opening interview with Baby Gammy's intended parents. In it, the host delved deep into the intended father's history of child abuse and the legal/social factors that, despite a criminal record, enabled him to 'commission' a baby. The interview posed hard questions on the humanity and ethics of refusing babies who don't meet the expectations of intended parents.[7] Unfortunately, Baby Gammy was not the only spur for examining the inadequate vetting of intended parents. Another scandal around the same time involved a Japanese businessman who fathered sixteen children with various gestational mothers in Thailand over one year (Rawlinson, 2014).

This coverage suggests a pattern where scrutiny, though improved in quality and quantity, is still triggered by and clustered around precipitating events, rather than around global problem-solving or consideration of regulatory response to current practice. In the past, cases like Baby M in the US (1985) and Baby Manji in India (Points, 2009) resulted in blitzes; more recently, Baby Gammy served the same short-lived purpose, as did the unveiling of Planet Hospital's shameful practices in countries like India and Mexico and the response of the Israeli government in the aftermath of the Nepal earthquake. On the other hand, lacklustre interest in Thailand's rapid policy response (after and as a direct fallout of the Baby Gammy debacle) is telling of the news media's distractedness once the related human-interest, breaking stories are yesterday's news.

It is also clear that coverage has shifted slightly over time from the 'women helping women' paradigm to the ways in which the practice denies or neglects the health and rights of gestational mothers and children. However, given the news media's ability to inform, educate and engage the public on important and emerging issues, its stature begs that it pay more attention to a few things: first, sustainability, so its coverage can ignite something more than fleeting public attention around specific episodes; second, cross-pollination with less visible news sources that can freely report and critically examine the practice without fear of reprisal; and third, cross-sectoral discussions with researchers and activists who have the data and can speak to the issues on the ground and with those directly engaged in the practice. A recent article by the *New York Times* (Najar, 2015) is a perfect example, citing the expertise and opinions of organizations like Sama and the CSR on India's latest bid to ban surrogacy for all foreigners. We need more of this.

Online: sorting through the internet noise

The second portion of our survey involved a random selection of websites of recruiting agents that often serve as public gateways to information on surrogacy. Through this sample, we aimed to document some of the practices of key transnational providers of commercial surrogacy, following a methodology of random selection that we believe reflects a process similar to that of a lay user interested in learning more about the issue and/or considering a transnational arrangement.

The internet is the foremost platform for social interaction/commentary and the sale/purchase of goods and services. It is priceless to intended parents, who seek gestational mothers online, and the facilitators in between, as a pathway to potential intended parents and payments across socio-economic, linguistic, cultural and physical boundaries. Because the 'products' and 'services' transacted involve the use and exchange of human bodies, especially in a commercial context, accountability and reliability of information are paramount. The internet's dual role in growing the business of and educating the public on transnational commercial surrogacy makes it an important study in any effort to tip the scales in the direction of independent and reliable information.

A basic search on the internet yields hundreds of hits for websites that offer fertility treatment and commercial surrogacy arrangements, including recruitment of gestational mothers and egg providers. The vast majority are sponsored by those in the business of assisted reproduction. While a few are databases that directly connect intended parents with gestational mothers and egg providers, others are websites for university-based clinics that blend service with research, freestanding clinics that provide direct fertility and surrogacy services, and support organizations that build networks for those seeking and providing services. Lastly, there are the concierge-style services that act as middlemen, intermediaries or brokers who facilitate arrangements between intended parents, gestational mothers and fertility clinics, taking care of every aspect of the negotiation and process, as well as needs related to an intended parent's travel, stay, entertainment and interaction with local legal and immigration officials. This last type, referred to as 'transnational agents/agencies' here, drives transnational commercial surrogacy.

Transnational agencies for destinations outside the US While our website survey focused on transnational agents, it also involved a brief but close examination of agents recruiting for surrogacy based in the US, another hub. These agents cater to intended parents living in the country or coming to the country seeking gestational mothers. While not without considerable problems themselves, we noticed a qualitative difference in the amount and type of information provided by these agencies, versus others that facilitate surrogacy arrangements outside the US, in countries like India and Mexico. Box 12.1 provides an overview and illustrations of key messages promoted by agents of US-based surrogacy. These agencies are very active online and, in the course of a lay person's search, might *also* reach intended parents interested in hiring gestational mothers outside the US, potentially leaving them with overly positive (and misleading) ideas of the transnational arrangements they are considering.

> **Box 12.1 Messaging on key websites promoting US-based surrogacy**
>
> - The US is an ideal destination because of automatic citizenship for children born here, quality medical care and good exchange rates.
> - Intended parents receive support on legal issues related to parentage and citizenship.
> - Gestational mothers are special, generous, committed and compassionate.
> - Arrangements stress the relationship cultivated between intended parents and gestational mothers.
>
> While not without problems, it is interesting to note that these websites detail the surrogacy process, including compensation, procedures and medications, and use images of predominantly Caucasian gestational mothers and intended parents. They offer complete criminal checks for both parties and emphasize the fulfilling nature of the arrangements and life-long relationships that are born from them.
>
> Sources: Growing Generations, Shared Conceptions, Circle Surrogacy and Conceivabilities.

The reality and presentations of transnational arrangements is quite different. For the purpose of our investigation, we focused on four key transnational players: Surrogacy Abroad, Surrogacy Beyond Borders, The Fertility Institutes and the former Planet Hospital.

One stark difference between transnational agencies and those involved in US-based surrogacy is the concierge style of service provided by the former. Websites for Surrogacy Abroad, Surrogacy Beyond Borders and The Fertility Institutes proudly advertise their '24/7' attendance on intended parents, all-in-one centres that not only include 'physicians, surrogates, donors and attorneys', but also list services that range well beyond ARTs to cover escorts to consulates, assistance with exit visas, travel and hotel reservations, tourism and pleasure. It seems that the intended parent's every need is addressed, from the start to the end of the process, by agencies that know how to work local systems to their own advantage and present attractive package deals that mix reproduction with comfortable travel.

> **Box 12.2 One-stop shopping for a baby**
>
> Surrogacy Beyond Borders is a 'one-stop-shop' for individuals considering transnational commercial surrogacy. Like others in the fertility business, the agency caters first and foremost to the needs of intended parents, explicitly advertising: caesarean sections for all births (unless intended parents prefer otherwise); contracts relinquishing parental rights and signed by gestational mothers before implantation; staggered payments to 'disincentivize' problems; 'reductions' (i.e. abortions) of one or more fetuses in cases of multiple pregnancies; and chaperoned contact between intended parents and gestational mothers to, it appears, protect the former from extortion. Gender selection is offered for an additional fee.

Aggressive marketing of discounted rates for the benefit of intended parents is another distinction from US-based surrogacy. Surrogacy Abroad advertises 'the cost for surrogacy in Asia and other countries are roughly a third of what it costs in the US' and the practice 'offers a unique opportunity for discretion, which would be difficult to achieve in the US'. Surrogacy Beyond Borders (see Box 12.2) claims to provide an 'affordable alternative' to the US system using the same procedures as its US-based counterparts use at 'two to three times the cost'. To outbid its transnational competitors, The Fertility Institutes claim their 'high quality services' are the best price and offer 'financing' to intended parents. Hard to find are any meaningful details on the compensation given to gestational mothers despite evidence that the majority are poor, socially and politically disenfranchised and driven by economic need; even when numbers are made public, like those by clinician Nayna Patel, it is impossible to verify promised payments, payment schedules and actual payments without asking surrogates or referencing the documentation of organizations working on their behalf.

Third, great care is taken to ensure detachment between intended parents and gestational mothers. This is in marked contrast with several key agencies of US-based surrogacy, where cultivating a relationship between the two is considered a desirable aspect of the arrangement. The detachment sought by transnational agents is achieved in a few different ways. One is the absence of images on their websites and promotional material that would serve to humanize gestational mothers and, instead, the use of images, such as headless belly shots, which portray these women as hosts or vehicles.

Another is by playing the role of 'gatekeeper' and the singular entity on which gestational mothers and intended parents must rely separately. Surrogacy Beyond Borders, for example, only arranges meetings once a pregnancy is confirmed. In an attempt at appearing protective of intended parents (and possibly scaring them in the process) its website includes the reassuring statement that 'all of our meetings or Skype calls are chaperoned' so their clients are not 'put in a position where they could potentially be leveraged for more money'. The Fertility Institutes 'do not accept surrogates who demand a post-delivery relationship with the couple' and 'contractually require that the surrogate not attempt to contact the couple after delivery', unless the intended parents want otherwise.

Another aspect that facilitates distancing of gestational mothers from intended parents is the minimal information provided to one about the other. Agency websites do not seem to give intended parents any personal information on gestational mothers, or details on the treatment procedures they undergo to artificially prepare their bodies to become pregnant. What is provided is primarily relevant to vetting and monitoring them as effective hosts for carrying a fetus and increasing choices for intended parents themselves. This includes, for example, a gestational mother's relationship status, physical and emotional health, prior birthing successes and medical testing/screening protocols.

Other advertised offers by transnational agencies go to great lengths to maximize consumer choice. For example, the now defunct Planet Hospital explicitly offered embryo reduction. One iteration of the agency's website had this to say: 'it is up to you to decide what you wish to do, you can choose to have all the children (which will cost slightly more of course ...) or you can request an embryo reduction'. This transnational agent also boasted offers like the 'India Bundle', which involved trying to impregnate two gestational mothers at the same time to increase 'the odds of pregnancy by more than 60 per cent'. If both women became pregnant, the intended parents had the option to decide if they wanted all the babies or an abortion. Gestational mothers do not have any control of the embryo transfers and, as a result of contracts they frequently cannot read, forfeit an independent ability to terminate (or continue) pregnancies. While terminations chosen by someone other than the pregnant woman may not be strictly legal, gestational mothers from resource-poor communities almost never have access to independent legal advice or the financial resources to repay the (often very small fraction) of the promised payment they have already received.

Planet Hospital has left its imprint on the practice of transnational commercial surrogacy, with many other agencies following suit. Surrogacy Abroad, for example, includes caesarean sections in its list of services. Surrogacy Beyond Borders, in a section on frequently asked questions, reassures intended parents that gestational mothers are constantly monitored, sign contracts 'relinquishing any and all rights to the baby', receive staggered compensation to disincentivize problems, and undergo fetal reductions if the commissioning parents are not interested in twins or higher order multiples. All their births are also performed by c-section unless intended parents prefer otherwise. These and other risks are well documented by organizations on the ground. They, along with medical providers, point to the benefits of vaginal births and the dangers of vaginal birth after caesarean sections in low-care settings, such as the environments to which gestational mothers are likely to return. Last, but not least, are concerns related to offers of gender selection as a gateway to eugenically motivated decisions.

The agility and growth of a business

In the absence of country-specific regulation or global policy, front-end marketing by transnational agents seems fearless in its advertising and promises. It is clear that a patchwork of law has forced the practice of transnational commercial surrogacy to adapt quickly to a changing landscape. For example, at the time of writing, The Fertility Institutes is rapidly expanding services in Mexico because India and Thailand now disqualify gay and single intended parents; and, at the time of writing this chapter, Surrogacy Abroad is looking at Nepal for the same reason. Surrogacy Beyond Borders has figured out the best way to use Mexican law to its own benefit and accommodate the comfort of intended parents, by starting the process in Cancun and ending it in Tabasco, which is the only state that recognizes commercial surrogacy in the country.

Targeted outreach to certain niche audiences, most notably gay communities, is a common and growing practice. The Fertility Institutes run multiple 'gay surrogacy centers' (touting as the 'largest providers of parenthood options to the worldwide gay community') and claim to understand the 'run-around' encountered by 'hopeful new parents when dealing with many other providers of similar services' (see Chapter 2). For those with financial limitations or concerns, this agency also offers a 'hybrid' programme with additional savings of US$10,000 to US$17,000 whereby intended parents receive all their medical care in the US while a 'well-screened surrogate' in India carries the pregnancy to term. In what is likely a case of frozen embryos being transferred across continents for implantation, this option is offered by the agency to intended parents who prefer not to travel.

These examples speak to the resilience and determination of transnational agents and the overall agility of the assisted reproduction business. Absent or inconsistent regulation will protect the status quo and the continued effects on gestational mothers and the children born of transnational arrangements, within a system that views women's bodies as a means to highly valued 'products' and is minimally motivated to act in their best interest. Other principles that can be observed operating in this emergent, unregulated market include:

- Downplay health risks to egg providers, gestational mothers and resulting children.
- Prioritize the delivery of acceptable 'goods' by one party to another, often with minimal contact.
- Rates of compensation to 'suppliers', i.e. gestational mothers, are set by demand and profit margins.
- Fail to impart evidence-based information or adopt 'best practices'.
- Promote marketing options that encourage eugenic decision-making by intended parents.
- Coopt the language of 'choice' and 'equity' into the simplified language of 'consumer options'.
- Disingenuously rely on and over-emphasize the language of 'gifts' and 'women helping women'.

For change to happen, it is imperative that greater attention be paid to voices on the ground. While this includes the individuals and organizations advocating on behalf of gestational mothers, egg providers and children, spaces must also be created for the narratives of gestational mothers and egg providers as well as intended parents and their call for improved practices.

One intended parent, for example, wrote on a community blog: 'after almost ten months ... we've been forced to accept that not only did [they] not pay the doctors in India ... [they have] a history of not paying surrogates ... .'[8] Another intended parent responds:

> When I read that all their surrogates in Mexico deliver by scheduled c-section, that just didn't sit well with me. Right there it felt like exploitation; the women don't even have a choice on how they deliver and have to have major surgery even if not medically needed.[9]

These narratives speak to the power of consumer voices, the singular ability of individuals who demand a service to act against it when the service fails or incorporates unsound or unfair practices, and must be included in any conversation around change. They also speak to the dangerous gap in reliable information encountered by intended parents, egg providers and gestational mothers when considering transnational commercial surrogacy as an option. Filling this gap is vital and complex. While the news media have been helpful in this process, they could certainly do more; and as transnational agents control the conversation on the internet, via websites and blogs with savvy marketing, the need for a response in their own backyard is also clear. Towards that end, researchers and advocates must continue to document and disseminate their findings and press for broader social discourse and action. Without this multi-pronged approach, a call for and implementation of best practices in this twenty-first-century landscape of childbearing will remain a pipe dream.

Surrogacy360: addressing the knowledge gap and expanding civil society discourse

Returning to our methodology and our effort to replicate the process and findings of lay users interested in learning more about the issues and/or considering a transnational arrangement, it seems clear that the vast majority of readily available information is sponsored by and/or sympathetic to ART providers or transnational agents. Evidence, where it exists, is often only available to select audiences, expensive to purchase or overly academic; it is almost always drowned out by marketing that overplays the altruistic benefits of what is essentially a contractual and financial venture.

As entities facilitating unregulated transnational third-party reproduction have come under scrutiny, the investigation by OBOS confirmed the need for an independent and fact-based resource. To that end, in December 2016, we launched a digital clearinghouse called Surrogacy360 to curate and disseminate reliable and well-rounded information on transnational commercial surrogacy. Surrogacy360 draws on information from many sources, including field and academic research that is generally inaccessible to the public, and feature the spectrum of debate on the issue. It is independent, with peer reviewed content, and complements the efforts of global partners advocating on behalf of gestational mothers in countries such as India, Nepal and Mexico.

Surrogacy360 does not facilitate surrogacy. As the platform gains momentum and reach, it will respectfully engage intended parents, especially those considering transnational arrangements, as an objective response to the flood of biased industry-sponsored information. And it will provide an examination of current practice for students, researchers, public health advocates, policy-makers and the wider public. It will be inclusive and probing to help our audience unpack and engage with an extremely complex and, when applicable, personal issue. Finally, it will serve as a bridge, in the absence of imminent change, to create a space for social discourse, an opportunity to forge partnerships and a call for better practices.

Conclusion

Women's health, human rights and public health educators and advocates have an important role to play in raising public awareness and addressing the challenges ahead. They need to identify, document and address the emerging health and human rights violations occurring quietly under the public radar in the global, largely unregulated business in assisted reproduction. They need to engage in public education on these issues and work with the media, policy-makers and clinicians to heighten visibility and call for appropriate practices and safeguards. Most importantly, they must connect the dots across the domestic and global spheres, the 'demand' and 'supply' sides of ART arrangements, and the short- and long-term implications of the new era in human reproduction.

Notes

1 The impact of recent restrictions on transnational commercial surrogacy in India (*BBC News*, 2015) and Nepal (Abrams, 2016) have yet to be seen.

2 <http://infoasaid.org/guide/nepal/radio-overview>.

3 Transcript: <www.oprah.com/world/Wombs-for-Rent/1>.

4 Thailand's crackdown on 'wombs for rent': <www.bbc.com/news/world-asia-31556597>; Thailand bans commercial surrogacy for foreigners: <www.bbc.com/news/world-asia-31546717>.

5 Readers are strongly recommended to watch the full clip: <https://drive.google.com/file/d/0B9qAYGzacgFBRFFrMXFrekZMdG8/view>.

6 An Australian couple abandoned a baby boy conceived using the husband's sperm and born with Down's syndrome. Taking the boy's healthy twin sister, the couple returned to Australia leaving 'Baby Gammy' with the surrogate who had given birth to him in Thailand (Pearlman, 2014).

7 The Australian parents of Baby Gammy speak on 60 Minutes. *60 Minutes* (2014): <http://sixtyminutes.ninemsn.com.au//stories/8887943/the-australian-parents-of-baby-gammy-to-speak-on-60-minutes>.

8 The reference here is to the malpractice of Planet Hospital, now defunct.

9 <http://community.babycenter.com/post/a44167630>.

References

Abrams R (2016) Nepal bans surrogacy, leaving couples with few low-cost options. *New York Times*, 2 May. <www.nytimes.com/2016/05/03/world/asia/nepal-bans-surrogacy-leaving-couples-with-few-low-cost-options.html?_r=0>

Ahmed A (2014) Offshore babies: the murky world of transnational surrogacy. *Al Jazeera*, 11 August. <http://america.aljazeera.com/articles/2014/8/11/offshore-babies-thebusinessoftransnationalsurrogacy.html>

BBC (2013) Interview with Nayna Patel, Akanksha Infertility Clinic. *Hard Talk*, 18 November. No longer available.

BBC News (2015) India to ban foreign surrogate services. 28 October. <www.bbc.co.uk/news/world-asia-india-34655084>

Bhalla N and Thapliyal M (2013) India seeks to regulate its booming 'rent-a-womb' industry. *Reuters*, 30 September. <http://www.reuters.com/article/2013/09/30/us-india-surrogates-idUSBRE98T07F20130930>

Boston Women's Health Book Collective (2011) *Our Bodies Ourselves*. 5th revised edition. New York: Touchstone.

Brooks JD (2007) Oprah on renting wombs in India: 'It's beautiful'. *Biopolitical Times*, 11 October. <http://www.biopoliticaltimes.org/article.php?id=3713>

Centre for Social Research (2010) *Surrogate Motherhood: Ethical or Commercial?* <https://drive.google.com/file/d/0B-f1XIdg1JC_Uio4RmlYUkNsTFE/edit>

Centre for Social Research (2012) *Surrogate Motherhood: Ethical or Commercial? Final Report.* <https://drive.google.com/file/d/0B-f1XIdg1JC_UGh5UTNxUGxMV1k/edit>

CNN (2013) Surrogate babies: 'Made in India'. 3 November. <www.cnn.com/video/data/2.0/video/world/2013/11/03/kapur-india-surrogacy-clinics.cnn.htm.l>

Cooper C, May A and Christiansen A (2014) Desperate for a baby: scammed in global surrogacy's newest frontier. *Al Jazeera*, 15 May. <http://america.aljazeera.com/watch/shows/america-tonight/articles/2014/5/14/desperate-for-a-babyscammedinglobalsurrogacysnewestfrontier.html>

Drennan J (2015) The future of wombs for rent. *Foreign Policy*, 2 March. <https://foreignpolicy.com/2015/03/02/the-future-of-wombs-for-rent>

Economic Times (2015) Blanket ban on NRIs, PIOs, foreigners having kids through surrogacy. 15 October. <http://economictimes.indiatimes.com/news/politics-and-nation/blanket-ban-likely-on-nris-pios-foreigners-having-kids-through-surrogacy/articleshow/49391832.cms>

Fox News (2007) Wombs for rent: commercial surrogacy growing in India. 30 December. <www.foxnews.com/story/2007/12/30/wombs-for-rent-commercial-surrogacy-growing-in-india>

Goodwin M (2015) Baby markets and the new motherhood: reproducing hierarchy in commercial intimacy. *Huffington Post*, 13 May. <www.huffingtonpost.com/michele-goodwin/baby-markets-the-new-motherhood_b_7263050.html>

Haberman C (2014) Baby M and the question of surrogate motherhood. *New York Times*, 23 March. <www.nytimes.com/2014/03/24/us/baby-m-and-the-question-of-surrogate-motherhood.html>

HCCH (Hague Conference on International Private Law) (2014a) *The Desirability and Feasibility of Further Work on the Parentage/Surrogacy Project.* Preliminary Document No. 3B. The Hague: HCCH <www.hcch.net/upload/wop/gap2014pd03b_en.pdf>

HCCH (2014b) *A Study of Legal Parentage and the Issues Arising from International Surrogacy Arrangements*. Preliminary Document No. 3C. The Hague: HCCH. <www.hcch.net/upload/wop/gap2014pd03c_en.pdf>

Huffington Post (2013) Celebrities who've used surrogates to conceive. 2 June. <www.huffingtonpost.com/2013/02/06/celebrities-who-have-used-surrogates_n_2624998.html>

Ilic A (2015) Nepalese court suspends commercial surrogacy. *BioNews*, 1 September. <www.bionews.org.uk/page_561682.asp>

Kamin D (2015) Israel evacuates surrogate babies from Nepal but leaves the mothers behind. *Time*, 28 April. <http://time.com/3838319/israel-nepal-surrogates>

Kumar R (2015) Trying to tame the wild west of surrogacy in India. *Al Jazeera*, 14 January. <http://america.aljazeera.com/articles/2015/1/14/the-wild-west-ofsurrogacy.html>

Lal N (2012) Risks flagged in India's fertility tourism. *Asia Times*, 1 August. <http://www.atimes.com/atimes/South_Asia/NH01Df01.html>

Lewin T (2014) A surrogacy agency that delivered heartache. *New York Times*, 27 July. <www.nytimes.com/2014/07/28/us/surrogacy-agency-planet-hospital-delivered-heartache.html?_r=0>

Najar N (2015) India wants to ban birth surrogacy for foreigners. *New York Times*, 28 October. <http://www.nytimes.com/2015/10/29/world/asia/india-wants-to-ban-birth-surrogacy-for-foreigners.html?smid=fb-nytimes&smtyp=cur>

National Public Radio (2014) Surrogacy storm in Thailand: a rejected baby, a busy babymaker. <http://www.npr.org/sections/goatsandsoda/2014/10/22/357870757/surrogacy-storm-in-thailand-a-rejected-baby-a-busy-babymaker>

Okwemba A (2012) A Kenyan surrogate mother speaks: 'I rented out my womb for $8000'. *Africa Review*, 8 February. <http://www.africareview.com/Special+Reports/Surrogacy+in+Kenya+gains+pace/-/979182/1322482/-/mf04pw/-/index.html>

Pandey G (2016) India surrogate mothers talk of pain of giving up baby. *BBC News*, Chennai, 15 August. <www.bbc.co.uk/news/world-asia-india-37050249>

Pearlman J (2014) Surrogacy case: the history of sex offences of the Australian accused of leaving surrogate baby in Thailand. *Daily Telegraph*, 6 August. <www.telegraph.co.uk/news/worldnews/australiaandthepacific/australia/11015898/Surrogacy-case-the-history-of-sex-offences-of-the-Australian-accused-of-leaving-surrogate-baby-in-Thailand.html>

Points K (2009) *Commercial Surrogacy and Fertility Tourism in India: The Case of Baby Manji*. Durham, NC: Kenan Institute for Ethics at Duke University. <https://web.duke.edu/kenanethics/casestudies/babymanji.pdf>

Rawlinson K (2014) Interpol investigates 'baby factory' as man fathers 16 surrogate children. *Guardian*, 23 August. <www.theguardian.com/lifeandstyle/2014/aug/23/interpol-japanese-baby-factory-man-fathered-16-children>

Ronan A (2015) Inside the dark realities of the international surrogacy industry. *New York Magazine*, 30 March. <http://nymag.com/thecut/2015/03/dark-side-of-international-surrogacy.html>

Sama Resource Group for Women and Health (2012) *Birthing a Market: A Study of Commercial Surrogacy*. New Delhi: Sama. <www.communityhealth.in/~commun26/wiki/images/e/e8/Sama_Birthing_A_Market.pdf>

Sama Resource Group for Women and Health (2013) *Can We See the Baby Bump Please?* New Delhi: Sama. For information regarding distribution contact: sama.womenshealth@gmail.com or sama.genderhealth@gmail.com.

Sloan K and Lahl J (2014) Inconvenient truths about commercial surrogacy. *TwinCities.com*, 1 April. <http://www.twincities.com/columnists/ci_25470963/sloan-lahl-inconvenient-truths-about-commercial-surrogacy>

Tuckman J (2014) Surrogacy boom in Mexico brings tales of missing money and stolen eggs. *Guardian*, 25 September. <http://www.theguardian.com/world/2014/sep/25/tales-of-missing-money-stolen-eggs-surrogacy-mexico>

Vogt A (2014) The rent-a-womb boom. *The Daily Beast*, 1 March. <http://www.thedailybeast.com/witw/articles/2014/03/01/the-rent-a-womb-boom-is-india-s-surrogacy-industry-empowering-or-exploitative.html>

13 | SURROGATE MOTHERHOOD: ETHICAL OR COMMERCIAL?

The Centre for Social Research

Introduction

The Centre for Social Research (CSR), based in New Delhi, is a non-profit NGO that aims to empower women and girls, promoting their fundamental rights and increasing public understanding of social issues from a gender perspective. Concerned about the lack of regulation surrounding the growing popularity of India as a destination for foreigners seeking to become parents through surrogacy, the National Commission for Women (NCW) and the Ministry of Women and Child Development (MWCD) commissioned the CSR to undertake two studies, in Anand, Surat and Jamnagar in the state of Gujarat (2010), and in Delhi and Mumbai (2012). The aim was to use our findings as a basis for formulating policy recommendations to protect the rights of the main three parties involved: surrogate mothers, children and commissioning parents.

This resulted in two reports, under the joint title *Surrogate Motherhood: Ethical or Commercial?* They include detailed profiles of the demographic and socio-economic backgrounds of around 100 surrogates, the decision to engage in surrogacy, experiences before and during pregnancy, and relinquishing the child; they also look at the role played by clinics. Incorporated into these findings is an analysis of the social and health protection rights ensured to surrogate mothers, the rights of the child in surrogacy arrangements and the rights and other issues pertaining to commissioning parents that existed at the time of the CSR studies.

After briefly discussing the inadequacies of the existing legal framework that triggered our studies, this chapter summarizes selected findings from the second project (conducted in Delhi and Mumbai). These focus mainly on the profiles of surrogate mothers in the two cities, with only brief findings related to commissioning parents, agents and doctors. We conclude with recommendations from the report of a two-day national conference, 'A Policy Dialogue on Issues around Surrogacy in India', which was organized by the

CSR in September 2014. Full copies of all three reports are at www.csrindia.org/surrogate-motherhood.

The landscape of surrogacy in India[1]

Surrogate motherhood raises difficult ethical, philosophical and social issues. Its transformation into a commercial transaction further complicates the picture. After the legalization of surrogacy in India in 2002, the practice of outsourcing pregnancy became a multi-billion-dollar business with a great deal at stake for all involved (CSR, 2014). This rapid expansion of the 'rent-a-womb' industry, which has drawn many hundreds of foreign childless couples to India every year, has unfolded against a backdrop of minimal regulation. Despite the drafting of the ART (Regulation) Bill 2010 (discussed below) little has changed.[1]

India saw the first successful birth through gestational surrogacy in 1994, in Chennai. In 1997, an Indian woman acted as a gestational carrier and received payment in order to obtain medical treatment for her paralysed husband. The numbers of births through commercial surrogacy escalated with estimates ranging from 200 to 350 in 2008 alone (Lal, 2008).

India soon became the most popular country for 'fertility tourists' outside the US (Pande, 2014). This is due to a number of factors. In 2002, the Confederation of Indian Industry (CII) published a study on the potential India has to develop a medical tourism sector. This was picked up on by the then Finance Minister who wanted India to become a global health destination. In order to stimulate this development he came up with measures to facilitate a medical tourism industry, including infrastructural improvements (Chinai and Goswami, 2007). Hospitals that treat foreign patients were to receive financial incentives including low interest rates on loans and low import duties on medical equipment. In addition, the Ministry of External Affairs introduced a medical visa that allowed patients and their families to stay in India for up to twelve months. Tourism departments teamed up with hospitals to attract foreign patients and not without success: the number of medical tourists increased from 150,000 in 2005 to 450,000 in 2008.

During this time, fertility tourism also increased in popularity. Ten years ago, the reproductive segment of the Indian medical tourism market was already valued at well over US$450 million a year (Ramesh, 2006). More recently a UN-backed study reported an estimated 3,000 fertility clinics established in both rural and urban areas in almost all states of India (Bhalla and Thapliyal, 2013). Fertility tourists do not all come from western countries; India is also a popular destination for infertile couples from Sri Lanka, Pakistan, Bangladesh, Thailand and Singapore.

While commercial surrogacy is also developing in other parts of the world, another contributing factor to the rise in popularity of surrogacy in India was that patients found it easy to communicate with the English-speaking doctors. This also enabled these doctors to promote surrogacy in the press (Ramachandran, 2006), glorifying success stories with no mention of all the failed attempts. Clinics sometimes used the media, particularly the internet, to deceive potential clients. Their websites often contained both facts and fiction as part of the marketing strategy (Mulay and Gibson, 2006) and it was not uncommon for them to encourage couples to ignore the laws regarding surrogacy in their home country.

The strongest incentive for foreigners to travel to India is most likely to be relatively low costs. The fees for surrogates are reported to range from US$2,500 to $7,000. The total cost can be anything between US$10,000 and $35,000. This is a lot less than what intended parents pay in the US, where rates fluctuate from around US$59,000 to $80,000 (Sharma, 2008). On average, most Indian surrogate mothers are paid in instalments over a period of nine months. If they are unable to conceive they are often not paid at all and sometimes they must forfeit a portion of their fee if they miscarry (*Insight*, 2006).

Jurisdiction in India

The ICMR Guidelines As an increasing number of childless couples from overseas come to India, legal experts express their reservations. Many foresee hurdles after the child is born because there is no law to control or regulate the process. The real problem arises after the birth of the baby since foreigners are unable to obtain legal assistance when it comes to taking their child back to their home country. There are also difficulties related to claiming parenthood, including a few rare cases when the surrogate mother has refused to relinquish the child. In order to deal with these problems, in 2006, the Indian Council of Medical Research (ICMR) published guidelines for the accreditation, supervision and regulation of ART clinics in India, the main points of which are listed below:

- DNA tests are compulsory to determine that the intended parents are indeed the genetic parents. If this is not the case the child must be adopted instead.

- Surrogacy should normally only be an option for patients for whom it would be physically or medically impossible/undesirable to carry a baby to term.
- The payments received by the surrogate mothers should be documented and cover all genuine expenses associated with the pregnancy.
- The responsibility of finding a surrogate mother should rest with the couple or a semen bank, not the clinic.
- A surrogate mother should not be over 45 years of age. The ART clinic should ensure that potential surrogates satisfy all the testable criteria to go through a successful full-term pregnancy.
- No woman may act as a surrogate more than three times in her lifetime.
- The surrogate mother must declare that she will not use drugs intravenously and not undergo a blood transfusion, except blood obtained through a certified blood bank.
- A relative or other known person, as well as a woman unknown to the couple, may act as a surrogate mother for them.

However, these guidelines do not hold any legal validity.

The Draft ART (Regulation) Bill 2010 A bill has long been in the works to regulate the practice of surrogacy. The 2010 Bill empowers a National Advisory Board to act as the regulatory body for laying down policies and regulations. It also seeks to set up State Advisory Boards that are, in addition to advising state governments, charged with monitoring the implementation of the provisions of the Bill once it becomes an Act, particularly with respect to the functioning of the ART clinics, semen banks and research organizations.

The ART (Regulation) Bill defines surrogacy as:

> an arrangement in which a woman agrees to a pregnancy, achieved through assisted reproductive technology, in which neither of the gametes belong to her or her husband, with the intention of carrying it to term and handing over the child to the person or persons for whom she is acting as surrogate. A 'surrogate mother' is a woman who agrees to have an embryo generated from the sperm of a man who is not her husband, and the oocyte from another woman implanted in her to carry the pregnancy to full term and deliver the child to its biological parents(s).

By this definition, all surrogacy arrangements that involve the woman bearing a child using her own egg (oocyte) and the commissioning man's sperm would be illegal. In addition, fertile surrogate mothers will necessarily have to use technology meant for the treatment of infertility. They will now be forced to use only in vitro technologies even though they can become pregnant using methods such as artificial insemination, which are much safer for them.

Further, in light of the ARTs practised today, the Bill reflects that there is no standardization of the drugs used, no proper documentation of the procedure, insufficient information for patients about the side-effects of such drugs and no limit to the number of times a woman may be asked to go through the procedure. In addition, clinics do not disclose the fact that a 'successful cycle' does not necessarily lead to a baby being born.

ART clinics are the central hub of all surrogacy-related activities. Some of their duties involve selecting the surrogate mothers (the Bill lays down the conditions that these women have to meet) and obtaining relevant information, informing all parties involved about their rights and obligations. The Bill specifies what is and is not allowed regarding these topics. ART clinics are also required to treat all the information they obtain with utmost confidentiality. In practice, this means that they are not allowed to provide any information about surrogate mothers or potential surrogates to any person. This creates a problem for intended parents since they have to turn to a middleman in order to find a surrogate. This is controversial, not just because of the involvement of agents, but also because it seems unfair that the intended parents, who are about to make a significant investment, have little control over the selection process. A better option might be to release personal information at the discretion of the surrogate.

The surrogate mother is entitled to receive monetary compensation from the couple or individual for agreeing to act as a surrogate. Owing to the increased risk of legal complications when the surrogate is also the genetic mother, traditional surrogacy is no longer allowed. Since several parties with dissimilar interests are involved in the surrogacy arrangement, controversy about someone's role can arise. The 2010 Bill draws clear lines to avoid these problems: the donors should relinquish parental rights at the time of donation while the surrogate does so shortly after birth.

Non-resident Indians and foreign couples are required to assign a local resident who is in charge of the surrogate's welfare until the act of relinquishment. For the same group, it is also mandatory to be able to document their ability to take the newborn back to their home country with them. The surrogate baby will be recognized as the legitimate child of the commissioning couple even if they divorce or become separated, with the child's birth certificate carrying both genetic parents' names. This stipulation was introduced in response to the Baby Manji case (see Box 13.1). This story generated intense media coverage and public debate in India, obliging infertility clinics to re-examine their purpose and practices in the light of evolving beliefs around commercial surrogacy in India.

> **Box 13.1 Baby Manji (Points, 2009)**
>
> In late 2007, a Japanese couple, Ikufumi and Yuki Yamada, travelled to India to hire a surrogate mother under fertility specialist Dr Nayna Patel. The doctor arranged a surrogacy contract with Pritiben Mehta, a married Indian woman with children, and supervised the creation of an embryo from Ikufumi's sperm and an egg harvested from an anonymous Indian woman. The embryo was then implanted into Mehta's womb. In June 2008, the Yamadas divorced and a month later Baby Manji was born to the surrogate mother. Although Ikufami wanted to raise the child, his ex-wife did not. As she saw it, she was unrelated to the baby biologically, genetically and legally. Under the terms of the agreement with the clinic, the egg donor's responsibility had ended once she provided the egg, and the surrogate's job was finished as soon as she gave birth. Suddenly, Baby Manji had three mothers – the intended mother who had contracted for the surrogacy, the egg donor, and the gestational surrogate – yet legally she had none.
>
> The surrogacy contract did not cover a situation such as this, nor were there any existing laws to help to clarify the matter. As far as Dr Patel was concerned, the clinic had fulfilled its promise to produce a baby. Both the parentage and the nationality of Baby Manji were impossible to determine under existing definitions of family and citizenship under Indian and Japanese law and the situation soon grew into a legal and diplomatic crisis. Yamada and his elderly mother launched a months-long campaign to secure the paperwork needed to bring the baby to Japan.
>
> Eventually, the Rajasthan regional passport office issued Manji an identity certificate as part of a transit document, paving the way for a travel visa for Japan. It was the first such identity

> certificate issued by the Indian government to a surrogate child born in India (Bhandari, 2008). As stated by *The Times of India* (2008), the certificate did not mention nationality, mother's name or religion, and it was valid only for Japan, according to the passport office. On 27 October, the Japanese Embassy issued the three-month-old a one-year visa on humanitarian grounds. Less than a week later, Manji Yamada and her grandmother, Emiko, flew to Osaka. Japanese authorities stated at that time that Manji could become a Japanese citizen 'once a parent–child relationship has been established, either by the man recognizing his paternity or through his adopting her' (*Hindustan Times*, 2008). However, nearly a year after her birth, no evidence had surfaced that Baby Manji's still precarious legal status in Japan had changed. Her one-year humanitarian visa was set to expire in October 2009.

The Rules of the 2010 Bill assume that ART is being used only by heterosexual infertile couples, so they specify indications for various techniques based on the nature of infertility. The side-effects are underplayed as 'ART procedures carry a small risk both to the mother and offspring'. This may be true in comparison with the pain and trauma of infertility, but the fact remains that the issue of using fertile women's bodies for egg retrieval or for surrogacy does not figure in the discussion on risk. The ART Bill has provided for numerous informed consent forms to be filled in and records to be kept, yet does not require that adequate information regarding potential side-effects be given to the surrogate mother.

Registration of surrogates with a 'sperm bank' further underlines the fact that she is seen as just another component of the technology: a womb. This ignores the fact that, while the donated egg or zygote becomes separated from the woman's body, the womb continues to stay inside her and therefore has to be looked at differently. Once again, a bill that is meant to safeguard the provider and the commissioning couples fails to protect the rights of the surrogate. She is the most marginalized and vulnerable one in this trade.

Surrogacy is both a threat and an opportunity: it offers infertile couples and surrogate mothers the possibility of fulfilling their desires – a child and the opportunity to take better care of their family. But there is a risk that, with the commodification of children and parenthood, women are exploited and turned into baby producers.

Although there are now some rules and regulations in place, not enough is done at a national level to protect the interests of Indian women who serve as surrogate mothers, the children they bear or those who travel considerable distances to commission pregnancies.

CSR study: Delhi and Mumbai

The following edited extracts are taken from the second exploratory study undertaken by the CSR. The sample size consisted of a hundred surrogate mothers and fifty commissioning parents and their families in Delhi and Mumbai. The research team also interviewed clinics conducting surrogacy, agents who facilitate such procedures (including travel agents who arrange for passports and other documents) and further stakeholders such as family and community members, and owners and caretakers of surrogacy hostels and guesthouses. The source of information for the surrogate mothers was mainly the agents who had approached them for surrogacy.

Methodology The methodology adopted for the study was based on exploratory research using situational analysis based on a survey. Tools included structured questionnaires comprising 75 per cent close-ended and 25 per cent open-ended questions. The gender aspect was kept in focus as personal observation and interviews included the husbands of surrogate mothers and, where possible, the male counterpart of the commissioning parents. Focus group discussions were also conducted with surrogate mothers, stakeholders and community members.

The surrogate mothers

Their profiles The surrogate mothers were mostly aged 26 to 30 (74 per cent of the respondents in Delhi and 58 per cent in Mumbai), and in both cases over half identified as Hindus. Many of the respondents in Delhi (72 per cent) were married, against less than half (46 per cent) in Mumbai.

Some of the respondents were educated up to primary level (54 per cent in Delhi and 44 per cent in Mumbai) and the majority were employed (68 per cent in Delhi and 78 per cent in Mumbai), mainly working as housemaids or domestic help and earning more than Rs.3,000 (approximately US$44) per month (50 per cent of the respondents in Delhi and 68 per cent in Mumbai).

The vast majority of the respondents came from nuclear families, belonged to male-headed households and had their own children (this was a prerequisite for infertility physicians/clinics/hospitals engaged in surrogacy as a proof of the fertility of the potential surrogate mother). Very few (12 per cent of the respondents in Delhi and 10 per cent in Mumbai) had experienced this before. Most (90 per cent of the respondents in Delhi and 96 per cent of them in Mumbai) were already pregnant and were in different stages of gestational pregnancy.

Why become a surrogate mother in India? The reasons to become a surrogate differed between the cities. In Delhi, under a third (28 per cent) of the respondents cited poverty as the reason, while in Mumbai, nearly half (47 per cent) said this. The decision was mainly taken by the surrogate herself, but under pressure from her husband. Only 36 per cent of surrogates in Mumbai and 14 per cent in Delhi had faced any resistance from their family and friends. Just over 30 per cent of the respondents in Delhi and 29 per cent in Mumbai said that they used the money for maintenance of their family. They also used it for the education of their children (23 per cent in Delhi and 34 per cent in Mumbai). Other priorities included building a new house and saving for a daughter's marriage.

The circumstances surrounding the surrogacy arrangements Few of the surrogates knew the commissioning parents prior to the surrogacy arrangement. This may be because the doctors/clinics matched the two parties, unless the commissioning parents had already homed in on a particular surrogate. Also, the commissioning parents usually came to India to sign the contract when the pregnancy had been confirmed and all abnormalities had been ruled out by the doctors dealing with the case – around the second trimester.

The surrogacy contract was signed between the surrogate mother (including her husband), the commissioning parents and the fertility physicians (sometimes). This way, the clinic authorities evade legal problems. More than 85 per cent of the contracts were signed around the second trimester of the pregnancy. This is because, after being informed about confirmation of pregnancy by the clinic/infertility physician, it takes one to two months more for the commissioning parents to arrange their visit to India. In some clinics/agencies, the contract is first signed by the surrogate mother and her husband and then sent either by email or post for the commissioning parents to sign and send a copy back to the clinic/doctor/agency dealing with the surrogacy arrangement.

Our research findings revealed that the majority of surrogate mothers had not received a copy of the written contract outlining the surrogacy arrangement: in fact, they were not even aware of the clauses outlined.

Regarding payment received by the surrogate mothers, under the surrogacy agreement, 46 per cent of the respondents in Delhi and 44 per cent of the respondents in Mumbai stated that they received Rs.300,000–399,000 (US$4,620–$6,144); 42 per cent of the respondents in Mumbai mentioned that they received payment between Rs.210,000 and 299,000 (US$3,234–$4,604). In Delhi, 26 per cent of the respondents said that they received Rs.4 lakh (US$6,160).

Experiencing surrogacy: health issues and when things go wrong
Anticipation (for 47 per cent in Delhi and 41 per cent in Mumbai) and fear (43 per cent in Delhi and 31 per cent of in Mumbai) topped the list of emotions experienced by surrogates before the pregnancy. This was because, unlike their own pregnancies, which happened naturally, an artificial procedure had been used to impregnate them about which they had no clue. Also, many knew that they would have to stay away from their families for nine months and were unsure about the payments they would be receiving.

The surrogacy contract rarely addressed issues related to the health and well-being of the surrogate. The ICMR guidelines suggest a maximum of three IVF sessions for a woman to become pregnant for a particular commissioning parent. But undercover, violations took place, as the surrogates were usually poor, illiterate/semi-literate and in need of immediate funds, and were not in a position to understand the medical procedures their bodies were being subjected to.

The health of the mother was considered only when the health of the fetus was an issue, and in cases where the intended parents did not wish to continue with the pregnancy due to fetal abnormalities or sex preference, the baby was aborted, often without consulting the surrogate. There was no fixed rule related to the amount of compensation she would receive: it was arbitrarily decided by the clinics.

Of the respondents in Mumbai, 80 per cent said that they hadn't undergone any test during pregnancy to determine the sex of the child. In Delhi, 60 per cent of the respondents had been tested to rule out any potential health abnormalities. The majority (71 per cent) stated that the child, if born with some deformity, would remain in the clinic/centre/agency until a solution was found regarding the next step. However, 6 per cent of the respondents in Delhi and 26 per cent in Mumbai expressed the view that the commissioning parents would accept the child even if an abnormality was detected. The clinic/hospital authorities said that in cases where the commissioning parents refused to accept the child or for some reason the pregnancy was aborted, the surrogate was often paid half of the amount she was supposed to receive under normal circumstances (56 per cent of the respondents in Delhi and 36 per cent in Mumbai), although some said they would not receive any money if the pregnancy went wrong.

There was no clarity regarding payment if the surrogate were pregnant with twins. The normal practice was that, when the doctor found out about a twin pregnancy, s/he consulted the commissioning parents, who in most cases were happy to take home two babies and wanted to continue with the pregnancy.

Relationships between surrogate mothers and commissioning parents
In most of the cases the relationship between the surrogate mother and the commissioning parents was described as harmonious but from a distance. Language was a barrier and the doctor was the sole communicator between them. Involvement of the commissioning parents was normally restricted to the initial stage of being introduced to the surrogate mother and making sure she delivered and relinquished the baby as agreed.

Handing over the baby Most of the surrogates we interviewed were not willing to answer questions on how they felt after relinquishing the child. However, field-level observations indicate that they felt attached to the babies even though they were not biologically their own. For those who were in the middle of their pregnancy, this was also an uncomfortable question for which they were not emotionally prepared. Only a very few expressed having a special bond towards the child (4 per cent in Delhi and 2 per cent in Mumbai), yet 44 per cent of the respondents in Delhi and 46 per cent in Mumbai stated that relinquishing the baby was the worst part of surrogacy. Other negative aspects were long and painful labour and having to live away from their families.

The commissioning parents

Here the amount of data collected was restricted by the extent to which clinics allowed the researcher to observe and the information they divulged. The CSR collected the maximum data it could from Delhi and Mumbai using findings from twenty-five respondents in each city.

Only 28 per cent of the respondents had been pregnant before and suffered miscarriages; 98 per cent of them said they had had no previous experience of surrogacy arrangements; 54 per cent had taken the decision to pursue surrogacy in India on the recommendation of other couples who had already done so.

The surrogacy contract basically deals with issues related to arrangements for relinquishing the child (27 per cent), compensation (19 per cent), the extent of supervision (13 per cent), etc. Although contracts include commissioning parents, the surrogate mother and the clinic as equal parties, only the commissioning parents and the surrogate are signatories. This way, clinics avoid being liable for any potential legal action against themselves.

The commissioning parents in our study seemed very desperate for the baby, so it hardly mattered to them whether the child was male or female (82 per cent of them said that the sex of the baby didn't matter at all for them and they were happy in any case).

All the major decisions related to the surrogacy arrangement were taken by the clinics and the commissioning parents. Surrogates were not involved in any decision-making and appeared to have no bargaining power at all.

Surrogacy centres/clinics/agencies in Delhi and Mumbai

The doctors felt that surrogacy was a good option since those who opted to be gestational surrogates are generally very fertile and surrogacy offers them an opportunity to improve their financial status. The coordinator of one agency mentioned that he felt the agency was doing humanitarian work where both parties in the arrangement, i.e. surrogate and intended parents, get something in their hand (the old win-win argument!). He also said that their success rate had increased since the surrogates had started residing in the surrogate homes. Being in such homes ensures that they eat nutritious food and take their medicines on time and that they do not run away. He also mentioned that the women realized they were answerable to the intended parents on account of all the money they had invested in the arrangement.

According to one doctor, contact between the two parties is not encouraged in his centre as this had been seen to put pressure on both sides. The centre's website mentions the option of hiring two surrogate mothers; when this question was raised, the embryologist said that 60 per cent of clients chose this route in order to increase their chances of begetting the child. It is also more economical for the intended parents: they can spend Rs.17 lakh (US$26,180) once – the rate for two surrogates – rather than spending Rs.13 lakh (US$20,020) – the rate for one surrogate – twice, in cases where the first attempt of surrogacy is unsuccessful. However, this is not allowed by the Draft ART Bill 2010.

As told by the embryologist, although a normal delivery would usually be possible in surrogacy, despite the fact that it can cause obstetric problems in the future, to avoid taking any chances the centre favours caesarean section. The embryologist mentioned that the surrogate child is immediately taken from the surrogate mother in order to avoid any emotional bond forming between her and the baby. This way the surrogate mother cannot breastfeed the child or even provide breast milk; either a donor mother or the intended mother are induced for lactation, using mechanical or hormonal induction.

One doctor mentioned a case where the surrogate mother had aborted the surrogate child. Therefore, she now makes sure that only those women are selected as surrogates who agree to stay in shelter homes. She also said that, although it is important for the surrogate mothers to stay in these homes, in their absence, some husbands start visiting commercial sex workers. Thus, she considered that surrogacy is 'spoiling the society'. The doctor called commercial surrogacy 'maid business'. She also emphasized that the amount of payment for surrogacy varies significantly according to the profile of surrogate mothers. Nowadays a lot of intended parents opt for educated and fair-skinned women to bear them a child.

More recent recommendations

In September 2014, two years after the publication of our report on surrogacy in Delhi and Mumbai, the CSR held a two-day national conference aimed at developing policy recommendations to strengthen the ART Bill from a human rights perspective.

Although the Draft ART (Regulation Bill) 2010 brought forth certain important points on which to base the legal framework, many crucial issues relating to surrogacy arrangements have been omitted and a number of questions remain unanswered. These include:

- Is it legal to become a surrogate mother in India?
- Will the child born to an Indian surrogate mother be a citizen of this country?
- Who arranges the birth certificate and passport required by the foreign couple at the time of immigration?
- Whose name will appear on the birth certificate? How will the commissioning parents claim parenthood?

- What happens if the surrogate mother changes her mind and refuses to hand over the baby or blackmails for custody?
- Who will take the responsibility of the child if the commissioning parents refuse to take the child?
- What would happen if the child is born disabled?
- What would happen if the sex of the child is not to the liking of the commissioning parents?

Such questions need thorough analysis before any policy related to surrogacy is designed and legal provisions are made. With this in mind, the conference came up with a number of specific recommendations (see Box 13.2).

Box 13.2 CSR conference recommendations (2014)

- The need for a rights-based legal framework to safeguard the human rights of each party involved in the agreement.
- The creation of an agency to act as a depository for all documents as well as a grievance redress cell.
- A central database or registration system of surrogacy arrangements for monitoring purposes.
- Mandatory insurance cover for surrogate mothers with US dollar benchmarks by overseas commissioning parents, as a prerequisite to the issue of medical visas.
- Videographic consent to be recorded to monitor informed/ forced consent of the surrogate.
- The intended parents should be legally bound to accept the custody of the child/children irrespective of any abnormality in the child. It should not be given to the surrogate and add to her problems or left in an orphanage.
- Surrogate mothers should have access to intensive care and medical check-ups of their reproductive organs for three months after pregnancy.
- Enforcement of the Pre-Conception and Pre-Natal Diagnostic Techniques Act, which forbids sex selection.
- Foreigners should only be allowed to opt for surrogacy in India if it is permitted by their country of origin.
- Police records regarding commissioning parents to be taken into consideration before any surrogacy agreement is signed.
- Deregulation of unscrupulous medical tourism agencies that offer surrogacy arrangements.

- Elimination of agents to avoid the commercialization of surrogacy.
- Anonymity should be maintained, if the surrogate so chooses. There should be zero tolerance of economic, social or legal exploitation.
- The introduction of a standardized bar of remuneration/compensation for the surrogate to control exploitation by the market.
- Surrogates bearing twins should be compensated accordingly.
- Hyperstimulation of gametes/embryos should be monitored and made punishable.
- The rights of the child must be protected.
- Contracts should be made in the surrogate's local language and she should be provided with a copy of the same.
- Delivery should not be undertaken at the expense of health.
- Termination of pregnancy should be considered in the case of potential trauma to the surrogate mother.
- Impose a check on black-marketing of frozen embryos and make it punishable by law.
- Counselling to be available to all the parties involved in the process, including doctors.
- Competition in the market to be regulated.
- A central database or registration system of surrogates for real information such as their permanent address, number of children, etc.
- Check on reproductive technologies for democratic and egalitarian use.
- Legislation in the case of the commissioning parents' death.
- Introduction of a mediation, arbitration and surrogacy ombudsman.
- Comprehensive consolidated surrogacy legislation, with extra-territorial application, such as the provisions of the Hindu Marriage Act, 1955.
- Illegal trading in gametes/embryos should be punishable.
- Aggrieved surrogate mother/immediate family members should be empowered to invoke the jurisdiction of the National Commission for Women (NCW) or appropriate state-level forums.
- Provision for mandatory coordination of NCW or appropriate state level forums with foreign missions, in case of default by erring foreign nationals/commissioning parents.

- Plea of data protection legislation by foreign missions in India should not be used to obstruct, thwart or stall the enquiry process
- Specific provisions ensuring protection of the fetus/child in case of abnormalities must be included.
- The law should not exclude LGBT, homosexuals, single parents and unmarried couples.
- Guarantee complete transparency between the doctor and the surrogate mother with respect to any medical practice applied.
- Strengthen doctors' criminal responsibility and accountability.
- No surrogacy arrangements should be carried out for the maintenance of beauty or career reasons, or if the couple already have one child of their own.

The conference was a massive success. It not only yielded concrete and substantial recommendations for policy-makers, but it was also an intellectual and rich experience for the researchers and other concerned parties, aiming to better the lives of fellow women and to help emancipate and empower them in the truest sense of the words.

Acknowledgements

With special thanks to Dr Manasi Mishra for permission to summarize some of CSR's findings and to Annabel Hendry for all her work in editing this chapter.

Note

1 As noted elsewhere in this volume, in August 2016, the Indian government approved the introduction of the Surrogacy (Regulation) Bill, 2016 in Parliament. This prohibits *all* commercial surrogacy arrangements but permits a limited form of altruistic arrangements. The outcome won't be known until this book has gone to press. Despite this major development, this chapter has largely retained the present tense to denote the state of affairs at the time when the CSR studies were carried out.

References

Bhandari P (2008) 'Identity' for Little Manji. *The Times of India*, 18 October. <http://timesofindia.indiatimes.com/city/jaipur/Identity-for-little-Manji/articleshow/3610725.cms>

Bhalla N and Thapliyal M (2013) India seeks to regulate its booming 'rent-a-womb industry'. *Reuters*, 30 September. <http://www.reuters.com/article/us-india-surrogates-idUSBRE98T07F20130930>

Chinai R and Goswami R (2007) Medical visas mark growth of Indian medical tourism. *Bulletin* of the World Health Organization 85(3): 164–5. <www.ncbi.nlm.nih.gov/pmc/articles/PMC2636228>

CSR (2014) *Report of the National Conference on 'A Policy Dialogue on Issues around Surrogacy in India'*. Delhi: Centre for Social Research. <https://drive.google.com/file/d/0B-flXIdglJC_ZmIsZXQwY3VvcW8/view>

Hindustan Times (2008) Surrogate baby born in India arrives in Japan. 3 November. <www.hindustantimes.com/world/surrogate-baby-born-in-india-arrives-in-japan/story-cIfjpEmKMowORsHNmwG7CP.html>

Insight (2006) Outsourcing to Indian surrogate mothers. CNN television broadcast, 17 October. <http://transcripts.cnn.com/TRANSCRIPTS/0610/17/i_ins.01.html>

Lal N (2008) A labour of love. *Khaleej Times*, 29 February. <www.khaleejtimes.com/DisplayArticle.asp?xfile=data/weekend/2008/February/weekendFebruary 116.xml&section=weekend&col=>

Mulay S and Gibson E (2006) Marketing of assisted human reproduction and the Indian state. *Development* 49(4): 84–93.

Niazi S (2007) Surrogacy boom. 14 October. <www.boloji.com/index.cfm?md=Content&sd=Articles&ArticleID=3056>

Pande A (2014) *Wombs in Labor: Transnational Surrogacy in India*. New York: Columbia University Press.

Points K (2009) *Commercial Surrogacy and Fertility Tourism in India: The Case of Baby Manji*. Durham, NC: Kenan Institute for Ethics at Duke University. <https://web.duke.edu/kenanethics/casestudies/babymanji.pdf>

Ramachandran S (2006) India's new outsourcing business – wombs. *Asia Times online*, 16 June. <www.atimes.com/atimes/southasia/hf16df03.html>

Ramesh R (2006) British couples desperate for children travel to India in search of surrogates. *Guardian*, 20 March. <www.theguardian.com/world/2006/mar/20/health.topstories3>

Sharma A (2008) Centre drafting surrogacy legislation. *The Times of India*, 9 August. <http://iaac.ca/en/commercial-surrogacy-in-india-exploitation-or-mutual-assistance-4>

The Times of India (2008) Identity certificate issued to surrogate Japanese baby. 17 October. <http://timesofindia.indiatimes.com/city/jaipur/Identity-certificate-issued-to-surrogate-Japanese-baby/articleshow/3609530.cms>

14 | SURROGACY IN MEXICO

Isabel Fulda and Regina Tamés (GIRE)

GIRE (Grupo de Información en Reproducción Elegida) is a non-profit, non-governmental organization founded in 1991 with the mission to promote and defend women's reproductive rights in Mexico, within the context of human rights. Our work is focused on promoting legal reform and changes in public policy that increase and guarantee access to reproductive health services and the exercising of reproductive rights. *GIRE* incorporated assisted reproduction, including surrogacy, into its list of priority issues in 2011 and has worked with legislators, lawyers in the field, reporters, surrogates and people involved in the practice of surrogacy ever since. See gire.org.mx for more information.

Surrogacy as a human rights issue

Among Assisted Reproductive Technologies (ARTs), surrogacy poses particularly difficult challenges as it involves a variety of controversial issues that remain unresolved from both a feminist and a human rights perspective. Moreover, the increasing number of people entering into surrogacy arrangements all over the world has led to complex theoretical and political discussions concerning issues such as the rights of the parties involved, the elements that should confirm informed consent, the rules surrounding parenthood and the international legal framework needed to respond to this global practice. In this regard, regulation of ARTS becomes crucial as a gender and human rights issue.

In November 2012, the Inter-American Court of Human Rights (I/A Court HR) pronounced its first ruling regarding ARTs: *Artavia Murillo et al. (In vitro fertilization) v. Costa Rica*. The case involved the Costa Rican Supreme Court, which in 2000 had declared in vitro fertilization (IVF) unconstitutional, arguing that it jeopardized 'the life and dignity of the human being'. The case was originally presented to the Inter-American System by nine infertile couples who, due to the ban, had not been able to undergo ART treatment. In its ruling, the I/A Court HR considered the Supreme Court's decision an arbitrary interference on the rights to privacy and family life. Furthermore, it established that this ban constituted a form of discrimination against infertile people in Costa Rica, as it impeded their access to a treatment that would have remedied their disadvantageous situation in relation to fertile couples, namely the possibility of having biological children.

The Court established Costa Rica's obligation to adopt measures that would overturn the prohibition of IVF and allow access to it without discrimination, as well as to establish quality control and inspection systems of professionals and institutions qualified to perform ARTs. Although it does not directly address the issue of surrogacy, this case represents a critical step towards the recognition of reproductive rights in Latin America and introduces crucial precedents, such as the acknowledgement that embryos should not be given legal personhood and that the protection of prenatal life requires protecting women's health. In Mexico, *Artavia Murrillo v. Costa Rica* is particularly important, as the rulings from the I/A Court HR oblige judges to interpret domestic cases in accordance with the principles presented in such cases.

ARTs in Mexico

Surrogacy arrangements became increasingly frequent in Mexico over the past decade, making the country a common destination for people seeking to become parents this way. According to Mexico's General Health Law, the sanitary regulation of organs, tissues and cells of which ARTs are part is a matter of federal jurisdiction. However, what is rarely known by people who travel here for surrogacy is that Mexico does not have any kind of federal regulation regarding ARTs in general, and the minimal framework concerning surrogacy that exists in certain states leaves many questions open to interpretation.

In the current situation, important issues such as the number of eggs transferred in an IVF procedure, donor confidentiality and the disposal of unused gametes or eggs remain undefined. This has allowed for the appearance of all types of arbitrary practices by private and public clinics alike. Moreover, it enables hospitals and clinics that provide ARTs to establish their own criteria for entry to their programmes, which leads to discriminatory practices against those seeking assisted reproduction services. GIRE has documented the various requirements stipulated by public hospitals and clinics that offer ART services in Mexico. These range from limiting them to married, heterosexual couples, to establishing a maximum number of previous children in order to apply for treatment. In the specific case of the Centro Medico Nacional 20 de Noviembre, one of Mexico's most important public hospitals, GIRE has challenged these criteria through the use of strategic litigation.[1]

In an attempt to regulate ARTs at the federal level, several legislators have submitted bills to both the Senate and the House of Representatives but none has been approved to date. Of significant concern is the fact that the majority of them look to regulate ARTs based on the two above criteria that violate the human rights protected by the Mexican Constitution and incorporate concepts contrary to medical science (GIRE, 2015). Simultaneously, several local congresses have introduced provisions regarding ARTs at state level. Some are related to the civil aspects of these techniques that pertain to local jurisdiction, such as the filiation of children born through surrogacy. Others, however, have included medical aspects of assisted reproduction in their civil legislations – provisions that do not correspond to the scope of powers of civil or family codes in Mexico and represent an infringement of federal jurisdiction in matters of general health.

Surely, a comprehensive surrogacy framework would imply aspects that go beyond the purely civil side of this practice and thus, local civil regulations would not be sufficient to provide thorough protection to all the parties involved. Nonetheless, state regulations should not interfere with federal jurisdiction on general health matters and, ideally, local and federal legislators need to work together to develop a comprehensive framework on the subject, as well as consult with experts to ensure that the regulation is compatible with science and human rights.

Surrogacy legislation in Mexico

To date, two Mexican states, Tabasco and Sinaloa, have introduced the question of surrogacy into their civil legislation.[2] Two more, Coahuila and Queretaro, have included articles in their Civil Codes that expressly disclaim any surrogacy agreement; they stipulate that the surrogate will always be presumed to be the mother of the child and that no agreement to the contrary will be acknowledged. This means that of Mexico's thirty-two states, two have explicitly recognized surrogacy arrangements and have formulated legislation accordingly and two expressly prohibit it. In the remaining twenty-eight states, where there is no mention of surrogacy in their normative framework, the practice is neither allowed nor prohibited. However, Mexican civil law generally recognizes the woman who gives birth as the child's mother and her husband, if she has one, as the father, which would lead to legal uncertainty in surrogacy cases performed outside the two states that regulate it.

Tabasco In Tabasco, the 1997 Civil Code sets forth strict stipulations regarding the filiation of children born through surrogacy based on the distinction between a 'gestational surrogate mother' who doesn't use her own eggs and therefore has no genetic link to the child, and a 'surrogate mother' who becomes pregnant for a commissioning couple or person using her own eggs. In the first case, the Code establishes that once they have produced a notarized copy of the surrogacy agreement before the Civil Registry, the intended parent(s) and not the surrogate will be the presumed parents of the child. In the second scenario, known as traditional surrogacy, the woman who gives birth using her own eggs is presumed to be the legitimate mother and only the process of full adoption can transfer filiation to the intended parent(s).[3]

Tabasco's regulation is minimal and leaves important issues, such as how much surrogates are paid, vague and open to interpretation.[4] Furthermore, it does not include provisions for cases where one of the parties changes their mind or when the pregnancy threatens the life of the surrogate, or any other health and legal protection for surrogates, intended parent(s) or children.

In December 2015, a bill was approved by Tabasco's Congress that restricts surrogacy to Mexicans. This bill is intended to limit the current international surrogacy boom in the state and respond to some of the public and media pressures to further regulate the practice locally. However, it introduces discriminatory criteria, for example restricting access to these arrangements to married heterosexual couples. The bill was published in January 2016, making it an official law in force. However, implementation of the law has yet to be seen and analysed since there is an open question as to what will happen with the current agencies and clinics that have been performing these services, especially those which direct their services specifically to international, gay and single intended parents. Given the flourishing surrogacy industry in operation at the time of writing, approval of these restrictions might well lead to the creation of a clandestine market in international surrogacy in Mexico that would leave surrogates, intended parent(s) and children even more vulnerable than they were before.

Sinaloa Unlike Tabasco, the regulation in Sinaloa is much more comprehensive and, in addition to the filiation of children born through surrogacy arrangements, includes issues related to health protections for surrogates, the obligations of intended parent(s), payments and even penal sanctions in case provisions are not followed. In principle, this more comprehensive regulation is desirable in terms of giving certainty to the parties involved and preventing abuses, particularly for surrogates.

However, some of the articles included in this framework interfere with federal jurisdiction to regulate general health matters concerning ARTs. Furthermore, the Code establishes that only Mexican couples can have access to such agreements and assumes that these couples will constitute a man and a woman, thus introducing implicit discrimination against both same-sex couples and single individuals. The few years during which this legislation has been in effect and the fact that international surrogacy is not permitted in the state have until recently limited the numbers of national and international surrogacy agencies in Sinaloa and not attracted significant media attention.

Surrogacy practices in Mexico

As there are no available public data regarding the number of children born through surrogacy agreements in Mexico, GIRE submitted information requests[5] to the Tabasco and Sinaloa Registry Offices. In Tabasco, the Civil Registry responded that five children born from traditional surrogate mothers have been registered since 1997. However, owing to privacy concerns for the children involved, there was no record of children born via gestational surrogacy.[6] In contrast, an interview with a surrogacy clinic lawyer revealed that in the previous month that clinic alone had facilitated fifteen surrogacy births. A member of staff from another clinic based in Cancun claimed to have witnessed at least fifty such births in the last year.

Protecting children's privacy may entail that there is no explicit mention of the surrogacy arrangements on their birth certificates, but this should not prevent the Civil Registry from having an internal registry of cases, thereby protecting the privacy of the parties and allowing the scope of the phenomenon to be noted. At present, the Mexican state does not know how many women have hired out their wombs for surrogacy procedures in Tabasco, how many foreign or Mexican couples or single persons have signed a contract of this kind and under what conditions these have occurred.[7]

The situation of surrogates The asymmetrical conditions of power in which surrogates enter into these types of agreements are of important concern for feminists and human rights advocates. Mexico's context of economic and social inequality cannot be ignored when discussing access to ARTs and surrogacy in particular. Although most women who become surrogates in Mexico do not come from a background of extreme economic poverty, they tend to be single mothers who, at the very least, are significantly less privileged than their intended parent(s) counterparts. Some come from other regions of Latin America and have migrated to Mexico in search of better opportunities; others have fled from the violence in other parts of the country, such as Guerrero. This does not negate their capacity as agents to decide over their own bodies and reproduction, but needs to be taken into account to understand the context in which they agree to become surrogates, the potential for abuses and the elements of informed consent that must be assured if these agreements are to take place.

Undoubtedly, a mere formal contract agreed to by signing a document is not enough to establish informed consent. For this, surrogates should have access to truthful, objective, impartial and unprejudiced information regarding the medical procedures involved as well as the legal implications of the contract.[8] The terms should be expressed in adequate and comprehensible language and signed without pressure or coercion (International Federation of Gynecology and Obstetrics, 2012: 317). To that effect, the parties to a surrogacy agreement must genuinely understand the risks they are running and their consequences, as well as the protection to which they are entitled should anything go wrong.

Yet, the experiences that some surrogates – as well clinical or agency staff – have shared with GIRE show that, in practice, informed consent is rarely respected and guaranteed.[9] In general, the surrogates we spoke to were only vaguely familiar with their contracts, the common practice being that a lawyer, hired by the agency and paid for by the intended parent(s), briefly explains the contents without necessarily ensuring that she has thoroughly understood it or giving her the option to negotiate certain clauses. This situation makes surrogates particularly vulnerable, as they have no independent legal counsel to represent their interests and no say in the clauses determined in the contract. This is illustrated by a surrogate interviewed by GIRE who reported being told by the lawyer: 'You have to obey the doctors. If you don't like it, don't sign.' This indicates the lack of influence women have in regards to the content of the contract, as well as the perception that the decisions and voices of surrogates will not be heard prior to a medical opinion.

According to current legislation in Tabasco, surrogacy contracts have to be signed in the presence of a public notary who attests to their validity. Although this is meant to act as a filter to protect the parties in the surrogacy contract, notarizing an agreement does not ensure informed consent. Unlike judges, public notaries are not accountable public servants and their services are costly. As these costs are generally covered by the intended parent(s), there is a conflict of interest for the notary that can become problematic and impede their role as a protective mechanism equally for all parties. In addition to the absence of legal counsel for surrogates, this leaves them in a particularly vulnerable position in relation to both intended parent(s) and agencies.

By interviewing several surrogates in Tabasco, Cancun and Mexico City, GIRE has documented the lack of clarity and complete information regarding the obligations and responsibilities to which surrogates agree when they sign an agreement of this type.[10] Such was the case of Maria,[11] a woman who lives in a surrogacy home in Tabasco.

> Maria is getting ready for her second embryo transfer after an unsuccessful one a couple of months ago. She was given a copy of the surrogacy contract she signed with the agency, which owns the house she now lives in with her five-year-old son, but nobody has taken the time to talk her through it and she has seen the agency's lawyer only once. For assurance, she sent her copy of the contract to her partner, a systems engineer who lives in Guerrero, on the other side of the country. She still has many questions, but nobody seems to be interested in answering them. The only documents she has with her are the loose papers that are posted by agency staff on the house's refrigerator to remind surrogates of their duties towards the agency and the intended parent(s).
>
> In addition, Maria related to GIRE that since signing the original contract a few weeks before the interview, she has decided to 'exchange' intended parents with Carmen, another surrogate in the home because one of the intended parents with whom Carmen signed is HIV positive. Unlike her friend, Maria trusts that the sperm that will be used for the transfer will be cleansed at the clinic prior to IVF, even though no one has explained to her how this works. Maria and Carmen informed the agency that they decided to exchange couples and the transfer is programmed to take place in a few weeks. However, she signed a contract with the

previous couple and she has no idea if she will be given a new one to sign before the procedure. From a legal standpoint, both Maria and the intended parents are in a significantly uncertain legal situation if this happens.

In another interview conducted by GIRE, staff from an agency in Tabasco emphasized the importance of careful and comprehensive matching between surrogates and intended parent(s) before any medical procedure or the contract is signed. According to them, this process takes at least seven months. During this period, the staff make sure that the surrogates, as well as their close relatives, understand the risks and implications of signing the contract and encourage them to form relationships with the intended parent(s). Once the contract is signed and the pregnancy begins, the surrogates stay in their homes for the duration of the process. (Unlike with some agencies they are not taken to a surrogacy house.) Certainly, good practice can exist in surrogacy arrangements whereby women are respected, protection of their life and health are ensured, and legal procedures are performed according to the law. However, the current framework lends itself to other types of practice and ultimately leaves the agencies and clinics to self-regulate, giving way to situations where problems occur.

The debate around surrogacy has centred on analysing whether women can decide to carry a pregnancy for other people with or without monetary compensation and, as previously mentioned, this aspect remains ambiguous in Tabasco's legislation. Furthermore, there is a common perception among people who take part in surrogacy in Mexico that women who sign such agreements 'give up' their ability to make decisions about their own bodies, including pregnancy termination and the conditions of birth. Some of the surrogacy contracts that GIRE has reviewed state that surrogates will not terminate their pregnancies even when they jeopardize their life – which would amount to a legal abortion in the state of Tabasco. Others establish that intended parent(s) will get to decide whether they want the surrogate to terminate a pregnancy in cases of fetal malformations, a practice that would constitute forced abortion and is penalized by law.

Some contracts lay down such provisions as the surrogate's obligation to follow a specific diet or refrain from having sexual intercourse for a given period or during the whole pregnancy. In other cases, although some of their obligations are not in writing, the surrogates' living arrangements constitute an important form of control over their bodies and activities: food at surrogacy homes is purchased and administered by home staff, visitors are not allowed and times to leave the house are prearranged.

Lastly, surrogates in Mexico face violations to their rights to privacy and health, which are widespread for pregnant women in the country but are made worse by the women's legal and economic situation in relation to agencies, clinics and intended parent(s). Fieldwork conducted by GIRE reveals that most children born under surrogacy agreements in Mexico are delivered by caesarean section, based on a concern for the preferences and comfort of intended parent(s), who can better plan their trip to the country and the state if the birth date has been established. This arrangement does not take into account the surrogate's wishes surrounding birth or the greater risk that caesarean sections entail to the surrogate's life and health. In fact, the rate of such births in Mexico (10–15 per cent) is significantly higher than that recommended by the World Health Organization (WHO, 2010). In 2012, of all the births occurring at public health institutions in Mexico, more than 50 per cent were caesareans; in the case of private hospitals, where surrogate births generally take place, this percentage increases.[12] Thus, although the number of unjustified c-sections is not the result of surrogacy agreements alone, it does worsen the situation of the already vulnerable surrogates and violates their right to privacy and health.

Arely's is a case in point. She was a surrogate in Quintana Roo, where her pregnancy jeopardized her health and life.

> Born in Colombia, Arely arrived in Mexico City in 2012 to rejoin members of her family living there. After unsuccessfully trying to find a job, a friend told her about the possibility of becoming a surrogate with an international agency in Cancun, in the state of Quintana Roo. After much thought, she finally agreed to it. She went to an assisted reproduction clinic in Mexico City to undergo IVF and a few weeks later, travelled to Cancun to live in a surrogacy home. She never signed a contract but was promised she would receive US$1000 upon confirmation of the pregnancy and 10,000 pesos (roughly US$600) monthly for every month of gestation.
>
> At the beginning, Arely lived comfortably in the home and made some friends. Soon she found out that she was carrying twins. Five months on, she began to experience discomfort but she never received help or a medical check-up. It was only when

her condition seriously deteriorated that she was taken to see a doctor, where she was informed that the fetuses had been dead in her uterus for more than a week. The next day, she was sent back to Mexico City.

She was not paid the agreed amount during the months she lived in the home and did not receive follow-up health care. Currently, she cannot even access her medical file and does not know if she will ever be able to get pregnant again. As she did not sign a contract whereby she could have demanded that the agency she contacted fulfil its obligations, she has no proof that she ever participated in a surrogacy arrangement.

The number of national and international surrogacy agencies and clinics that operate in the country is steadily increasing.[13] Although an important number of them are based in Villahermosa, the capital of Tabasco, many others have been established in cities outside the state, mainly Cancun, Mexico City and Puerto Vallarta. The agencies set up elsewhere benefit from the ambiguity in the law by which only the birth has to occur in Tabasco in order for it to be recognized as a surrogacy arrangement. Hence, it is common practice to carry out the contract, embryo transfer and pregnancy in another city and then transport surrogates to Tabasco a few months – or even weeks – before the birth. This, of course, poses several health and legal risks and, in addition to the absence of a comprehensive normative framework around surrogacy and the economic and social conditions of surrogates in relation to intended parent(s), can give way to various problems and human rights violations for all the parties involved. Arely's story is terrifying but not surprising given the total lack of protection to women in Cancun, where surrogacy is commonly practised.

Situation of intended parents and children born through surrogacy Even though most problems arising from surrogacy in Mexico impact surrogates, intended parent(s) and children born through surrogacy arrangements are also affected by the lack of an adequate regulatory framework and the problematic practices this enables. The main recurring problem faced by intended parent(s) is the difficulty of obtaining both birth certificates and passports for the children.

Tabasco's Civil Code stipulates that if intended parent(s) present a notarized surrogacy contract to the Civil Registry following the birth they will be recorded as the child's parents on the birth certificate, which should be produced diligently by this office. However, in practice, arbitrary obstacles have been placed in the way of obtaining these documents. Birth certificates used by the Registry Office in the state of Tabasco and in most other states (in spite of local legislation that recognizes same-sex marriage and adoption as well as precedents by the Mexican Supreme Court regarding non-discrimination based on sexual orientation) continue to include fields only for a mother and a father. Thus, other types of families, particularly single men or same-sex couples, are faced with public officials who refuse to fill out these forms, especially if no woman is to be attested as mother of the child.

According to agency staff and lawyers involved in surrogacy in Tabasco, in the last two years the length of time in which a birth certificate is issued, once all the documents required by law have been submitted to the Civil Registry, has increased greatly, sometimes taking twice as long. Rather than the expected two days, some parents have had to wait up to two months. In response, the common practice related to GIRE in interviews with both surrogates and intended parent(s) seems to be to include the surrogate as mother on the birth certificate (even though she and the baby share no genetic tie) and, later, to establish a process whereby she renounces maternity in favour of the intended parent(s). However, this imposes legal risks on all parties, including the child, and is in no way ideal for anyone.

After successfully obtaining a birth certificate, the next obstacle commonly faced by intended parent(s) becomes procuring a passport for the child, without which they cannot leave the country. Unlike birth certificates, which are issued by local offices and in cases of surrogacy pertain to the Civil Registry of Tabasco, providing passports is the responsibility of the Ministry of Foreign Affairs, a federal institution. Hence, cases have been documented whereby the Ministry has denied passports to the children of male couples, arguing that a woman always has to appear on the birth certificate, and instigating investigations for child trafficking. While protections against child trafficking are paramount, both at local and federal levels, the Foreign Ministry's failure to recognize the existence of legal surrogacy agreements in the state of Tabasco has resulted in discriminatory practices that not only affect intended parent(s), but most importantly leave children born through surrogacy arrangements in legal limbo. Jorge and Esteban's case illustrate this problem.

> Jorge and Esteban met in Madrid. After living together for
> many years, they married and then decided to have children.

They investigated the places offering surrogacy services, the requirements and the costs entailed. They looked for an affordable option that would provide the service to same-sex couples and respect the rights of the surrogates. They chose a clinic in Tabasco and signed a surrogacy agreement with Mercedes, a single mother from the locality. With Jorge's genetic material and a donor's egg, an IVF procedure was performed.

Mercedes had an uncomplicated pregnancy. After the birth, the baby was registered only as Jorge's son. According to the lawyer who advised them, this was easier than trying to have their same-sex marriage recognized in the state of Tabasco. Since the passport office in Villahermosa was closed for the holidays, the couple travelled to Mexico City with the birth certificate, a copy of the surrogacy agreement, and a letter from the hospital to obtain the baby's passport. In the passport office they were told that the passport could not be issued because the birth certificate did not include the mother's name. The officer concerned even suggested that they invent and enter one in the appropriate field to solve the problem but they refused. A few weeks later, the couple travelled back to Tabasco to request the passport, only to be told by the presiding officer that she disagreed with surrogacy and would refuse to help them. She said that, instead, they should abandon their baby in Mexico and return to their country. Esteban flew back to Madrid alone and Jorge lost his job while he remained in Mexico with the baby. Seven months later, they were able to obtain a passport and travel back to Spain.

This case demonstrates the serious problems that emerge when surrogacy regulations do not adequately protect all the parties involved and, particularly, how children born under such agreements can be left without any legal security. The international human rights framework regarding children's rights encapsulated by the United Nations Convention on the Rights of the Child (1989) emphasizes the importance of considering the best interests of the child. In surrogacy cases, this would mean assuring that children born through these types of agreements are able to obtain legal documents that recognize their filiation and nationality. The recent cases presided over by the European Court of Human Rights in *Mennesson v. France* and *Labassee v. France* are a case in point: failure to recognize parenthood in surrogacy arrangements is a violation of children's rights. Given that surrogacy contracts are recognized in certain normative frameworks in

Mexico, administrative procedures must adapt to these requirements and federal institutions respond accordingly.

Final remarks

Without doubt, surrogacy is a complex issue and its importance in international discussions on reproductive rights will continue to grow. In Mexico, absence of federal regulation in relation to ARTs leads to legal uncertainty for the parties involved and opens the door for arbitrary acts and discrimination against those seeking assisted reproductive services. The minimal regulation surrounding surrogacy in the country is not adequate to respond to the increasing numbers of people travelling to Mexico to engage in surrogacy agreements. Thus, a federal sanitary regulation of ARTs as well as a comprehensive framework on the civil aspects of surrogacy seem necessary in order to prevent human rights violations against the parties involved. In the meantime, surrogacy will continue to be practised mostly without supervision, giving rise to serious problems, particularly for surrogates who, in the current situation, are most vulnerable to abuses.

Notes

1 For more information regarding this case, as well as the requirements for obtaining public ART services in Mexico, see GIRE (2015).

2 A number of bills have been presented in other states with this same aim, as is the case of Coahuila, Guerrero and Mexico City, but none are in effect. In the case of Mexico City, the Legislative Assembly passed the Surrogacy Law on 30 November 2010; the law, however, has not been published and is currently not in effect.

3 This fact and the obstacles to adoption in Mexico, especially for single persons and same-sex couples are, according to an interviewee, the main reasons why surrogacy clinics and agencies prefer gestational surrogacy and rarely establish agreements that include using the surrogate's eggs.

4 The Civil Code as such makes no mention of payment to surrogates. However, a common perception exists that paid surrogacy is illegal in the state of Tabasco and that only altruistic surrogacy is permitted (although in practice, surrogates are paid for their services in hidden contracts which are not shown to the public notary). This interpretation is based solely on an article in the General Health Law prohibiting the sale of bodily organs, which some interpret as analogous to the practice of surrogacy. However, the truth remains that current legislation does not address the issue of payment to surrogates and it is left as a matter open to interpretation.

5 Information requests are a legal practice whereby individuals can request public information that is not widely available but that public officials have an obligation to respond to in a limited amount of time.

6 Government of the State of Tabasco, General Direction of Civil Registry, System for Access to Public Information: Infomex. File 06560814.

7 In the case of Sinaloa, the Registry Office responded by saying it had no record of any child born through a

surrogate agreement since the Family Code was published in 2013. To a certain extent, this can be explained by the short time the Code has been in effect as well as the restrictions imposed on same-sex couples and non-Mexicans, which seriously limit the scope of the practice.

8 See *AS v. Hungary*, where the CEDAW Committee indicates what should be understood by informed consent, especially in the area of reproductive health. <http://bit.ly/1RXe4Xq>.

9 The information that GIRE has been able to obtain by performing fieldwork interviews as an advocacy group has been limited by the availability and willingness of the parties, particularly surrogates, to participate in them, given the highly stigmatized and legally ambiguous status of surrogacy in Mexico. Although access to these testimonies is limited and often difficult, we believe the experiences we were able to obtain are most useful in shedding light on an area that has been little explored in Mexico and whose practices cannot be uncovered without first-hand testimonies from surrogates themselves. Some surrogates' contacts were provided by agencies themselves, others through academics, reporters and organizations with whom GIRE has contact.

10 Information that GIRE has been able to obtain via fieldwork.

11 All the names have been changed in order to protect the privacy of those involved.

12 See graph created by GIRE (2015).

13 As the legislation regarding surrogacy in Tabasco is not new, this recent significant expansion of the surrogacy industry has been attributed to many factors, among which the recent restrictions in Indian surrogacy legislation stand out.

References

GIRE (2015) *Women and Girls without Justice: Reproductive Rights in Mexico*. <http://informe2015.gire.org.mx/en/#/Home>

International Federation of Gynecology and Obstetrics (FIGO) (2012) *Recommendations on Ethical Issues in Obstetrics and Gynecology by the FIGO Committee for the Ethical Aspects of Human Reproduction and Women's Health*. London: FIGO. In English, French and Spanish: <www.figo.org/sites/default/files/uploads/wg-publications/ethics/FIGO%20Ethical%20Issues%202015.pdf4893.pdf>

WHO (2010) *The Global Numbers and Costs of Additionally Needed and Unnecessary Caesarean Sections Performed per Year: Overuse as a Barrier to Universal Coverage*. World Health Report, Background Paper 30. <www.who.int/healthsystems/topics/financing/healthreport/30Csectioncosts.pdf>

15 | A REPRODUCTIVE JUSTICE ANALYSIS OF GENETIC TECHNOLOGIES: REPORT OF A NATIONAL CONVENING OF WOMEN OF COLOUR AND INDIGENOUS WOMEN

Generations Ahead

Generations Ahead was founded in 2008 with the aim of building a multi-movement coalition to address the ways in which new genetic technologies affect women, people of colour, people with disabilities and the LGBTQI community. During the four years in which it operated (up to 31 January 2012), the organization used a comprehensive social justice framework to increase awareness and activism on concerns related to assisted reproductive technologies (ARTs), prenatal genetic screening, egg and sperm donation, surrogacy, DNA forensic databases, sex selection, personalized genomic medicine, genetic trait selection and race-based medical therapies. This work took the form of organizational briefings, conference presentations, white papers and public events that reached upwards of 2,000 leaders, advocates and activists. Generations Ahead also convened a number of meetings designed to foster dialogue among different groups.

One such initiative, in September 2008, gathered together women of colour and Indigenous women leaders from across the US to share and discuss their diverse viewpoints on reproductive genetic technologies. This chapter is an edited version of the report of that meeting, reproduced with kind permission from Sujatha Jesudason, former Executive Director of Generations Ahead.[1]

Introduction

Reproductive and genetic technologies are critical social justice issues that can have lasting effects on how individual identity, family relations and community connections are defined. Many of these technologies offer enormous potential for treating infertility and allowing women and men, who in the past were not able to have biologically related children, to do so. At the same time, these very technologies can be used in ways that are potentially harmful to some groups of people, particularly communities with the least amount of power and resources.

Given the numerous ways in which structural inequality and racism shape the reproductive decisions of all women, many advocates are concerned either that women of colour and Indigenous women will be systematically excluded from the benefits of ARTs, or that these technologies may be used to 'design' babies, further deepening racial bias against certain physical features. The voices, values and perspectives of women of colour and Indigenous women are not only critical for a robust public debate, but also to ensure that the many uses of genetic technologies benefit all women, their families and communities, without causing harm or deepening existing social inequalities.

To include the leadership and voices of those historically marginalized in reproductive health and rights debates, Generations Ahead convened a group of twenty-one women of colour and Indigenous women leaders from across the US for two days in September 2008. The convening, in Philadelphia, was co-sponsored by seven reproductive rights and justice organizations: Asian Communities for Reproductive Justice, Black Women's Health Imperative, California Latinas for Reproductive Justice, Indigenous Peoples Council on Biocolonialism, National Asian Pacific American Women's Forum, National Latina Institute for Reproductive Health, and SisterSong Women of Color Reproductive Health Collective. The majority of leaders in the reproductive justice movement were present, as well as four leaders from the Indigenous peoples' rights movement. In this new millennium, when technologies are being offered faster than policy-makers and the average citizen can keep up, this group began a discussion about the social and ethical implications of using these technologies from the perspective of affirming the value of all human beings, all types of families and a diverse range of communities. This report documents the core of that discussion.

Need for the convening In the four years of its existence, Generations Ahead found that the groups represented express unique concerns about the relationships between genetic technologies and their communities. Among these concerns are:

- higher rates of infertility among women of colour but less access to reproductive technologies;
- government attempts to control the reproductive rights of women of colour and Indigenous women;

- the potential for eugenic applications of the technologies to breed 'better' babies;
- the impact of genetic research on Indigenous peoples' cultural responsibilities and values;
- concern about the impact of biotechnologies on whole communities – not just women – and consequences for future generations;
- the resurgence of scientific racism and accompanying 'geneticization' of social and environmental problems;
- targeted advertisements for sex selection in Asian immigrant communities.

In previous conversations these women leaders often spoke of the diversity of histories, experiences and perspectives among the groups they represent. These histories can lead to varying experiences with genetic technologies. The differences between African American, Latina, Asian and Indigenous groups are further complicated by factors such as class, ability, sexual orientation, gender identity, age, geography and immigration status. This convening was deliberately designed to provide participants with the opportunity to share these distinctive and diverse perspectives and learn about each other's experiences.

In addition, Generations Ahead wanted to use a reproductive justice methodology and perspective to document a different approach to genetic technologies. This starts with the voices of those from historically less powerful groups, who have the potential to be the most adversely affected by these technologies. A traditional *reproductive rights* framework is grounded in a civil rights model and relies primarily on legal and legislative strategies. It also tends to prioritize freedom of choice traditionally associated with the legal right to abortion. *Reproductive justice*, on the other hand, uses an intersectional analysis that recognizes the multiple factors that impact people's lives. It contextualizes reproductive choices and decisions by including the intersecting economic, social and political forces that shape the lives of women, their families and their communities. In contrast to the traditional strategies used by the reproductive rights movement, reproductive justice organizing centralizes the voices and concerns of marginalized communities, particularly women of colour and low-income women. It goes beyond securing abortion rights to advocate for a more comprehensive agenda.

By the end of the two days the participants had generated a specific analysis and distinct set of values to guide the development and use of genetic and reproductive technologies. These values form the beginning of an alternative framework based on notions of collective human dignity rather than the individual right to privacy and profit, the valuing of all human beings, respect for all types of families and all communities, and decision-making by those most affected.

Section 1 of this report articulates the unique impact genetic technologies have on different communities and the particular perspective each group brings to their analysis of them. Section 2 documents some of the discussion about specific technologies with examples from three of five case studies. Section 3 summarizes the group's recommendations for next steps, and section 4 gives a concrete example of how this work of identifying shared values and principles was translated into concrete policy advocacy.

1. Genetic technologies in different communities

To identify and acknowledge the different ways in which genetic technologies benefit and raise concerns in different communities, participants were asked to divide themselves into constituency-specific affinity groups from the beginning. This resulted in five groups: Indigenous women, Asian women, women of African descent, women with disabilities and Latinas in the US.

Indigenous women While most of the participants were somewhat aware of the effects of genetic technologies on Asians, Latinas and African American women, few knew anything about their impact on Indigenous peoples. The only formal presentation was on the relationship between Indigenous peoples and biotechnologies, which was new to most of the women of colour in the room.

The Indigenous women explained three terms that define this relationship: *bio-colonialism* is a new form of colonization affecting Indigenous peoples that imposes foreign belief and legal systems and attempts to claim ownership over biological and genetic material; *bio-prospecting* is the search for potentially profitable or useful genetic resources, including human, plant, animal, micro-organisms and associated traditional knowledge; and *bio-piracy* is the theft of genetic resources and associated traditional knowledge. They described experiences of exploitative and/or unethical research on Indigenous peoples in the areas of medical, behavioural and anthropological genetics. Through these various examples, they identified the following common problems:

- the assumption of open access to Indigenous communities by researchers;
- top-down and outside-in approaches to research in Indigenous communities, rather than working with them and leaders on community research priorities;
- Indigenous peoples bearing the risks but rarely, if ever, having access to the benefits of the research;
- researchers making false promises of economic and non-economic benefit sharing with Indigenous communities;
- lack of informed consent, particularly from tribal leaders for research done within the community;
- widespread secondary uses of samples without additional consent;
- unwillingness by researchers to repatriate misappropriated genetic material.

Based on these experiences, the group explained that they had more concerns than confidence in the benefits of genetic technologies. They declared that the scientific framework underpinning their development is based on 'an ideology of progress' and undermines Indigenous peoples' self-determination and sovereignty. The move towards industrializing childbirth and women's reproduction fails to recognize women as the 'first environment' and amounts to manipulating the natural process of reproduction. The group asserted that genes are not the cause of problems, so genetics is not the solution.

These women stated that the full effects of genetic and reproductive technologies are unknown and therefore need further discussion among Indigenous peoples. They pointed to the technologies as intentional genocidal practices, undermining tribal sovereignty, manipulating life and affirming ownership of sacred property. They shared how scientific knowledge rejects and denies the existence of many other ways of knowing, including Indigenous creation histories and tribal stories of belonging and migration. Genetic ancestry testing can also be used to undermine tribal rights to determine community membership and sovereignty for Indigenous Nations by shifting to a biological/genetic definition of citizenship/membership rather than a social, political and cultural definition of community.

Within their framework for addressing bio-colonialism, Indigenous peoples have a comprehensive approach that does not distinguish between human and non-human (plant or animal) genetic technologies. Their cultural perspective is based on sacredness of the body and body parts, respect for life force, guardianship of community and the environment, sacredness of the ancestors and responsibility to future generations.

In their own words:

> We have our own medicines, practices and ceremonies regarding reproduction. These have always been there and we've always used them. The new ways are counter to what we've done.
>
> We are a cultural, social, spiritual and political group, and this makes us different from the groups of women of colour at the convening. Indigenous people are considered nations within a nation (in the US). This is based on a colonial past.
>
> Our rights are collective rights protected in international and national law. Our responsibilities are to the collective; we operate as a collective and not as individuals who can make decisions for the whole group.
>
> Bio-colonialism is part of the ongoing colonization that is happening to all Indigenous people.

The group articulated a comprehensive perspective on community and the connection between plant, animal and land, with stewardship and respect for all life as core values. The recognition of and respect for Indigenous peoples' culturally based values, worldview, cultural responsibilities and customary laws are critical to their perspective on these technologies. The concept of the 'Seventh Generation', which teaches that one must take into consideration the impact of every decision and action on the seventh generation yet to come, was identified as a guiding principle in decision-making related to research, development and utilization of genetic technologies.

Asian women Keenly aware of the high cultural value placed on children and family, the group stated that many Asian women feel pressured to use genetic technologies to have children or certain types of children – primarily sons. While these technologies are sometimes seen as an answer to the pressures of having to bear children, there is, at the same time, shame about having to use fertility treatment as the way to achieve this. Furthermore, the technologies are not socio-economically accessible to all women. They described the ways in which access is constrained by language, culture, ethnicity, immigration status and economics; also how the market for eggs from Asian donors places them on the 'supply side' of the spectrum in troubling ways.

The group highlighted concerns about the ways in which the availability of genetic technologies not only allows but also can promote sex selection. They noted the disproportionate marketing of pre-pregnancy sex selection techniques to Asian communities and in Asian community media. They spoke about the potential for selecting traits such as intelligence and the impact this might have on Asian communities where intelligence is highly prized.

The group recognized international linkages, such as buying and selling reproductive services across borders – surrogacy, reproductive tourism, etc. – and the ways in which cultural norms, such as son preference in home countries, can be carried over to the US.

Finally, the group explained that a respect for science in many Asian communities means that it is often not questioned. In addition:

> Asians are often more accustomed to prioritizing family and community needs in the face of individual needs and rights, which can lead to acceptance of a broader perspective on genetic technologies, or more problematic policies like population control policies and 'one-child' policy in China.

These Asian women highlighted the diversity of perspectives and approaches to health within Asian communities, and suggested that traditional approaches to health and health care should be included in this discussion. They identified a need for disaggregating health data rather than lumping different ethnic communities together. And they discussed the importance of valuing differences in linguistic and cultural practices in health and wellness, along with being mindful of transnational connections and the ways in which cultural practices and values can travel globally.

Women of African descent These African American women decided to identify their group as women of African descent in recognition of the diasporic and mixed race experiences of Black people in the US. They expressed concern about the potential for increased commodification and exploitation of Black women's bodies given the long history of slavery and eugenics in that country. They pointed to trends towards genetic determinism where families, intelligence and inherent value could be based on one's genetics, not on one's humanity. The group explained that the technologies create an environment that equates parenthood with biology and challenges Black women's notions of family and community. Participants emphasized that addressing the high rate of infertility among Black women means focusing on its causes rather than solely on access to the technologies to address or 'fix' it. They also stressed the importance of connections to family, community and nation over seeing oneself individually. Comments included:

> We have a healthy critique of these technologies based on our historical mistrust of the medical establishment and science.
>
> We acknowledge linkages to other racial and ethnic groups: there is a feeling of community and inclusivity.

Women of African descent highlighted that individuals, families and communities should be in a relationship of mutual responsibility. They valued inclusiveness, a commitment to social and structural transformation, and gender equity in addressing concerns raised by genetic technologies.

Women with disabilities Women with disabilities started by pointing out the historical abuses of women with disabilities, including coerced sterilization. They explained how the medical model of disability[2] supports a eugenic outlook and that the increase in genetic testing could lead to more and more people being defined as disabled, accompanied by a mentality of 'personal responsibility' that places the task of living with disability on individuals, absent of any state or community responsibility.

They valued inclusiveness, a commitment to social and structural transformation, and gender equity in addressing concerns raised by genetic technologies. They identified the perspective of the (not possible) 'extinction' of disability as a viewpoint that could encourage declining support for services and resources for people with disabilities, while further devaluing them. The 'benefits' of the technologies are based on a paternalistic paradigm that assumes such people need to be helped and considers certain lives to be expendable.

They connected disability oppression with queer oppression in two ways: the normalization of non-disabled and heterosexual people, and the fact that both disability and queer communities are discouraged from reproducing. They observed a critical need to carefully examine the oppressive language around disability that is used when talking about genetic technologies (e.g. abnormality, fetal anomaly and birth defects). And they reiterated the point made by several other groups, that with these technologies attention shifts to the biological roots of what are really social problems and conditions.

In their words:

> Because many in our community depend on [health care] technology for survival, we hold both contradictions and complexities in our analysis. We can embrace the good in technology without the oppression and ensure that the technology is helpful.
>
> It is hard for people with disabilities, who are political, to be part of the pro-choice and reproductive health community because of the controversial nature of abortion following genetic testing.
>
> We bring a social critique of ableist systems, including a call for alternative institutions and models of support.
>
> We recognize that everyone has to confront disability at some time in their lives.

The group emphasized the importance of critiquing systematic oppression rather than individuals and the importance of using a social model of disability. They affirmed the leadership of people with disabilities in these discussions as providing a critically needed perspective and voice. And they recommended using a justice framework that integrates an ableist analysis to ensure the valuing of all bodies.

Latinas living in the US Latinas spoke about the need to examine their complex relationship to notions of fertility, particularly the myth of the hyper-fertile Latina woman, the lack of information and research about who uses ARTs in the Latino community and how that intersects with class and immigration privilege. They shared anecdotal stories of Latinas who came to the US to be surrogates for other families and were then able to obtain a Green Card, illustrating an intersection between the technologies and immigration. The group discussion focused primarily on how much was still unknown about Latinas' use of these technologies.

Even while they highlighted many values shared by other groups – including the importance of family, parenting, spirituality and community – the group mostly felt that it was just the beginning of this conversation for their community. They wanted a deeper discussion about fertility and family that is grounded in research and current data about community attitudes and uses of reproductive and genetic technologies.

2. Identifying shared values and perspectives

Each group identified specific values and perspectives that the group collectively affirmed as forming a nuanced and comprehensive picture of what is at stake for women of colour and Indigenous women. Through further discussions, everyone then worked to clarify an inclusive list of shared values. These included valuing interdependence and intersectionality with a strong focus on community rather than just the individual. All agreed that family was vital, even as they stated that family was not to be defined by genetics alone but rather by shared lived experiences.

In order to deepen their analysis and refine their perspectives, participants discussed a wide range of genetic technologies. These included prenatal genetic testing, assisted reproduction, race-specific medicine and DNA collection for research and for forensic testing for criminal investigations. In small groups, they examined the ethical and social questions raised in different situations and the particular implications for women of colour and/or Indigenous women, families and communities in five case studies: reproductive tourism; genetic determinism related to the high mortality rates among African American women with breast cancer; research in relation to the Genographic Project; prenatal screening for Down's syndrome; and the use of DNA dragnets[3] for solving crime. Recommendations for how to address the complex issues in the first three of these areas are summarized below.

Reproductive tourism Discussion focused on transnational commercial surrogacy whereby US, European and other overseas citizens hire surrogates in India for a fraction of what it would cost in their home countries. Recommendations:

- Find real solutions to poverty: most Indian surrogates have limited options and surrogacy is not a solution to poverty.
- Protect human rights: surrogacy can create a system of servitude based on the idea that one can purchase a womb. These women can be seen as commodities and intensely monitored in this arrangement for another's benefit.
- Ensure reproductive autonomy: how do we distinguish between informed consent and coercion based on financial need and poverty? Are these women exercising their rights or being exploited?
- Ensure access to health care and social protections against stigmatization for being a surrogate.

- Pay attention to long-term health consequences.
- Recognize the imbalance of money and power: these Indian women are paid less than those who are providing the same service in the US.

Genetic determinism: African American women and breast cancer This refers to the high rates of mortality among African American women with breast cancer even though they have lower incidence of the disease. Recommendations:

- Assess the real benefits of genetic research for marginalized communities by examining the links between environmental toxins and cancer, and the way toxins can cause biological changes in genes that are then explained only as genetic conditions.
- Articulate immediate versus long-term needs and solutions to address health disparities in communities of colour and Indigenous communities.
- Those most impacted must be involved in the process, strategy and solutions.
- Build alliances with environmental health and justice movements locally and nationally.
- The attention to genetics perpetuates the notion that race is biological destiny and an individual's own burden.
- More data and resources are needed to address other theories that explain health disparities other than genetics.

DNA collection for research: the Genographic Project This refers to the National Geographic Society's project to collect DNA samples from 100,000 Indigenous people around the world to study ancient human migration. The group identified the following concerns and advocated a boycott of the Genographic Project. Recommendations:

- The project undermines Indigenous peoples' cultural, social and political approach to identity, community and origins. It promotes the non-Indigenous collection and ownership of oral histories related to creation stories, migration, family histories and languages.
- It treats Indigenous people, their genes and their ancestral remains as historic artefacts to be collected on genetic 'safaris' in the name of honouring them.
- The project was created without community input and buy-in.
- It reinforces corporatization and privatization of genetic research.

The significance of case studies The small group discussions on these topics illuminated the intersections between genetic technologies and a variety of pressing issues: disability oppression; globalization, commodification and exploitation; scientific racism and environmental justice; bio-colonialism; and criminal justice and racial profiling. While some technologies or practices directly affect only one community, their implications can be far-reaching. Bio-colonialism opens the door to genetic exploitation of communities of colour, such as the creation of DNA databases through ancestry testing. Allocating research dollars to determine the genetic link to breast cancer among African American women diverts resources away from addressing environmental impacts on all low-income communities of colour who are most affected by exposure to toxins. Outsourcing surrogacy to women in India may normalize the exploitation of women of colour for reproductive services.

If genetic technologies are to be used to benefit rather than harm communities, the perspectives articulated here must be taken into account by researchers, policy-makers, advocates and society as a whole. In a time when so many areas of life are dominated by a focus on genetics, the analysis put forward by women of colour and Indigenous women offers a new framework that affirms interdependence and community well-being, not just individual benefits.

3. Next steps

The women at this convening identified several next steps for advancing a reproductive justice approach to genetic technologies.

Community-based education was identified as a priority. Most of the leaders felt they lacked the knowledge, resources and time to develop the kinds of popular education tools that they could take to their grassroots membership. And until their members started identifying genetic technologies as a high priority issue, most of these organizations would not be able to engage more robustly in the public debates and policy-making. They asked for public education materials related to ancestry testing, DNA forensics, reproductive technologies and fertility/infertility in culturally specific contexts for Latinas, Asian, Pacific Islander and African American women.

Several participants stated the need for more research for their communities to deepen their own knowledge on these issues. They wanted more information about policies in other countries, international standards and opposition research on the right with regards to genetic technologies. They also advocated more community-based research that included qualitative and quantitative questions about knowledge, beliefs, attitudes and usage rates of genetic technologies in different communities.

Given the way this convening was set up to identify specific community perspectives and shared values, many participants expressed a strong interest in intersectional and cross-movement discussions and dialogues, particularly on abortion as it relates to reproductive genetic technologies. It was also thought that deeper conversations with the LGBTQ movement, environmental justice and Indigenous people's rights movement would be helpful.

Ultimately, the participants highlighted the importance of using a reproductive justice and movement-building approach in policy advocacy and messaging. They reiterated the value of utilizing proactive (as opposed to reactive or defensive) strategies to reshape any debate on abortion and reproductive genetic technologies.

4. Application of analysis and strategy in response to federal legislation

One week after the convening, Congressional Representative Trent Franks (R-AZ) introduced a bill that would ban abortions for sex selection and what he termed 'race selection'.[4] At the convening, the group had discussed this bill, recognizing it as a strategy to limit access to abortion and limit some (Asian and African American) women's decision-making authority about their reproductive health. They saw it as an attempt to divide communities and create a wedge between like-minded groups – including feminist, pro-choice, Asian and Black communities. The bill targeted Asian women without naming them, using language about son preference 'within certain segments of the US population, primarily those segments tracing their ethnic or cultural origins to countries where sex-selection abortion is prevalent'.

When the bill was introduced, Generations Ahead, SisterSong and the National Asian Pacific American Women's Forum (NAPAWF) reached out to other movement leaders in reproductive rights and justice, domestic violence, racial justice and Asian communities to host a conference call and form an alliance to craft a different kind of message to respond to this bill. Using the kind of contextual and intersectional analysis that they had refined at the convening, they highlighted the double standard embedded in the issue of sex selection in the US. While Asian Diaspora communities are condemned for practising sex selection, non-Asian individuals and couples using it for 'family balancing' or 'gender variety' are free from this judgement. They discussed the underlying factors of sexism, son preference and reproductive autonomy, and actively engaged South Asian and Asian domestic violence prevention leaders in the discussion.

Rather than respond with a traditional defence of abortion as an individual choice premised on privacy, the group wrote an opposition letter to Congress incorporating the values and principles established at the convening. They reiterated a commitment to social justice and intersectionality, and pivoted to a call for a deeper engagement with racial and gender equality in this situation, with a focus on eliminating health disparities without limiting access to abortion. Instead of leading with a message of individualized decision-making devoid of a broader, complex lived reality, they called for a more community oriented and community led solution. The group ensured that women of colour leaders (particularly from the Asian and South Asian anti-violence movement) would be the most visible spokespeople and messengers.

The growing awareness of shared commitments identified at the Generations Ahead convening was the starting point for a longer discussion to develop deeper strategies to reach out to other movements, including disability rights and LGBTQ rights, and create an advocacy plan that includes more community participation. Their goal was not simply to defeat this legislation, but to use it as a movement-building opportunity led by those who would be most affected by the bill.

On 8 December 2008, Generations Ahead, SisterSong and NAPAWF held a day-long strategy meeting with reproductive rights and justice organizations and South Asian domestic violence prevention organizations to build awareness and organize momentum on this issue. Twenty-seven leaders came together for this important gathering of both mainstream reproductive rights organizations, such as the Center for Reproductive Rights, American Civil Liberties Union and Planned Parenthood, and leading reproductive justice organizations like the National Latina Institute for Reproductive Health and the Black Women's Health Imperative. Working groups formed at this meeting are continuing to work in several areas, including development of a legislative package educating Congressional leadership on issues of sex selection and the way this particular bill seeks to drive a wedge between Asian and African American groups and reproductive rights groups.

Conclusion

Several important successes emerged from this meeting. Now more than twenty organizations appreciate the benefits and dangers of emerging genetic technologies. They have a political framework in which to locate and analyse the issues, which no longer appear as a concern of only affluent white women seeking fertility services. Based on the values and principles they identified, they are better equipped to engage in public debates and respond to policy proposals in ways according to their core values and strategies. In addition, they are now part of a network of allied organizations and leaders shaping a social justice response to these issues, and have had a successful experience putting their learning into action with the proposed sex selection and 'race selection' abortion ban. While genetic technology is still not at the top of the priority list for their organizations, they are now prepared and able to engage when necessary. They will be seen as the early leaders on this issue, potentially shaping future debates and policy advocacy.

The marvels of genetic science and the new world of possibilities suggest that we need new ideas, theories or paradigms to understand and govern them. However, we also need to remind ourselves of our historically held values. These values and principles orient us towards unity, collaboration, mutual responsibility, shared purpose and the prioritization of human beings, in all our diversity, over profits. These women envision a world in which those affected have a seat at the decision-making table, and in which policies governing responsible uses of genetic technologies integrate a complex and interdependent understanding of social life.

Reproductive justice theory and methodology provide a critical framework within which to analyse the potential impacts of reproductive and genetic technologies on women of colour, Indigenous women, young women and girls, economically vulnerable women, women with disabilities, lesbians, bisexual women and transgender people. The potential benefits and risks lie at the intersection of multiple social and political forces. The reproductive justice movement fights for the rights of all women to decide to have children as well as not to have children, and to parent with dignity and respect. Reproductive justice offers a vision of justice for all women in reproductive decision-making – justice that includes balancing individual desires with collective needs, human rights and shared responsibility, and including multiple stakeholders in the decision-making.

Notes

1 The full report is available at: <www.generations-ahead.org/files-for-download/articles/GenAheadReport_ReproductiveJustice.pdf>.

2 In the medical model, disability is seen as an individual medical problem that needs to be 'fixed'. In the social model of disability, the problem is not the disability but rather negative social attitudes towards it and the lack of accessible built environments for people with disabilities.

3 Dragnet is a police term meaning a system of coordinated measures for apprehending criminals or suspects. This may include road barricades and traffic stops, widespread DNA tests and general increased police alertness. The term derives from a fishing technique of dragging a fishing net across the sea bottom, or through a promising area of open water.

4 Representative Franks claimed that the high rate of abortions among African American women amounts to 'race selection', disregarding the root causes leading to unintended pregnancies and disparities in abortion rates.

16 | I DONATED MY EGGS AND I WOULDN'T DO IT AGAIN

Ari Laurel

The following personal account was originally posted on beyoungandshutup.com and weareeggdonors.com; this updated version was retrieved from the-toast.net on 4 March 2015.

My desire to donate my eggs came from my desire not to use them for myself. I didn't want kids. Asians don't donate as often as other women, but there are Asian couples out there who want children and can't have them. I was a healthy, young, college-educated woman in my early 20s. Why not get compensated for helping someone else start a family?

But the application process was a *process*. The application itself had eugenic qualities, I noticed as I filled it out. I was supposed to note my skin colour as 'fair', 'medium', 'olive/light brown', 'dark brown', 'ebony', 'freckled' or 'rosy'. I was asked if I would be comfortable taking an IQ test, what my philosophy on life was, what my goals were and if I had achieved them. I was asked what talents ran in my family and whether I was in any gifted and talented programmes. I answered each question to the best of my ability and sent in flattering pictures of myself as well as a copy of my college transcript.

The next step was to wait for a match. In the meantime, I contacted *We Are Egg Donors*, a donor advocacy resource forum where several hundred women have shared their experiences and collective knowledge. There were many women who, like me, were starting this process for the first time. There were women who had chosen to donate up to eight times. There were women concerned about Ovarian Hyperstimulation Syndrome (OHSS), one possible and serious result of taking fertility medications, with an increased risk as the dosages increase. Of those who had experienced health issues, they couldn't say for certain if their problems were related to the repeated use of fertility medications. Why? Because there isn't adequate research. (A range of typical symptoms and clinical advice on how to respond to them is listed in Box 16.1.)

Box 16.1 Coping with symptoms: information for egg donors

Signs and symptoms	Why it happens	What to do
MILD You may experience: • Abdominal bloating and feeling of fullness • Nausea • Diarrhoea • Slight weight gain.	**This may be due to:** • Ovaries are larger than normal, tender and fragile. • High levels of oestrogen (E2) in your bloodstream may upset your digestive system and fluid balance, causing bloating.	**Recommended treatment:** • Avoid sexual intercourse. • Do not have a vaginal (pelvic) exam other than by one of our physicians. • Reduce activities, no heavy lifting, straining or exercise. • Drink clear fluids, flat coke, ginger ale, cranberry juice, Gatorade or Ensure. • If you're unable to drink for more than 24 hours, call your primary nurse.
MODERATE You may also experience: • Weight gain of greater than 2lbs per day (excessive weight gain) • Increased abdominal measurement causing clothes to feel tight • Vomiting and diarrhoea • Darker urine and less • Dry skin/hair • Thirst.	**This may be due to:** • High levels of hormones in the bloodstream upset the digestive system. • Fluid imbalance causes dehydration because body fluid collects in the abdomen and other tissues. • The fluid collection causes severe bloating.	**As above plus:** • Call your primary nurse. • You may well be seen by a physician who will do an ultrasound. • Do daily weights in the morning. • Measure around your abdomen while lying flat (just below the belly button) before getting out of bed. • You may need blood tests.

SEVERE	This may be due to:	As above plus:
In addition, you may experience: • Fullness/bloating up above the belly button • Shortness of breath • Urination has reduced or stopped and become darker • Calf and chest pains • Marked abdominal bloating or distention • Lower abdominal pain.	• Ovaries are extremely large. • Fluid collecting in lungs and/or abdominal cavity, as well as in tissues. • The risk of abnormal blood clotting increases now.	• Call your primary nurse or, after hours, the physician on call as soon as possible. • You may need to be assessed at the hospital or our clinic. • Hospitalization may be necessary. • It may be necessary to remove excess fluid at our office or hospital.

There were women who had scheduled back-to-back donations, only having recently recovered from a previous cycle. There were women who had decided to stop after their third or fourth donation, but found themselves feeling guilty when they were matched again, worried about letting down another couple that the agency said 'needed' them.

One of the most disturbing things I noticed was that doctors would tell some women that their ovaries were 'overachievers', using the word jokingly after retrieving more eggs than the recommended twelve to fifteen. The use of this language was suspect, first because it was so widely used among many different clinic doctors, and second, because it put such a positive spin on having fertility drugs forcibly stimulate a woman's ovaries to produce more eggs than they should. Ovaries aren't designed to overachieve. The 'overachieving' was artificial. The doctors did not note: 'You produced more eggs than typical, so if you decide to donate next time, we'll lower your dosage so you won't be at risk for OHSS.' Instead, donors were congratulated for their hard work. Some, to their dismay, experienced similar or increased dosages in their next cycle.

In egg donor databases, you will see headshots of young women with carefully groomed hair, bright smiles and white teeth. Alongside each potential donor is her age, location, height and any other notable information. Prospective parents may feel more like they are browsing a dating website.

Ads target college-aged women who may have just graduated with loans to pay back. Officially, donors don't get paid for their eggs (that would be illegal, silly!). So they get compensated for their time, and their pain and suffering. This doesn't explain the disparity between those whose eggs are more desired (Asian, Jewish, redheads, Ivy League, gorgeous people, etc., etc.) and those who are 'run of the mill'.

Clinics and agencies often use feel-good and altruistic language. As a 'donor', even if you are not feeling wholly altruistic you will act accordingly, knowing what's expected of you. I found myself answering each application question with the kind of thoughtful and upbeat attitude found only in the most successful of job interviews. In my meeting with the psychologist (part of the process is a psychological evaluation and genetic screening), I dressed business casual to impress, but after I had signed the contract, I wore my snapback, t-shirts and sports bras. When asked about whether I wanted to disclose my sexuality, I declined for fear of not being chosen. As a potential donor, I had an acute sense of when the stakes were higher or lower.

If you apply to be an egg donor, you will be asked quite often why you want to donate. Sperm banks often emphasize compensation when reaching out to donors. While egg donors are also presented with tempting compensation, most will also encounter discussions in which they have to prove that they are not entirely in it for the money.

Sometimes the desire to help may come into conflict with the desire to self-advocate. You don't want to feel like a difficult donor. When I stuck to my guns about my compensation, my agency said, 'We're not in the business of trying to just take money from parents.' It was a subtle accusation, but I couldn't shake the idea that that is *exactly* the business they were in. My agency would be making a lot of money off my body from a couple who could afford to pay the fee.

I asked a lot of questions throughout the process. What was my follicle count? How high were my estradiol levels? Would I be taking cabergoline to mitigate OHSS symptoms? I compared notes with other donors, relieved to find that my own numbers were conservative. In the end, I wasn't afraid of the drugs. If you've gone to college, you've woken up in the morning cognizant (or not) of your mistakes. I was more afraid of being lied to.

This is how I gave myself shots: I went into the clinic and a woman explained to me in a sing-song voice (so as to show how fun it is) how to mix your drugs in the tiny bottle provided, and how to measure 225 IUs into a syringe and how to get all the air bubbles out. Needles didn't make me particularly nervous, but I'd never poked myself before, and yeah, I was nervous. At home the next evening, I read the instructions over and over and then mimicked the demonstration. I pinched the fat in my lower abdomen, just beneath and a few inches left or right of the belly button, and poked. It really didn't feel like much.

My breasts got bigger, which is par for the course when on hormones. It always happened when I was on birth control and it's the last thing I maybe still dislike about my body, and of which male affirmations only make me feel more despairing. Leading up to the days of retrieval, I felt bloated and uncomfortable, and could walk at the same pace as my grandmother. The injection sites became bruised. Damn, I was sick of it.

Though nervous, I was relieved when my retrieval date finally arrived. The doctor told me the anaesthesia would work in ten seconds and I didn't even get a chance to start counting. In the end, the clinic retrieved twelve eggs. The next day, another donor shared that her clinic had retrieved a drastic fifty-two eggs from her – three-and-a-half times the recommended amount. Floods of support and tips rushed in for her and I found myself thinking of her during recovery.

Every donor is different, has different motivations and is willing to take different calculated risks. Several of the donors at *We Are Egg Donors* made connections with the intended parents and personally saw and experienced the difference they made. Others felt cast off and unsupported.

I never met the intended parents who got my eggs. I'm happy if they're happy, but I didn't feel like a 'hero' the way many agencies or clinics will often tell donors they will. I felt like I was giving away something that I didn't particularly need and receiving something in return. I learned to exercise self-advocacy. But still, I participated in a transaction I was critical of the whole time. I signed the contract and stayed the course out of some abstract feeling of commitment and obligation, like clinging to a marriage you don't believe in.

Would I do it again? Doubtful. I saw what happens when an industry is almost entirely unregulated. You can do your research, take precautions, self-advocate, and even come out with an optimal experience as I did. But to me the process will always feel exploitative, too.

At this age (early 20s), my body feels resilient, but the money doesn't seem worth the possible and expensive health complications faced by many repeat donors whose collective knowledge highlights some shady business practices, manipulation and a lack of transparency. The promise of being well compensated to help others achieve their dreams is sweet, but not even the fine print can give you the full picture.

17 SWEDISH FEMINISTS AGAINST SURROGACY

Kajsa Ekis Ekman, Linn Hellerström and the Swedish Women's Lobby

The first part of this chapter reproduces extracts from Chapter 5 of Kajsa Ekis Ekman's (2013) book, *Being and Being Bought: Prostitution, Surrogacy and the Split Self*, reprinted with kind permission from Spinifex Press.

In likening surrogacy to prostitution, Ekman argues that both practices entail a woman selling her body and with it the 'division of the Self and the body, person and function, mother and child, soul and sexuality' (p. 190). This split, where in surrogacy the womb becomes a container or 'oven' for the gestation of someone else's child, not only negates the psyche of the woman to whom it belongs, but demonizes her as a potential obstacle who may lay claim to the baby she has been commissioned to produce. As a mother she is a commodity to be bought, used and abandoned.

Ekman's contribution is followed by a statement from Linn Hellerström and the Swedish Women's Lobby (*Sveriges Kvinnolobby*) with whom she launched the Swedish Feminist No to Surrogacy campaign in 2013.

THE STORY OF THE HAPPY BREEDER

Kajsa Ekis Ekman

Organizations and lobbyists have begun to demand that surrogacy is legalized in Sweden. These proponents include associations of childless couples, queer theorists and politicians from both right and left. Surrogacy is still relatively unfamiliar territory but the Swedish Federation for Lesbian, Gay, Bisexual and Transgender Rights (RSFL) has taken a stand in favour of commercial and altruistic surrogacy. All political parties, except the Left Party and the Christian Democrats, voted in 2012 to open an investigation on the matter. Some, like Birgitta Ohlsson of the Liberal Party of Sweden, are only in favour of 'altruistic' surrogacy, in which no money changes hands. Others, such as philosopher Kutte Jönsson from the Swedish Association for

Surrogacy and conservative politicians like Christer G Wennerholm, advocate commercial surrogacy as well. We have started seeing a whole arsenal of texts take shape – from family stories to debates, political proposals and philosophical dissertations: all attempt to establish an ethics for the acceptance of a pregnancy contract. Two parallel stories have developed from this discourse: 'the happy family' and a 'norm-breaking practice' of 'revolutionary acts'.

Happy families

In lifestyle sections of the daily press and in magazine articles about surrogacy, the longing of 'childless' people to have children always takes centre stage. The articles have headlines like: 'A happy family thanks to a surrogate' and focus on surrogacy as a solution to a problem. They describe how celebrities, such as Sarah Jessica Parker, Angela Basset, Michael Jackson, Elton John, Ricky Martin and Nicole Kidman, have had children via surrogate.

Some examples An article in *Expressen* begins with the words: 'André, 20 days old has come home' (Kazmierska, 2009). A Swedish couple had hired a woman in Ukraine to bear a child for them, but the child could not get a Swedish passport since he was legally from Ukraine. The article expresses no doubt about whether the Swedish couple are the child's real parents, or that Sweden is his home country. The central issue is a 'family' that should 'be united'. The parents were 'confused about why *their* newborn baby didn't get a Swedish passport' (my emphasis), until the previous Conservative Party leader, politician Bo Lundgren, intervened. When the child was allowed to enter the country, it was 'an enormous relief'. The article ends, as they usually do, happily: 'For John, Sara and André, a happy ending. The family is back home in Sweden ...' The mother who gave birth to the child does not have a voice in the story, it is only briefly mentioned that she is from Ukraine, had two children previously and had to give birth to André via caesarean section because the placenta was misaligned in the uterus.

The surrogate is generally presented as happy and the buyers as well-established, stable, upper middle-class couples who will give the child the best possible upbringing. There is never any question: it is the couple that pays for the baby who comprise the 'true' family. The woman who gives birth is never presented as the child's mother or even a person with a background and a will of her own – she is just a kind soul, a fairy godmother, who helps the people who pay for the child get want they want.

Her function is to create this family – but she is prohibited from being part of it. What characterizes surrogacy is the requirement of an absent mother. It engages a woman whose only function is a physical one.

In the newspaper *Aftonbladet*, father through surrogacy Daniel Szpigler (27 July 2009) writes a thank you note to himself – in his daughter's name!

> My dear dads, I am so glad you decided to have my brother and me via surrogate. I know it wasn't an easy decision for you. You didn't want to share me with a lesbian couple or a heterosexual woman. You wanted to be full-time dads. Raise me full time. Love me full time.

While the daughter in question is not even 2 years old and obviously oblivious to having written to *Aftonbladet*, Szpigler clarifies on her behalf that 'it is completely okay for me' not to have a mom. Szpigler not only takes the liberty of writing a declaration of love to himself in his daughter's name, he even arms her with political opinions. That a mother otherwise tends to be automatically seen as a parent 'should be changed, I think'. And what about the fact that they paid money for her? 'It's not strange I don't think. People pay to adopt a child, do *in vitro* fertilization or egg donation. What's the difference?' He signs the article: 'A daughter of two dads through Daniel Szpigler, the driving force of surrogat.nu'. The surrogate is illustrated with a child's drawing.

Words such as 'whole' and 'complete' are constantly repeated in this story of happy families. We are meant to see that surrogacy creates families that would otherwise be incomplete. All of the children's drawings, talk of wonderful walks with baby carriages and families that are 'reunited' in the 'homeland' portray an image that something that was broken has now been fixed; something unfinished has been completed. But this 'wholeness' presupposes an absent mother. If she meets the child or takes part in the child's upbringing, it is understood to be a division or split. It is the dream of the nuclear family – but one in which the mother is suddenly a threatening figure.

A 'revolutionary act'

Parallel to the newspapers' sweet stories, another legitimising story of surrogacy is being constructed by queer theorists, cultural analysts, liberal politicians and organizations like RFSL.

The very same activity that paved the way for the perfect family in the magazines changes face completely. In this version, surrogacy has become a 'norm-breaking' and subversive practice that challenges outdated conservative models. Philosopher Torbjörn Tännsjö writes that surrogacy 'dissolves the "natural" idea of motherhood, of fatherhood and what a family is' (1991: 147). Fellow philosopher Kutte Jönsson writes that surrogacy can 'challenge the norm of biological parenthood' and function as 'a battering ram against conservative family traditions where the heterosexual nuclear family represents the norm' (2003: 117, 13). Similarly, Ulrika Westerlund and Sören Juvas from RFSL claim that the prohibition of surrogacy is proof that we have a 'biological, heteronormative, couples-oriented view of parenthood and family' (Juvas and Westerlund, 2008). Alesia Goncharik writes in the same vein that the prohibition is 'simply an expression of the conservative view of gender roles and traditional motherhood we still find today' (2009).

In spite of the fact that people who want to have children through a surrogate mother stress that they *don't* want to adopt because they want to have a child who is genetically their own, the arguments presented in favour of surrogacy in the cultural arena are often anti-biological. The rhetoric is borrowed from social movements, where the concept of 'social parenthood' is emphasized and set in opposition to biological parenthood. Szpigler (2009) writes: 'It is not the biological connection that is important, but just the desire to become a parent' (2009). In an essay from 2006, Sarah Vaughan-Brakman and Sally J Scholz criticize the 'biological paradigm' that stipulates that there is 'a natural connection or a natural bond between mother and child'. Kutte Jönsson (2003) also questions 'the myth of the sacrosanct relationship between biological mother and child' and believes that it is important to 'challenge the norms of biological parenthood' (p. 117).

Nevertheless, they don't consider *all* of the biological connections to be unimportant. What they are criticizing is the birth mother's biological connection – that is called a 'norm' and a 'sacrosanct myth'. The father's biological connection is not questioned at all. Despite the fact that he lays claim to the child for the same biological reasons as the mother, he is not accused of defending biology or the nuclear family. In other words, this criticism of the biological connections is directed at only one sex. What is never addressed is the fact that if *all* biological claims were rejected, it would be incredibly difficult to decide whose the child is. And while the argument speaks of the importance of social parenthood, it is silent about the fact that surrogate motherhood isn't about giving a child more parents; it is about keeping one of the parents away from the child.

The story of the surrogate resembles the story of the sex worker in many ways. It is a story that connects a practice – in this case pregnancy as work – to a multitude of contemporary social concepts.

Prostitution

Surrogacy can be seen as an extended form of prostitution. Someone, most often a man, pays for the use of a woman's body. In both cases, his needs take centre stage, while the woman is only the means to achieving this end. Andrea Dworkin points out that the difference is that in surrogacy, it is the woman's uterus that is sold rather than her vagina, which keeps her from being stigmatized: she is a Madonna and not a whore (in Corea, 1985: 275). These arguments have strong similarities to those put forward in the prostitution debate. Sistare wants surrogacy to be seen as work. She believes that there is nothing inherently wrong with selling one's body (Sistare, 1994: 397):

> [W]e certainly allow people to treat their bodies as property in a variety of ways, e.g. the selling of blood, of antibodies, and (most apropos) of sperm. A fortiori, in our society, we permit people to sell their labor and even think well of them for it. In fact, the surrogate is more a laborer than a seller of body parts, since she really only sells her services while renting out her body ...

Malm claims, in contrast, that it is not about selling one's body. He thinks the difference is that, in surrogacy, it is not the *buyer* who uses the woman's body; it is the women *themselves* who use their bodies to satisfy the buyer (Malm, 1992: 297):

> There is no need to view the payments to the woman as payments for the use (i.e. rental) of her body – the customer does not acquire a space over which he (or she) then has control. He may not paint it blue, keep a coin in it, or do whatever else he wishes provided that he does not cause permanent damage. Instead, the woman is being paid for her to use her body in a way that benefits him – she is being compensated for her services. But this does not treat her body as an object of commerce, or her as less than a person, any more than does my paying a surgeon to perform an operation, or a cabby to drive a car, or a model to pose for a statue.

His argument works on two levels and has a double effect: on the one hand, he denies the objectification of women; on the other, he compares a woman's body with an object. He experiments on both a literal level and a deeper, figurative level. On the literal plane, he uses concepts such as freedom, independence, individuals, free will and work. On this level, he claims that surrogacy is not exploitative, that it is not human trafficking, that it does not compromise women's integrity. On the figurative plane, he does the opposite. When he wants a metaphor, he uses a taxi driver who drives a car, a surgeon who performs an operation ... in other words, he creates a metaphor that *de facto* compares the woman's relationship with her body with a taxi driver's relationship to his car, even as he, on the superficial level, distances himself from these comparisons: 'To illustrate it, suppose that you own a lawnmower.'

Malm continues his comparison by claiming that if you pay someone to mow the lawn, you don't make a claim on the lawnmower but on the service of having the lawn mown. That is, lawn mowing is a service but not the purchase of a lawnmower. On a figurative level he draws an analogy between a woman and her body and a gardener and his lawnmower. It is this analogy that drives his argument forward; it is this association we are urged to make: women relate to their children in the same way as men relate to their lawnmowers. Being a surrogate is like mowing a lawn. Still, Malm assures us that he *doesn't* mean that women's bodies are comparable to machines.

Thus the surrogacy story works on two levels simultaneously. It accustoms us to the idea that women are objects in the marketplace at the same time as the arguments for surrogacy deny this. We are supposed to become accustomed to being objects, but we are not supposed to understand what that means, because *naturally* we are not objects.

It is just like prostitution all over again, coming back to haunt us. It is the same division of the Self and the body, person and function, mother and child, soul and sexuality. And the same fear that the two will be reunited. The division is made sacred while the unity is demonized. What everyone in surrogacy longs for – whole families, happiness, sacredness, Virgin Mary status, forgiveness and atonement – is the diametric opposite of the functionalization and commodification that is actually taking place. What Daniel Szpigler (2009) calls 'the creation of the whole' is in actuality a compulsory divorce. We all know it, exactly as we know when we are lying, but we convince ourselves that if everyone agrees with the lie, it becomes truth.

A FEMINIST 'NO' TO SURROGATE MOTHERHOOD
Linn Hellerström and the Swedish Women's Lobby

Surrogacy is currently not regulated in Sweden. There is no legislation to regulate the phenomenon of Swedish citizens using surrogate mothers abroad and bringing children born this way back to Sweden. In the last couple of years the issue has been up for debate and the Swedish government has commissioned an investigation to examine the possibilities of legalizing altruistic surrogacy in Sweden.

The women's movement in Sweden has a long tradition of working for sexual and reproductive rights for all women, and surrogacy is the current big issue on our agenda. The Swedish Women's Lobby (*Sveriges Kvinnolobby*), which gathers forty-five women's organizations, opposes all forms of surrogacy and calls on the Swedish government not to open up for this harmful practice.

As Kajsa Ekis Ekman demonstrates in the previous part of this chapter, surrogate motherhood is often portrayed in the media as a new and progressive method of reproduction, a welcome solution for infertile couples, singles and gay men seeking parenthood. On the contrary, we believe that like prostitution surrogacy builds on the ancient perception that women's bodies exist for other people's enjoyment and benefit. It is a violation of fundamental human rights as it reduces the surrogate mother and baby to commodities that can be regulated by a contract.

Surrogate motherhood in Sweden

Scandinavian countries are commonly referred to as some of the 'most gender equal nations' in the world. Sweden owes this fortunate position to the continuous struggles of the women's movement and to brave politicians who dared to implement political reforms on behalf of women's rights at a time when this was seen as controversial. For example, in 1999, Sweden was the first country to introduce a Sex Purchase Act to combat sex purchase and the demand for women in prostitution. This is a unique law in that it criminalizes the person who buys sex, not the person who sells it. The law works to fight the demand for prostitution, while at the same time establishing that women are not mere commodities in a market. The law has had a clear positive effect with the number of men buying sex between 1999 and 2010 dropping from one in eight to one in thirteen. The law has had a normative effect on society. Neither does there appear to be a significant increase in underground prostitution (Ekman, 2013: xiv–xv).

Drawing on the Swedish understanding of prostitution as a form of violence, it would have been natural for a subsequent debate on surrogacy to focus on women's human rights and for a long time this seemed to be the case. But during the last decade the Swedish debate about surrogacy and artificial reproduction in general has changed dramatically, and the notions and arguments have shifted away from the human rights perspective. Voices in favour of legalizing 'altruistic' surrogacy have been raised as lobby organizations and interest groups have grown stronger.

In early 2013, the Swedish National Council on Medical Ethics declared a positive view towards opening up for altruistic surrogacy in Sweden. Shortly afterwards, in June 2013, the Swedish government issued a commission to investigate the possibilities for allowing altruistic surrogacy. In February 2016 the government study Different Paths to Parenthood produced its concluding report and recommendations. Although the title has the perspective of the childless client, the report recommends the prohibition of surrogacy in any form. At the time of writing, the government has yet to put any such regulations into practice.

Why feminists say 'no' to surrogacy

The Swedish feminist movement has openly criticized the neglect of women's rights in the political process and debate surrounding surrogate motherhood. In 2011, a group of feminist organizations, professionals and other activists came together and formed the network Feminist No to Surrogacy. The campaign takes a strong stand against surrogacy on feminist grounds and supports items 20 and 21 of the European Parliament (EP) resolution of 5 April 2011 on priorities and the outline of a new EU policy framework to fight violence against women (2010/2209(INI)):

> 20. Asks Member States to acknowledge the serious problem of surrogacy, which constitutes an exploitation of the female body and her reproductive organs.
>
> 21. Emphasises that women and children are subject to the same forms of exploitation and both can be regarded as commodities on the international reproductive market, and that these new reproductive arrangements, such as surrogacy, augment the trafficking of women and children and illegal adoption across national borders.

The EP later also adopted another resolution condemning the practice of surrogacy. In its resolution on Human Rights from December 2015, the EP states:

> [it] condemns the practice of surrogacy, which undermines the human dignity of the woman since her body and its reproductive functions are used as a commodity; considers that the practice of gestational surrogacy which involves reproductive exploitation and use of the human body for financial or other gain, in particular in the case of vulnerable women in developing countries, shall be prohibited and treated as a matter of urgency in human rights instruments.

Rejecting all forms of surrogacy, we seek to raise public awareness concerning the risks and consequences involved and how this increasingly popular practice relates to the structural discrimination against women.

There is no such thing as 'altruistic' surrogacy

The debate in Sweden is mainly focused on 'altruistic' surrogacy. Unlike commercial surrogacy, altruistic surrogates are expected not to ask for any compensation for sacrificing their bodies, but to do so out of mere compassion. Altruistic or 'non-compensated' surrogacy relies on the goodwill of other women, the self-sacrifice and disposition of their own bodies and reproductive organs without any remuneration for the duration of the pregnancy through to handing over the child to the buyers.

However, it is difficult, if not impossible, to separate so-called altruistic from commercial surrogacy. There are very few ways of ensuring that no money or bribes are involved. It is also virtually impossible to distinguish between compensation for extra expenditures or loss of income and an actual wage payment. Furthermore, social pressure, expectations and class and socio-economic inequalities between the concerned parties have to be taken into account.

In debates about altruistic surrogacy, carrying children for others is often portrayed as a natural wish on the part of the surrogate mother – a longing to be pregnant and produce a baby for someone who cannot conceive or carry a child to full term that should not be denied. These stereotypical notions of womanhood are used to defend the commercialization of women's bodies. Making surrogacy sound like a mutual desire from both sides of the arrangement successfully shifts the focus away from the realities of going through a pregnancy and relinquishing the baby to its 'real' parents after nine months. By emphasizing the emotional/supportive aspects of the arrangement, altruistic surrogacy is frequently described by its promoters as being of a different nature than commercial arrangements. But no matter how you refer to it, surrogacy still amounts to the violation of a woman's right to bodily integrity that cannot be negotiated by any form of contract; whether or not money is transferred is irrelevant. In the words of our policy paper: 'Having a feminist approach to surrogacy means rejecting the idea that women can be used as containers and their reproductive capabilities can be bought' (Swedish Women's Lobby, 2013).

To make altruistic surrogacy legal in Sweden would be to ignore all of the aspects above. It is naïve to argue that it would not lead to similar patterns of increased commercial surrogacy that have been seen globally. Experiences from countries such as the UK, the Netherlands, Australia and the US show that when altruistic surrogacy has been legalized, commercialization has ensued as global interests in the form of lawyers, agencies and even governments step in and more and more prospective parents are encouraged to turn their attentions overseas. For example, India, with its ready-made infrastructure of medical tourism has become perhaps the leading country providing gestational surrogacy services, US and UK citizens among the most prominent clients. Even when it is permitted in their own country, economic incentives drive many buyers to seek cheaper services in poorer parts of the world.

Swedes using transnational surrogacy

Despite surrogacy not being legal in Sweden, there is currently no legislation prohibiting Swedish citizens from using surrogate mothers abroad and bringing the children back home. The exact figures are unknown, but it has been estimated that at least 100 children born via surrogate mothers overseas have been transferred to Sweden. Again, the most common destination countries for Swedes are the US, especially California, and until recently India, where the procedure is legal and therefore the infrastructures are in place.

As shown in the first half of this chapter, media coverage of Swedish couples using international surrogacy often focuses on the childless couple's side of the story. This type of idealized coverage risks overshadowing any discussion about the rights of the surrogate mother and the children. Representing the women's movement in Sweden, we regard it as highly important not to let the national surrogacy debate be led by one-sided interests and emotional illusions. Investigating surrogacy needs to involve leveraging knowledge and evidence that comes from the surrogate mothers and children themselves. If we do not closely examine the issue from a women's and children's rights perspective and learn from real experiences, we are at risk of enabling a detrimental practice that will be hard to reverse.

Conclusions

Surrogate motherhood is one of the most critical feminist issues of our time. It embodies yet another example of women's rights being neglected in favour of more powerful interests. Surrogacy is not about empowering women and it has nothing to do with women's self-determination. In reality, it comes down to reproducing the patriarchal view that women and women's bodies exist for the pleasure and benefit of others.

Sympathy and respect should be given to childless couples, but their wish should not be used to legitimize the trade with women's bodies and children. Opposing surrogacy on feminist grounds is not about trivializing the longing for children. No matter if it involves a sister or an unknown woman's reproductive organs, it is about acknowledging that children are not an entitlement through which we can justify exploiting other human beings.

The rights of women and children to freedom from exploitation need to be the focus of all decisions around assisted reproduction. It would be shameful if Sweden, a nation with a history of defending women's rights, promoting gender equality and standing at the forefront of battles against the demand for prostitution, were to legalize surrogacy. As feminists, we say 'no' to surrogacy in all its forms.

References

Corea G (1985) *The Mother Machine: Reproductive Technologies from Artificial Insemination to Artificial Wombs.* New York: Harper Collins.

Ekman K (2013) *Being and Being Bought: Prostitution, Surrogacy and the Split Self.* Melbourne: Spinifex Press.

European Parliament (2011) Resolution of 5 April 2011 on priorities and outline of a new EU policy framework to fight violence against women (2010/2209(INI)). <www.europarl.europa.eu/sides/getDoc.do?pubRef=-//EP//TEXT+TA+P7-TA-2011-0127+0+DOC+XML+V0//EN>

European Parliament (2015) Resolution of 17 December 2015 on the Annual Report on Human Rights and Democracy in the World 2014 and the European Union's policy on the matter (2015/2229(INI)). <http://www.europarl.europa.eu/sides/getDoc.do?type=TA&reference=P8-TA-2015-0470&language=EN&ring=A8-2015-0344>

Goncharik A (2009) JA till surrogatmammor! *ETC*, 21

May. <http://orebro.etc.se/blogg/ja-till-surrogatmammor>
Jönsson K (2003) *Det förbjudna mördraskapet*. Malmö: Bokbox Publishing.
Juvas S and Westerlund U (2008) Tillät surrotgatmödrar i Sverige – annars åker folk utomlans. *Expressen*, 17 July. <www.expressen.se/debatt/tillat-surrogatmodrar-i-sverige----annars-aker-folk-utomlands>
Kazmierska N (2009) Bebisen som väckt debatten om att få hyra en livmoder. *Expressen*, 6 April. <www.expressen.se/nyheter/dokument/bebisen-som-vackt-debatten-om-att-fa-hyra-en-livmoder>
Malm HM (1992) Commodification or compensation: a reply to Ketchum. In: Bequaert HM and Purdy LM (eds) *Feminist Perspectives in Medical Ethics*. Bloomington, IN: Indiana University Press.
Sistare CT (1994) Reproductive freedom and women's freedom: surrogacy and autonomy. In Jaggar AM (ed.) *Living with Contradictions: Controversies in Feminist Social Ethics*. Boulder, CO: Westview Press.
Swedish National Council on Medical Ethics (2013) *Assisted Reproduction: Ethical Aspects: Summary of a Report*. <www.smer.se/wp-content/uploads/2013/03/Slutversion-sammanfattning-eng-Assisted-reproduction.pdf>
Swedish Women's Lobby (2013) *Surrogacy Motherhood: A Global Trade with Women's Bodies* [sic]. Policy paper. <http://sverigeskvinnolobby.se/wp-content/uploads/2013/08/POLICY-PAPER-SURROGACY-MOTHERHOOD.pdf>
Szpigler D (2009) Surrogatmamma maste bli laglit. *Aftonbladet*, 27 July. <www.aftonbladet.se/debatt/article11938880.ab>
Tännsjö T (1991) *Gora barn: en studie I reproduktionsetik*. Stockholm: Sesam Publishing.
Vaughan-Brakman S and Scholz SJ (2006) Adoption, ART, and a re-conception of the maternal body: toward embodied maternity. *Hypatia* 21(1): 54–73.

PART FIVE
LOOKING AHEAD

18 | MAPPING FEMINIST VIEWS ON COMMERCIAL SURROGACY

Emma Maniere

Introduction

Leslie Morgan Steiner's 2013 *New York Times* bestseller, *The Baby Chase*, presents a profile of commercial cross-border surrogacy that many people may find familiar, framed around a middle-class couple from Arizona who want nothing more than to have a baby. After a vasectomy reversal, IVF, attempted domestic adoption and unyielding disappointment, the Wiles turn to the next most affordable option: surrogacy in India. After yet more tribulations (infertility is a 'battle that requires courage, wile and determination', Steiner reminds us), they fall in love with India and the two surrogates who help complete their family (p. 93). Of course, the surrogates are well cared for, the clinic is compassionate and the doctors care about their patients rather than profit; the couple even names their two Indian physicians their son's godparents. The Wiles likewise care for their surrogates: they give their first surrogate, Shashi, US$1000 to make the final payment on her family's new home and assure the reader that 'she did not feel exploited' (p. 228). Shashi greets the birth of the Wiles's son, Blaze, with a 'smile' that, Steiner remarks, the critics of surrogacy never see (p. 226).

Beneath Steiner's fairytale depiction of surrogacy lie problematic suppositions that reek of US paternalism and India's colonial past. The author repeatedly refers to India's simultaneous 'overpopulation' and booming surrogacy industry as 'ironic'. She dubs the country's gender roles backward and characterizes the rapidly industrializing nation as 'growing up' (p. 257). Steiner entertains the possibility that Indian surrogates are being exploited, but ends her analysis by asserting that their apparent emotional gratification is more important than the fact that they are paid one-fifth to one-tenth the sum of their counterparts in the US (p. 226).

Steiner's reluctance to engage seriously with the ethical issues raised by commercial surrogacy is typical of journalistic accounts. Feminist scholars writing about the topic, on the other hand, have grappled with the ways in which surrogacy interacts with important concerns including the commodification of female bodies, the public versus private sphere, liberalism and neoliberalism, agency and autonomy, informed consent and reproductive rights.

Unsurprisingly, feminist scholars do not share a single position on the growing practice of commercial surrogacy. In this chapter, I offer a survey of mostly academic feminist views, seeking to explore the range of their opinions. This overview is by no means comprehensive; rather, it offers a sample of influential works and viewpoints.

I have divided feminist perspectives into two major categories – *abolitionists* and *reformists* – each of which encompasses subtle differences and some overlap. I also address a third approach that I characterize as *libertarian* and which is less common among feminist scholars.

The abolitionist view is closest to the dominant policy situation on commercial surrogacy globally. While many jurisdictions have no codified policy on surrogacy, of the seventy-one countries that do, sixty-two prohibit its commercial form (Allan, 2015: 140). Reformists accept the existence of commercial surrogacy, at least in some jurisdictions, and seek to mitigate the abuses they recognize.

Among the positions I examine, abolitionists and reformists have more in common than one might think. Both groups share a myriad of concerns about the practice and repercussions of surrogacy. Abolitionists, who advocate for (commercial) surrogacy to be prohibited altogether, are anxious about the commodification of women, their bodies and babies. They are also concerned about the meaning of genetics and biology, the reinscription of gender and race hierarchies, and the particular form of alienated labour that surrogacy entails. Reformists, who believe that surrogacy need only be regulated, share these concerns. Additionally, they question the meaning of 'choice' and 'agency'; they are attentive to the daily realities that surrogates encounter and sometimes offer policy recommendations.

Mapping this complex terrain will build an appreciation of the diversity of feminist opinions expressed in the course of what is now a thirty-year-old and ongoing debate about commercial surrogacy.

Before discussing the views of those who favour abolition versus reform, I briefly consider arguments for a libertarian approach through the works of two legal scholars: Kimberley Mutcherson (2012, 2013) and Judith Daar (1997).

The libertarian approach

While many feminist scholars approach commercial surrogacy from either an abolitionist or reformist viewpoint, not all fit neatly into these two categories and some endorse a very different perspective. Mutcherson (2012: 316), for example, challenges the notion that the US is the 'Wild West' of fertility treatment and instead stresses that the fertility sector is regulated by the same laws as all other medical care in the US. She believes that because there is no global consensus on the desirability of surrogacy, international regulation is neither feasible nor advisable. That individual countries can create laws that reflect their own values, Mutcherson asserts, is a positive good; in fact, it allows nations with comparatively little regulation (i.e. the US) to serve as a 'moral safety valve' (2012: 390). For example, same-sex couples who are not permitted to receive fertility care in Australia can come to the US to achieve their goals (2012: 390). She argues that 'the United States should feel that its role in leading nations toward more inclusive policies is justified and productive' (p. 391). However, Mutcherson overlooks the fact that this failing to regulate assisted reproductive technologies (ARTs) is *not* tantamount to supporting diverse family structures.

Mutcherson's thesis in her later (2013) article, 'Transformative reproduction', is that ARTs allow for the creation of 'transformative' (i.e. non-heteronormative) families. This is unarguably true, and important: ARTs allow people to become biological parents who could not have done so forty years ago. She also emphasizes that at least some surrogates attest to the positive financial and/or psychological impacts of surrogacy on their lives. Further, she claims that ARTs can 'shatter' racial hierarchies by decoupling a parent's phenotypic race from his/her child, challenge gender norms and alter the very meaning of reproduction (p. 209). In short, Mutcherson believes that 'some reproductive choices may de-emphasize and de-stabilize mechanisms of reproductive oppression', and when this is the case, 'opportunities for transformation should be properly balanced against other legitimate concerns about exploitation and subjugation of others' (p. 233). In other words, regulation must proceed with caution.

Given their shared libertarian ethos, Judith Daar might agree with Mutcherson on many counts. She is a bit less clear in assessing the ART regulatory landscape in the US; she both acknowledges that it was 'quite bare' and asserts that it is sufficient (Daar, 1997: 615). Much like Mutcherson, Daar suggests that current reporting and regulatory mechanisms in the US adequately guard against abusive practices.[1] But Daar fails to consider the imbalance of power between patients/consumers, who are often desperate to have genetically related children, and the medical and legal professionals who arrange and provide ARTs. More convincingly, she argues that the dearth of direct regulation is due not to legislators' careful consideration of ARTs, but to their reluctance to wade into this policy area because of its connection to the intractable abortion debate that exerts a 'chilling effect' (1997: 640). Daar also argues that legislative support for a body along the lines of the UK's Human Fertilisation and Embryology Authority (HFEA)[2] in the US is unlikely because public opinion would not support the creation of a federal agency to oversee ARTs. In her opinion, this is not a problem: 'Instead of creating new schemes for regulation, let [the US] put to work those we have already built' (p. 664).

Mutcherson and Daar, then, contend both that current regulations suffice *and* that a free market facilitates reproductive choice in important ways. This perspective stands in contrast to the majority of feminist scholars who view federal or international regulation of ARTs and (commercial) surrogacy as urgently needed.

Reformists

Feminist scholars such as Gupta (2014), Marwah (2014), Nayak (2014), Pande (2014) and Teman (2010), who take a reformist approach to commercial surrogacy, tend to express concern about at least some of the practices associated with it, but do not believe it should be abolished. Many contend that while surrogacy presents ethical pitfalls – at least as currently practised – it could benefit all parties if properly regulated by state or international bodies. That is not to say that these scholars find surrogacy completely unproblematic; in fact, they often raise similar objections as those who believe in prohibition.

A theme that runs throughout the writings of reformists is that surrogates' 'choice' to commission their bodies must be evaluated with some nuance incorporating attention to the conditions of surrogates' lives. Another important theme in their work is that state regulation in the realm of reproductive decision-making – despite the inclination of many reproductive rights advocates to the contrary – does not necessarily infringe on individuals' autonomy and should sometimes be supported.

Three key aspects of the reformist position on commercial surrogacy are: (1) choice and agency; (2) the daily realities of surrogates; and (3) proposed policy solutions.

1. *Choice and agency* Many reformist scholars note the drawbacks of applying the idea of choice to surrogacy. Most caution that while

women's decisions must be honoured, they should also be considered in the context of women's lived reality. In other words, the choice to serve as a commercial surrogate cannot be separated from pressures created by persistent sexism, racism and economic hardship. To consider surrogacy as a simple opt-in or opt-out choice then erases the layered complexity of such choices.

Amrita Pande, who carried out a major ethnographic study of commercial surrogacy in India, notes that surrogacy is evolving into a survival strategy for some poor rural women for whom the earnings from one contract pregnancy are often equivalent to approximately five years of total family income (2014: 8, 20). Surrogacy is thus a rational economic strategy. In less dire financial situations, the choice to carry a surrogate pregnancy is unlikely to be made or even considered.

Many reformist scholars contend that while a decision to engage in surrogacy cannot be seen as a pure and unfettered choice, neither is it likely be wholly coerced. To quote Vrinda Marwah (2014: 292):

> Too much 'choice talk' obscures the structural and systemic forces acting on apparently free choice; but at the same time, focusing only on how a particular context has compelled a particular choice ignores the negotiation, fluidity and complexity in choices, and reduces the woman in question to a passive victim. The coercion versus choice argument set up a binary of its own, when in fact it may be more appropriate to argue that there is no such thing as an absolutely non-coercive context, just as 'free' in 'free choice' is relative. Thus, all choices are restrained, and what we are all always confronting is a difference of degree, not kind.

Similarly, Preeti Nayak (2014: 5) calls choice rhetoric a 'trap', a diversionary tactic that pulls our focus away from the true issues at hand. She describes surrogates' agency as hampered by 'crushing constraints' (p. 17).

Feminist legal scholar Mary Lyndon Shanley (2001) suggests that another reproductive rights axiom, 'autonomy', is also complicated due to the fact that a surrogate mother and the fetus she is carrying are inherently physically intertwined. She writes that 'to speak of the "freedom" of the mother as residing in her intention as an "autonomous" agent misunderstands both the relationship between woman and child and of the woman to her ongoing self' (p. 113). Writing about the global fertility market, anthropologist Jyotsna Agnihotri Gupta (2014) notes that terms like 'choice' and 'agency' cannot be separated from the western context in which they originated, and that both terms 'operate within the neoliberal epistemology' (p. 193). Thus, liberal notions of individualism and accompanying choice cannot be unproblematically applied to surrogacy.

Other reformist scholars take the analysis of choice and agency in a different direction, and suggest that commercial surrogacy *enhances* surrogates' sense of agency. After studying surrogacy in Israel, anthropologist Elly Teman (2010: 5) concluded that women 'make surrogacy more about personal agency, gift giving, heroism, and birthing a mother' than other theorists have suggested. Thus, rather than signalling a *lack* of agency, surrogacy *produces* agency. Similarly, Pande's lengthy research in India prompted her to warn against 'dismissing the labor market as inherently oppressive and the women involved as subjects of this oppressive structure'. She argues for the 'need to recognize, validate and systemically evaluate the choices that women make in order to participate in that market' (Pande, 2014: 9).

It is perhaps significant that both Teman and Pande studied surrogacy on the ground, while many abolitionist scholars come to their conclusions purely as theorists. Ethnographic methods could be seen as providing a more subtle and realistic picture of a practice like surrogacy; alternatively, they can unduly colour or constrain researchers' perspectives. For example, in the introduction of *Birthing a Mother*, Teman (2010: 3) forthrightly admits that she is 'not concerned with making an argument for or against surrogacy or entering into the debate over whether it is right or wrong'.

While scholars tend to complicate ideas of agency and choice, surrogates often present their decisions in straightforward terms. For instance, Laxmi, an Indian surrogate interviewed by Marwah (2014: 269), asserts, 'Whatever I did, it was my choice.' Laxmi paid for her daughter's wedding with the money she earned. Similarly, a surrogate interviewed by Varada Madge (2014) defends the practice as an equal trade: 'I do not think there's anything wrong with surrogacy because the couple wants children and we want money. It's as simple as that' (Madge, 2014: 53). These scenarios – and presumably many others like them – guide us into the murky waters of false consciousness. Should we respect the restrained choices of women in challenging socio-economic circumstances, or question their decisions because their roots lie in systems of sexism and colonialism?

Sayantani DasGupta and Shamita Das Dasgupta (2014) discuss this dilemma in 'Shifting sands: transnational surrogacy, e-motherhood, and nation building' (2014). They find traces of the legacies of imperialism and colonialism in the online conversations of intended parents who engage in cross-border commercial surrogacy, noting that these conversations, in which such parents imagine themselves 'helping' Third World women, constitute 'a reenactment of India's colonial past' (DasGupta and Dasgupta, 2014: 84). Importantly, surrogates' narratives are absent in these chatrooms. The authors describe the Indian surrogates as 'both defended as agents of their own destinies, and simultaneously silenced in the dialogue about their lives' (p. 84).

2. *The daily realities of surrogates* While both abolitionists and reformists raise a multitude of concerns about the practice of commercial surrogacy, reformists tend to highlight the daily realities of surrogates' lives, especially the myriad disadvantages they encounter that pre-exist and inform their decisions about surrogacy. Simply put, women who work as surrogates generally have few prospects for economic growth and are likely to be impoverished. Rather than work in a factory or clean houses, they opt to carry a gestational pregnancy to term. They are told and come to accept that the child will not belong to them, and deem this preferable to the physical or emotional exploitation that may accompany their alternative options, especially because surrogacy often offers far more lucrative economic prospects (Madge, 2014: 49; Pande, 2014: 20). Reformists, too, conclude that surrogacy may be the lesser of two evils. Some note that the social stigma often encountered by surrogates may not be very different from the stigma experienced by domestic workers (Madge, 2014). In other words, in the context of surrogates' lives, a contract pregnancy is a rational choice.

In the words of one surrogate: 'This work is not ethical, it's just something we have to do to survive' (Allan, 2015: 129). It is not completely clear whether this is a value judgement about surrogacy or an assertion that because she is engaging in this work to survive, ethical qualms are irrelevant. The bottom line is that surrogacy offers unparalleled economic gain. Pande notes that all the surrogates whom she met in a large Indian city 'were motivated by the sheer need for money' (2014: 61).

Feminist bioethicist, Laura Purdy, offers a slightly stronger analysis, asserting that the critique of the economic exploitation of poor women via surrogacy 'depends upon ignorance of the kinds of risks working-class people routinely face ... What needs to be shown here is that contract pregnancy is more exploitative than other services the rich now buy from the poor' (1992: 315). Purdy encourages us to dial down academic abstraction in favour of a more practical approach to understanding surrogates' possible decision-making processes. She asks whether a 26-year-old woman with a husband and two children might prefer to carry a child to be relinquished to someone else to raise rather than work in a sweatshop where exploitation is *unquestionably* part of the job. In a similar way, Teman (2010: 293) counters the surrogacy-as-necessarily-exploitative model by suggesting that surrogates in fact attain a sense of gratification that is unavailable to them in any other type of employment given their likely limited skills. Perhaps the question of one surrogate herself is most important here: 'Why am I exploited if I am paid, but not if I am not paid?' (Shanley, 2001: 109).

3. Proposed policy solutions For reformists, the answer to the problems presented by commercial surrogacy falls between the hands-off approach of libertarians and the prohibition of surrogacy that abolitionists support. Many view prohibition as detrimental, making the questionable argument that they would foster unsafe and/or underground markets (ironically, a number of egregious crimes have occurred in jurisdictions where ARTs are strictly regulated). Recent legal changes restricting cross-border surrogacy have demonstrably led to shifts in the market from one country (e.g. India) to another (e.g. Nepal or Mexico) (Kohli, 2015).

Both reformists and abolitionists are uncomfortable with market control of an intimate sphere of life like human reproduction, and often suggest that public policy is needed to regulate surrogacy. Teman (2010: 292) explicitly argues that state intervention can be positive; she asserts that her ethnography 'challenges the idea that state control of reproduction is always antithetical to women's and children's interests ... in this arena at least, the benefits of state control outweigh the costs'.

While reformist solutions usually involve some type of state or inter-state regulation, they often lack detailed policy proposals. Shanley, for example, argued in 2001 that while altruistic surrogacy (in which the surrogate is paid only for medical and living expenses) is permissible, additional payment for gestational surrogacy is not. She bases this position on her critique of libertarian notions of individualism, which she believes are reinforced by legally sanctioned commercial pregnancy. But she fails to offer any details delineating how payment ought to be monitored. Similarly, Pande cautions against a ban of surrogacy in India, and instead supports 'policies based on the real lived experiences of the surrogates' as revealed in her book (2014: 25) and reiterated in her contribution to this anthology (Chapter 19). Teman, too, requests 'policy decisions on surrogacy that [are] based on the perspectives and experiences of those who have been through this process' (2010: 295). But neither account includes specific prescriptions.

Debora Spar (2006), in her landmark book, *The Baby Business*, also calls for regulation. She argues that the market for reproduction must first be acknowledged (overcoming the tendency to see babies and commerce as separate entities), and then regulated, in no small part due to the inequities upon which the baby market hinges: 'Bluntly put, the book suggests that governments need to play a more active role in regulating the baby trade' (Spar, 2006: xviii). Spar suggests that a system of contracts and property rights be codified in the interest of bringing order to the currently chaotic market. She also advocates for a public discussion about these tricky and emotionally laden topics in order to inform the political process. The tenth anniversary of the publication of *The Baby Business* has passed, yet still no such public discussion has ensued. Perhaps the same sense of discomfort or moral ambiguity that prevented recognition of the baby business in the first place continues to stymie political debate.

One point on which there appears to be wide agreement is the need for cooperation on issues raised by transnational surrogacy among national and subnational governments. In 'Biocrossings and the global fertility market', Jyotsna Agnihotri Gupta (2014: 199) suggests that

> a meaningful response to the global biocrossings for reproduction will require transnational co-operation across various sectors, international government organizations, state and non-state actors to deal with this phenomenon and protect the rights of vulnerable individuals and groups.

Legal scholar Sonia Allan (2015) encourages international and domestic prohibitions on commercial surrogacy but, short of this, proposes stop-gap regulations to deal with the present legal situation of surrogacy wherein global agreement remains 'elusive' (p. 130). One may summarize her recommendations (greatly elaborated in the final chapter of this book) as follows (Allan, 2015: 137–9):

1. Require independent legal advice and counselling for (potential) surrogates and intended parents.
2. Ensure uniformity and transparency of any payments made.
3. Consider who 'brokers' surrogacy agreements (and consider prohibitions on payments to them).

4. Establish screening and eligibility requirements.
5. Establish high standards of practice for health professionals in relation to the medical treatment and care of women, children, and providers of human eggs, sperm or embryos.
6. Create legal provisions that address the legality and enforceability of contracts.
7. Guarantee information recording and sharing.

Allan's recommendations serve as methods to combat the inequality that drives the surrogacy market. She presents such methods recognizing that while most jurisdictions prohibit commercial surrogacy, for as long as some jurisdictions allow it, there must be protections for all those involved. Her view, however, emphasizes that the focus cannot just be on the end points of the agreement, i.e. legal parentage and nationality of the child born as a result, but must first and foremost confront the human rights issues raised, as well as the structural inequalities and market forces that drive commercial surrogacy. Her ultimate solution, therefore, would be to address such dilemmas, perhaps ending the practice of commercial surrogacy altogether.

Abolitionists

Rather than create legal stipulations to monitor commercial surrogacy, many feminist writers have averred that these arrangements ought to be banned altogether, particularly in the wake of the infamous 'Baby M' case of 1985. Although since then surrogacy has expanded far beyond US borders, many of the same themes underlie contemporary arguments that seek to prohibit it. Three key themes regularly arise in the writings of abolitionists: (1) the commodification of women, reproductive organs and babies; (2) the reinscription of gender and race hierarchies; and (3) alienated labour and market logic.

1. The commodification of women, reproductive organs and babies
Those who cite commodification as a reason to prohibit commercial surrogacy argue that its 'product' is very different from other products rightly subject to market forces. By buying and selling babies as we do cars or computers, these authors suggest, we risk losing what distinguishes human beings from commercial goods and jeopardize the human bond that connects a baby and its parent(s) with little understanding of the long-term consequences of such disruption. Writing just a few years after the 'Baby M' case, for example, sociologist Barbara Katz Rothman asserted, 'Biological motherhood is not a service, not a

commodity, but a relationship' (1989: 238). In her view, the 'nurturant relationship' between a surrogate mother and the fetus she carries in and of itself constitutes motherhood (p. 254). Hence, surrogacy cheapens motherhood because it severs a relational (not genetic) bond. In 1993, lesbian feminist author and activist Janice Raymond likewise concluded that motherhood is only partly biological and is more accurately described as 'relational' (p. 38). She described surrogacy as the product of the combined forces of capitalism, technology and patriarchy driving 'the commodification of children and the proletarianization of motherhood' (Raymond, 1993: 66).

Reproductive technologies scholar Gena Corea, writing in the 1980s, agreed that patriarchy has played the key role in commodifying children and leading women who serve as surrogate mothers (whom she dubbed 'breeder women') to be treated as 'incubators, receptacles, "a kind of hatchery", rented property, plumbing' (Corea, 1985: 214, 222). For Marxist feminist Kelly Oliver (1992), on the other hand, the role of the free market more than patriarchy has accounted for the commodification of children. She contended that when babies are exchanged, they are rendered merely commercial products. More than two decades later, in 2013, Swedish journalist Kajsa Ekis Ekman also argued that surrogacy is wrong because it constitutes commodification: 'When a child is produced via surrogacy, the market is pivotal to *the child's very existence*' (Ekman, 2013: 160).

2. *The reinscription of gender and race hierarchies* A number of feminist scholars have pointed out that the commercialization of pregnancy is intertwined with the inequities along lines of gender, race and citizenship that the free market has historically produced. Anthropologist Sarah Boone (1992) articulates these dynamics in her article, 'Slavery and contract motherhood: a "racialized" objection to the autonomy arguments', which likens slave mothers' lack of legal rights to the children they bore to the similarly amorphous rights of surrogate mothers. Boone (1992: 351) argues that what she deems 'commercialized contract motherhood' (CCM) 'reinforces the multi-tiered oppression of all women and devalues both women and people of color'. In fact, CCM produces a hierarchy that divides 'top women', who purchase the services of surrogate mothers, from 'bottom women', who serve as surrogates. In addition, she argues, gestational surrogacy allows mostly wealthy, likely white, individuals to produce a genetic heir and thereby assigns a higher value to their reproduction (p. 363; also see Twine, 2015).

Australian feminist Heather Dietrich (1992) makes a similar point. She regards the unequal power dynamics inherent in the surrogate/contracting parent relationship as antithetical to feminist interests. She writes (p. 374):

> The ultimate irony of surrogacy is that, while it may provide some women with their heart's desire, it can only do this by reducing others to their biological function, and putting them socially at risk in their families and places of living. The practice of surrogacy contains the seeds of injustice for women and children.

In much the same way, Oliver states that surrogacy contracts are only possible due to the wealth disparity between the parties. In the words of Janice Raymond (1993: 44–5): '"No woman would do this only for the money" is the cry of surrogate brokers. The other side of the coin is that few women would do it without the money.' Simply put, if socio-economic equity existed between contracting parents and surrogates, the contract would not.

3. *Alienated labour and market logic* Many scholars who urge that surrogacy be prohibited criticize the application of the logic of wage labour to human reproduction and refer to Marx's theory of alienated labour. Like a factory worker, they say, surrogate mothers are expected to remain detached from the product of their labour, but gestating a fetus for nine months generates a bond that cannot be devoid of intimacy. Pregnancy involves a woman's entire body twenty-four hours a day, with no breaks or lunch hours, yet a surrogate must always remain mindful that the fetus she is carrying is not hers. Ekman (2013: 191) asserts that 'a part of the Self is made into "something else" that belongs to "someone else"' and that '[w]omen all over the world are denied their complete humanity'. Abolitionists find this split consciousness troubling.

Surrogacy abolitionists have closely interrogated the meaning of choice and the notion of 'reproductive liberalism' in the context of contract pregnancy and argue that the constraints of poverty and subordination must be acknowledged even as we continue to value women's choices. Raymond (1993) avers that reproductive liberalism assumes equality between men and women, and fails to acknowledge women's collective subjugation. She claims that 'reproductive liberals also *reduce complexity to relativism*' (Raymond, 1993: 106), by which she means that when people are assumed to have full self-determination, analysing the complexity of their choices becomes irrelevant. Ekman, too, objects to the moral relativism associated with market ideology, asking: 'How can we justify a situation in which wealthy people use poor people as breeders, inject them full of hormones, take children away from them and leave pocket money in exchange?' Her answer? 'A good dose of relativism' (2013: 150).

Ekman also takes up another facet of liberalism: contracts. Rational beings are expected to uphold the agreements outlined in contracts, but she claims, they serve a symbolic function as well: '[V]ia a contract the economic power differential between the wealthy and the proletariat is "cleansed" and remade as an equal relation' (Ekman, 2013: 151). Thus, in a variety of complex ways, the market erases the very economic and gendered forms of inequality that give rise to surrogacy in the first place.

Conclusion

Feminist scholars have expressed a range of views about commercial surrogacy from the time it emerged as an extension of IVF procedures. Though calls for prohibition were more common in writings published during the 1980s and 1990s, they are still heard. For example, a 'Stop Surrogacy Now' campaign involving both pro-choice and anti-choice organizers, women and men, has recently been launched (www.stopsurrogacynow.com) and, in 2016, far fewer national and subnational jurisdictions permit commercial surrogacy than allow it.

Yet between the 1980s and now, commercial surrogacy has become more widespread, and some feminists seem to have concluded that its eradication is unlikely. As Spar wrote in 2006 (p. 196): 'It's hard to imagine that we could ever put this particular genie back in its bottle.'

The difference between calling for surrogacy's prohibition and its regulation is apparently sharp, but the concerns expressed by scholars who urge abolition and those who advocate for reform are in fact quite similar. Both camps are deeply concerned with the ethical implications of commercial surrogacy: they both fear the exploitation of women facilitated by economic inequality, lament the commodification of bodies and question the supple meaning of choice and agency in the context of surrogacy. Another similarity between them is that their admirable concern for women sometimes overshadows consideration of the best interests of the children created through surrogacy arrangements. I would urge more feminist scholars to take up this topic urgently and without compromising their dedication to reproductive justice.

Notes

1 For example: the 1992 Fertility Clinic Success Rate and Certification Act; guidelines issued by the American Society for Reproductive Medicine (ASRM); civil and criminal laws; self-regulation by ART providers; and patient demand for quality care.

2 The HFEA is the UK's independent regulator overseeing the use of gametes and embryos in fertility treatment and research. Its work includes licensing fertility clinics and centres carrying out in vitro fertilization (IVF), other assisted conception procedures and human embryo research (see <www.hfea.gov.uk/index.html>).

References

Allan S (2015) The surrogate in commercial surrogacy: legal and ethical considerations. In: Gerber P and O'Byrne K (eds) *Surrogacy, Law, and Human Rights*. Aldershot: Ashgate, pp. 113–44.

Boone SS (1992) Slavery and contract motherhood: a 'racialized' objection to the autonomy arguments. In: Holmes HB (ed.) *Issues in Reproductive Technology: An Anthology*. New York: Garland, pp. 349–66.

Corea G (1985) *The Mother Machine: Reproductive Technologies from Artificial Insemination to Artificial Wombs*. New York: Harper & Row.

Daar JF (1997) Regulating reproductive technologies: panacea or paper tiger. *Houston Law Review* 34: 609–64.

DasGupta S and Dasgupta SD (2014) Shifting sands: transnational surrogacy, e-motherhood, and nation building. In: DasGupta S and Dasgupta SD (eds) *Globalization and Transnational Surrogacy in India: Outsourcing Life*. Lanham, MD: Lexington Books, pp. 67–86.

Dietrich H (1992) Social control of surrogacy in Australia: a feminist perspective. In Holmes HB (ed.) *Issues in Reproductive Technology: An Anthology*. New York: Garland, pp. 367–80.

Ekman KE (2013) *Being and Being Bought: Prostitution, Surrogacy, and the Split Self*. Melbourne: Spinifex Press.

Gupta JA (2014) Biocrossings and the global fertility market. In: Sarojini N and Marwah V (eds) *Reconfiguring Reproduction: Feminist Health Perspectives on Assisted Reproductive Technologies*. Chicago, IL: University of Chicago Press.

Kohli N (2015) Outsourcing motherhood: India's reproductive dystopia. *Hindustan Times*, 26 July. <www.hindustantimes.com/india/outsourcing-motherhood-india-s-reproductive-dystopia/story-iCG1IuJJYMV994Gus2LZuK.html>

Madge V (2014) Gestational surrogacy in India: the problem of technology and poverty. In: DasGupta S and Dasgupta SD (eds) *Globalization and Transnational Surrogacy in India: Outsourcing Life*. Lanham, MD: Lexington Books, pp. 45–66.

Marwah V (2014) How surrogacy is challenging our feminisms. In: Sarojini N and Marwah V (eds) *Reconfiguring Reproduction: Feminist Health Perspectives on Assisted Reproductive Technologies*. Chicago, IL: University of Chicago Press.

Mutcherson KM (2012) Welcome to the Wild West: protecting access to cross border fertility care in the United States. *Cornell Journal of Law and Public Policy* 22(2): 349–94.

Mutcherson KM (2013) Transformative reproduction. *Journal of Gender, Race, and Justice* 16(1): 187–233.

Nayak P (2014) The three Ms of commercial surrogacy in India: Mother, Money, and Medical Market. In: DasGupta S and Dasgupta SD (eds) *Globalization and Transnational Surrogacy in India: Outsourcing Life*. Lanham, MD: Lexington Books, pp. 1–22.

Oliver K (1992) Marxism and surrogacy. In: Holmes HB and Purdy LM (eds) *Feminist Perspectives in Medical Ethics*. Bloomington, IN: Indiana University Press, pp. 266–83.

Pande A (2014) *Wombs in Labor: Transnational Commercial Surrogacy in India*. New York: Columbia University Press.

Pollitt K (1987) The strange case of baby M. *Nation* 244(20): 667–88.

Purdy LM (1992) Another look at contract pregnancy. In: Holmes HB (ed.) *Issues in Reproductive Technology: An Anthology*. New York: Garland, pp. 303–20.

Raymond JG (1993) *Women as Wombs: Reproductive Technologies and the Battle over Women's Freedom*. San Francisco, CA: HarperSanFrancisco.

Rothman BK (1989) *Recreating Motherhood: Ideology and Technology in a Patriarchal Society*. New York: Norton.

Shanley ML (2001) *Making Babies, Making Families: What Matters Most in an Age of Reproductive Technologies, Surrogacy, Adoption, and Same-Sex and Unwed Parents*. Boston, MA: Beacon Press.

Spar DL (2006) *The Baby Business: How Money, Science, and Politics Drive the Commerce of Conception*. Boston, MA: Harvard Business School Press.

Steiner LM (2013) *The Baby Chase: How Surrogacy Is Transforming the American Family*. New York: St Martin's Press.

Teman E (2010) *Birthing a Mother: The Surrogate Body and the Pregnant Self*. Berkeley, CA: University of California Press.

Twine FW (2015) *Outsourcing the Womb: Race, Class and Gestational Surrogacy in a Global Market*. 2nd edition. New York: Routledge.

19 | TRANSNATIONAL COMMERCIAL SURROGACY IN INDIA: TO BAN OR NOT TO BAN

Amrita Pande

The year 2015 witnessed a flurry of activities around commercial surrogacy in India. Though the Indian government has been reluctant to pass any concrete laws governing surrogacy, an affidavit was placed before the Supreme Court in October 2015, which, in a nutshell declared that the Indian government 'does not support commercial surrogacy' and the scope of surrogacy would be now limited to 'needy Indian married couples only'. This ban on commercial cross-border surrogacy falls in line with the Union government's previous attempts, in 2012 and 2013, to restrict commercial surrogacy to married couples of Indian origin. The government's latest affidavit, which ultimately aims to 'prohibit and penalise commercial surrogacy services' and ban commercial surrogacy *per se*, while allowing only altruistic surrogacy, is far more surprising.[1]

India is not the only country to propose a ban on cross-border surrogacy. Other popular surrogacy destinations in Asia – Thailand and Nepal – recently imposed similar bans, limiting surrogacy services to their nationals. Another popular destination, the Mexican state of Tabasco, has also voted to 'prevent foreign couples and gay men from having children through surrogacy' (Ochert, 2015; US Embassy, Kathmandu, 2015).

This chapter analyses the rationale and outcomes of a ban on the industry of paid contract pregnancy. In the first section I unpack the implications of a ban on commercial surrogacy and situate it within national imperatives as well as a global political context. In the second section, I use data from my decade-long ethnographic work in surrogacy clinics in India, together with the recent developments in the surrogacy industry, to argue against such a ban for two connected reasons: the effect of such a ban on the most vulnerable in the supply chain (the surrogates or womb mothers); and the utter naivety of trying to resolve a global problem merely through restrictive national legislations.[2] Finally, as an alternative I propose 'fairtrade surrogacy'

– cross-border surrogacy founded on transparency and dialogue on three fronts: in the structure of payments; in the medical process; and in the relationships forged within surrogacy.

Surrogacy scandals and surrogacy laws

The practice of surrogacy has long troubled people. Some are repulsed by the commodification aspect – what they argue are 'acts of love like mothering and pregnancy' and 'priceless' children increasingly entering the market. Dystopic imageries in the form of reproductive brothels, baby machines and baby farms were associated with this industry long before it reached its current proportions. Others are troubled by its potential to be utterly exploitative of women, especially women of particular race and class. In recent years, this anxiety has reached panic levels since the technology and the related industry spread to the global south and the 'wombs *sans frontières*', started belonging to women there (Sengupta, 2010: 8). The commissioning parents take on the role of evil avatars in the form of 'reproductive tourists', using their privileges to fulfil their 'right to a child' borne by a poor woman in the global south. The media report cases where commissioning parents 'abandon' their newborn, allegedly 'sell' their babies born out of surrogacy and have even exposed a case where an intending father had a history of child abuse. India, labelled by some as the 'mother destination' of cross-border surrogacy, has become pivotal in all such debates and discussions. Despite the burgeoning and nuanced ethnographic literature on the surrogacy industry in that country,[3] sensationalist media reportage continues to dominate public opinion and has ultimately pushed the Indian government to take a prohibitory stance.

The government's reluctance to pass any concrete laws in India does not mean that the issue of surrogacy has received no official attention until now. The delays and discrepancies merely highlight the conflict of interests embedded in taking any legal stand. The Indian Council of Medical Research (ICMR), as an institution of the Ministry of Health and Family Welfare (MoHFW), was the first to suggest a set of guidelines, published in 2005 as the National Guidelines for Accreditation, Supervision and Regulation of ART Clinics in India. This was later revised and prepared as a Draft ART (Regulation) Bill in 2008 and again in 2010. Curiously, the subsequent 2013 draft was not made public for a while and was even classified as 'top secret' by some agencies. In 2015, it was made accessible and available for public comment. Apart from the ICMR guidelines, the Law Commission of

India published its 228th *Report on the Need for Legislation to Regulate Assisted Reproductive Technology Clinics as well as Rights and Obligations of Parties to Surrogacy in 2009*, which presented a critique of the Draft ART Bill.[4]

The report recommended taking a 'pragmatic' legal approach that would prohibit commercial surrogacy in its entirety but allow altruistic surrogacy. For the Law Commission, and as per the 228th Report, surrogacy is not necessarily immoral and may in fact be a desirable way to deal with 'infertility'. The problem is its commercialization. Despite these recommendations, the subsequent Draft ART Bill (2010) yet again proposed the legalization of commercial gestational surrogacy. This dissonance continued to divide the ICMR and the MoHFW from not just the Law Commission but also the Union government. In 2013, however, the MoHFW started toeing the Union line and a 2014 draft bill put forward by the Health Ministry and the National Commission for Women (NCW) proposed to ban surrogacy for all foreigners. This reversal was most likely precipitated by several factors: the Supreme Court of India admonishing the government for delaying laws and allowing the 'business' and the 'tourism' to continue, and a spate of international 'surrogacy scandals' making headlines.[5]

Since the inception of commercial surrogacy, 'surrogacy scandals' have been pivotal in bringing about legal changes across the world, the most famous being the 1986 Baby M case in the US state of New Jersey.

India had its own Baby M – the much publicized 'Baby Manji' case. This was an unusual kind of custody battle with a biological father from Japan fighting for custody of a baby girl whom no one else really wanted (*The Hindu*, 2008). The couple from Japan had hired the services of a surrogate mother in India and used the eggs of an anonymous donor. Just a month before the baby, Manji, was born, the couple separated. When his ex-wife refused to travel with him to take possession of the baby, the intended father flew to India alone. The Indian authorities, however, refused to give Manji to her father because the Guardian Wards Act of 1890 bans single men from adopting girls in India. The next few weeks saw the drama unfold with a weeping grandmother making her appearance from Japan to convince authorities to give her custody over her grand-daughter. Manji was being declared the first surrogate orphan. Ultimately there was a happy ending, with the Indian Supreme Court stepping in and directing the government to give Manji a travel certificate for Japan.

A more recent 'surrogacy orphan' tale in India involved an

Australian couple abandoning the twin boy and taking the girl home. This case echoes the famous baby Gammy case in Thailand, where Australian parents decided to bring back the healthy girl and leave the twin brother diagnosed with Down's syndrome behind. The Gammy controversy pushed the Thai government to outlaw international surrogacy. In the Indian version, the couple decided to leave the boy behind because they could not afford him. They announced that they already had a son at home and wanted to 'complete their family' with a girl. The case nearly caused a diplomatic crisis between Australia and India, with each blaming the other for creating a stateless child. The case remains unresolved.[6]

It is worth recognizing that for countries like Thailand and India, which were garnering substantial revenue from medical tourism, there are enormous costs in closing their borders to surrogacy. But one cannot but wonder: should tabloid stories be the driving force behind a country's surrogacy laws? The problem with such legislation is it often misdiagnoses the root cause of a problem, and so recommends inadequate and inappropriate remedies. For instance, Indian governments' responses to these international scandals have been typical, a defensive and myopic reaction with an obvious priority – to avoid any more international legal battles. But is that all that needs to be debated? What is the problem that the legislation is attempting to remedy – assisted reproductive technologies like surrogacy, the commodification of pregnancy or the fact that it has started crossing borders?

In its enthusiasm to avoid international scandals over 'stateless babies', the Union government ultimately deprioritized another vital part of the story: the welfare of the womb (gestational) mothers. This prohibitory affidavit also diverts attention from the series of consultations and criticisms of the ART Bill. Feminist and health activists have been criticizing the Bill for a variety of reasons that I have discussed previously (2014, 2015), the critical one being that it is totally inadequate in addressing the concerns of the women who give birth, or in protecting their health and well-being (Qadeer, 2010; Sama Resource Group for Women and Health, 2010). The Bill is especially hazy on critical issues such as the rights of the surrogate, details of the contracts, the role of different intermediaries, the nature of 'informed consent', nature of compensation, and legal, medical and post-partum assistance for the surrogates. While many suggestions made by feminists and health activists in India are yet to be implemented, prohibitory Home Ministry stipulations are accepted and implemented without any appraisal or consultation.

A national prohibitory approach

The frame through which we analyse surrogacy will shape the ultimate policies and regulations devised. If we use the lens of morality, we might well come to the conclusion that commercial surrogacy is inherently immoral and undesirable. It defies laws of nature, family and religion and represents a commercialization of motherhood, the act of giving birth and of children. An obvious policy corollary for a class of action considered intrinsically wrong is to prohibit it by imposing a formal ban. I have previously expressed my discomfort with the 'inherent immorality' claim, especially since it reifies the dichotomy between production and reproduction, and universalizes and naturalizes the so-called 'sacred' bond between mother and child (Pande, 2014).

As surrogacy shifts to countries in the global south, there is an urgent need to revisit the frames for analysing the industry. Instead of the immorality or commodification frame of viewing surrogacy as an unnatural vice and the womb mothers as victims, the reality on the ground demands an updated analytical lens. Once the industry is systematically studied as an empirical reality, we realize that surrogacy in countries like India has been a rapidly expanding labour market, with characteristics not unlike other gendered and informal markets in the global south. Unarguably the limited range of Indian women's alternative economic opportunities undermines the voluntary nature of this labour. But instead of dismissing the labour market as inherently oppressive and the women involved as subjects of this oppressive structure, it makes sense to recognize, validate and systematically evaluate the choices that women make in order to participate in that market. Once we comprehensively and sensitively assess these choices, we can actually start discussing the many intersecting layers of structural, economic, political and cultural domination that shape these choices and can then effectively move towards a discussion of appropriate policies and laws.

While the 'surrogacy is immoral' argument continues to inspire several contemporary campaigns, another popular frame for understanding commercial surrogacy is one of reproductive rights. In *Discounted Life: The Price of Global Surrogacy in India*, Sharmila Rudrappa (2015) convincingly argues that the reproductive rights frame cannot capture the dilemmas of transnational surrogacy. Those against surrogacy can use it to pitch clients, often privileged individuals from the global north, against the womb mothers. The same frame is used by advocates of surrogacy to argue that all individuals, whether gay men (with their right to have a child) or surrogates (with the right to choose what they want to do with their bodies) have a right to have their reproductive rights met! Rudrappa extends legal scholar Dorothy Roberts's argument to clarify that 'markets in life' may indeed empower women and further working-class women's rights. Yet, given social and economic realities in India, for reproductive justice to prevail we need to consider the 'totality of women's experiences ... and alter power relations in their favour' (Rudrappa, 2015: 173). But what can the various actors involved in surrogacy do for reproductive justice to prevail?

Contemporary examples have made it amply clear that state actors cannot live in the naïve hope that the market will empower the women working in the womb industry. There are two possible policy options: an outright ban or a regulatory framework. Whatever our stance on surrogacy may be, I would caution against an outright ban on surrogacy. People's desire for genetic babies is unlikely to diminish in the near future. Development in relevant assisted reproductive technologies cannot be reversed and, with globalization, clients will continue to cross borders to make use of these technologies. A *national* ban is not just unrealistic but also undesirable. Banning surrogacy in India will just push it underground, further stigmatizing the profession and the women involved and undermining their rights as workers. If there is one thing that can be learned from the experience of sex workers, the abolitionist tendency can only be calamitous for working women, whether in sex work or commercial surrogacy. To quote Debora Spar (2006: 305):

> Unless one posits, however, that the existence of global inequality renders all economic choices moot; and until there is any path by which these inequalities can feasibly be addressed, denying women this particular choice seems oddly counter-productive. It also does not square with the kind of logic applied to other areas of the global labour market ... where concerns about global inequality lead toward international rules and regulations, not a total prohibition of the activity involved.

Given that countries like India will most likely lack the political will to implement effectively a ban on surrogacy, the more probable outcome of prohibition would be to make surrogates even more vulnerable and without any protection from brokers and clients. A 2012 news report on the surrogacy industry in China confirms this prediction. Although there is no specific law regulating the industry in China, in 2001 the Ministry of Health banned any trade in fertilized eggs and embryos, which in turn forbade hospitals from performing any gestational surrogacy procedures. The ban is regularly flouted by clinics and clients and has effectively driven the industry underground. While there is no official count of this fledgling industry, a 2011 study estimates that, to date, more than 25,000 children have been born in China through surrogacy arrangements. The article reports that, in fact, people of higher economic classes use surrogacy practices to bypass the one-child rule (Davison, 2012). A similar controversy was unearthed in Taiwan, where surrogacy is illegal. A surrogacy company based there was charged with human trafficking for allegedly holding Vietnamese women in hostels after confiscating their passports. In Guatemala, surrogacy seems to be replacing the industry of international adoptions, which has been featured in the media because of rampant human rights abuses. A *Washington Times* investigation reports that 'some of the same people who were arranging international adoptions are acting as surrogacy brokers in Guatemala' (Ehrlich, 2011).

Imposing a blanket ban on surrogacy in India is likely just to shift the business to another country in the global south. We need not go that far to hunt for proof but just have to peer over the Indian borders into Nepal and further to Thailand. The 2013 stipulations restricting surrogacy in India to married heterosexual couples effectively pushed all cases of 'gay surrogacy' to Thailand. After a spate of international surrogacy scandals, Thailand banned cross-border surrogacy in 2014 and now only married heterosexuals with at least one Thai partner are allowed to use surrogates. Some gay surrogacy clients pushed out from India in 2013 resorted to another neighbouring country: Nepal. This industry flourished unnoticed before the earthquake brought media attention to the 'scandal' of gay Israeli men supposedly abandoning the Indian surrogates and rescuing only their child after the earthquake. But these media reports revealed another scandal, which ironically no one discussed: the 2013 ban on gay surrogacy made the Indian surrogates even more vulnerable (see Chapter 3). Most of the Indian women who were in Nepal after the earthquake reported feeling most abandoned not by the Israeli clients but by the Indian government. The ban had pushed them to make their living in Kathmandu instead of in Delhi, Anand or Mumbai. Their status in Nepal was para-legal and most did not have money to purchase a flight ticket home. Indian authorities would not sign release papers for a child commissioned by gay parents. So what would happen to the child they were gestating, their contract and their payment even if they managed to return home? The Indian state banning their labour option is what made the India women more vulnerable, not the fact that their clients were international or gay.

The idea of imposing a ban on just the cross-border aspect of surrogacy as it, arguably, increases the likelihood of exploitation, is not new. In fact scholars in several sending countries (where the clients of surrogacy come from) have been debating the costs and benefits of permitting cross-border reproductive travel for services like surrogacy. Some believe that cross-border reproductive travel is an obvious and fair solution to restrictive national legislation. It promotes moral pluralism in democratic states, as it 'prevents the frontal clash between the majority who imposes its view and the minority who claim to have a moral right to some medical service' (Pennings, 2002: 338). Others see this kind of travel as not only a poor solution to moral and political pluralism but also counterproductive. It allows only a certain class of people – the ones with the economic means to travel – the option to escape the restraints of the law. Moreover, in effect, the availability of cross-border options allows national governments to enact stricter laws at home than they might otherwise have the political will to enact. Strict national laws, in turn, export the morally contentious industry to some other country, very often a country in the global south.

With the rise in transnational surrogacy, most sending countries have started recognizing the need to incorporate these new complexities into their policies around surrogacy. Some countries, for instance Turkey and Malaysia, have extended their prohibitive approach to cross-border surrogacy and ban their citizens from obtaining these procedures abroad. Others, such as France, the UK, Germany, Spain and Japan, attempt to discourage their citizens from doing so by withholding legal recognition to such cases (Storrow, 2010). Children born out of surrogacy arrangements abroad, for instance, may not be given travel documents or not be granted citizenship status. With the rise in international legal disputes regarding the citizenship of children born out of surrogacy in India, other countries are contemplating a different strategy – making their domestic surrogacy laws less restrictive so that their nationals need not travel outside their borders to access this technology. Iceland and China, for instance, are currently debating a shift towards a less restrictive approach at home to discourage their citizens from going abroad in search of surrogates. With more than fifty Australian families who had babies born through surrogacy caught in a bureaucratic limbo in Nepal after the government passed an interim ban on surrogacy, the Australian government is under pressure to open up discussions on the domestic ban.[7]

These recent events highlight the ultimate ineffectiveness of restrictive national laws; a global and complex issue like surrogacy cannot be resolved or regulated within national borders but urgently needs a global dialogue. Much like intercountry adoptions that have been regulated and discussed internationally (for instance, by The Hague Convention on Protection of Children and Co-operation in Respect of Intercountry Adoption 1993), cross-border surrogacy needs a global platform. In my recent works I proposed a step towards such a global regulation by discussing the provocative notion of 'fairtrade surrogacy' – cross-border surrogacy founded on openness and transparency on three fronts: in the structure of payments; in the medical process; and in the relationships forged within surrogacy (Pande, 2014; Pande and Bjerg, 2014). I connect the notions of free and ethical trade surrogacy in the following section.

'Fairtrade surrogacy' and the dignity of labour

The reality is that surrogacy cannot be resolved as a national issue or by closing borders. Nor can it be left for state actors to resolve. As already stated, given the nature of this industry, it would be naïve to expect that any national law will be enforced and effective on its own. As Wendy Chavkin (2010: 7) surmises: 'With increasing globalization, a country's policy decisions on reproduction are not contained by national borders, as people, products, body parts, technologies and ideas move across borders.' A more practical step might be to have an open international dialogue on the nature of this industry.

Medical practitioner Casey Humbyrd (2009) proposes a move towards such an international dialogue and regulation in her guide to 'fairtrade practices' in international surrogacy. Humbyrd provides a provocative argument in favour of 'applying Fair Trade principles to international surrogacy' in order to ensure that the benefits of surrogacy 'are justly shared between the participating parties' and that it is beneficial to those who are the 'weakest in the supply chain' – the surrogates (Humbyrd 2009: 116).[8] Although Humbyrd fails to address how this regulatory and compensation framework can be implemented, I find it constructive to evaluate and extend some of her policy insights based on my ethnographic findings. For instance, Humbyrd briefly mentions that a 'fair price in the regional or local context' is 'one that has been agreed through dialogue and participation'. She goes on to add that there is a need for 'transparency and accountability ... of financial transactions between surrogacy brokers, prospective parents and surrogate mothers' (2009: 118). I extend Humbyrd's insights and propose an international model of surrogacy founded on openness and transparency, not just at the 'price' end but on three fronts that relate more to dignity of labour: in the structure of payments, in the medical process and in the relationships forged within surrogacy.

Financial transparency Transparency in financial transactions and allowing wage settlements through dialogue between the surrogates and intended parents are valuable recommendations, highlighted by the surrogates themselves. Some clauses in the Draft ART (Regulation) Bill 2010 attempted to address concerns about financial transparency but these were completely inadequate. Oddly, while the Bill seemed to promote the 'business' of surrogacy and other ARTs, it was strangely myopic in its understanding of the realities of this industry. Social scientist and community health activist Imrana Qadeer (2010) has highlighted many instances of this. For instance, the Bill paid very little attention to details of administration of the contract between the surrogate and the intended parents. There is little information on how the money transaction would actually take place and no mechanism to ensure the enforcement of other financial aspects of the contract. The Bill failed to lay out clearly the details of the financial arrangement between the surrogate and the intending parents. Although it emphasized the need to have a legally binding contract, it did not clarify whether the intended parents would reimburse all prenatal and postnatal care expenses as well as the loss of opportunity to work after surgery. It did not require that surrogates be provided with legal assistance in case of any conflicts during the surrogacy arrangement. The payment structure reflects that priority is accorded firmly to the intended parents. For instance, the latest draft of the Bill before the ban recommended that payment be made to the surrogate in five instalments with the majority (75 per cent) to be paid on the delivery of the baby. This structure would clearly disadvantage surrogates, especially in the event of a late miscarriage.

A meaningful discussion on transparency in financial transactions needs to consider the distinctive attributes of this work. Surrogacy involves an intense amount of body and emotion work and often forges relationships, arguably more intimate, than between the buyer and the seller in many other markets. Consequently, national or international laws cannot exclude the potential for change through dialogue and negotiations at the local level. The intimate and personal relationships that surrogates build with their clients are not just a source of potential exploitation for the worker but can be a basis for negotiating everyday advantages. For instance, scholars have indicated that the personalized employer–employee relationships forged in the provision of reproductive services like domestic caregiving work, often portrayed as disempowering and archaic, are not necessarily perceived as negative by the workers themselves. Workers may well see these intimate relationships as a way to gain extra benefits.[9]

The latest ruling may, of course, render moot much of this discussion on payments as the Indian government seems to be moving determinedly towards altruistic surrogacy. While, at some level, this form of surrogacy may seem ideal for erasing the alleged commodification of bodies, emotions and children within the industry, it is indeed that – a naïve ideal that does nothing to reduce the exploitative potentials of this industry or empower its workers. In essence, altruistic surrogacy reinforces the stereotype of women as 'naturally' nurturant and selfless by making their labour and hardships free of charge. Sharyn Anleu (1992) and Janice Raymond (1990) have argued that the distinction between commercial and altruistic surrogacy is 'socially constructed' and, in essence, altruistic surrogacy oppresses women under the guise of a 'moral celebration' of their altruism. Others have used the 'vulnerability of source' indicator in organ donations to demonstrate that due to gender imbalances and power inequalities within families and households, women are often 'encouraged' to be altruistic donors. For instance in the US, a study indicated that more than two-thirds of kidney donors are women; another revealed that while more than 30 per cent of wives who were able donated to their spouses, fewer than 7 per cent of husbands eligible to donate did so (Liberto, 2013). This becomes particularly critical in India, where altruism and gendered notions of familial duty have often been forced onto female relatives, or those in positions of relative vulnerability such as domestic workers.

Medical transparency For surrogacy in India, transparency and control in the second arena – medical process – needs to be much more than a signature indicating informed consent. For women who have little experience with bio-medical technologies and professional medicine, being 'aware' of the medical requirements and implications of ARTs should be a continuous process of explanation and interaction over a period of time. Beyond transparency, there is a need for surrogates to have control over the medical interventions, whether it be abortions, selective terminations in cases of multiple births or c-sections. The current unregulated environment allows those with more power – mostly the doctors and the clients – to take all medical decisions. I have previously discussed the first two aspects; I want to end with a focus on the third front for transparency – that of relationships.

Transparency in relationships If we are indeed in the midst of a 'biological century', with bodies, body parts, organs and gametes entering the market, we need to reimagine how we define and value relationships forged by these bio-markets. What could fairtrade surrogacy mean for the relationships forged within surrogacy? For many surrogates, for surrogacy to be 'fair' what is required is not just an increase in the payments they receive for their labour, but as critically, an affirmation of their dignity as labourers. Almost all respondents in my research emphasized the desire that their efforts at forging relationships with the fetus/baby are acknowledged and reciprocated, and clients continue to respect the ties that they have forged across seemingly impossible borders of religion, race, class and nation.

This call for openness and transparency is not as idealistic as it may sound. Legislations and policies around national and intercountry adoption have, for long, made this a central concern. Some recent reports on the growing industry of surrogacy indicate the urgent need to make productive comparisons between intercountry adoption and transnational surrogacy laws. For instance, social work scholars Karen Smith Rotabi and Nicole Footen Bromfield (2012), who primarily focus on intercountry adoptions and 'adoption frauds' in Guatemala, predicted that surrogacy may well be replacing adoption in countries like Guatemala. Rotabi and Bromfield argue that the consistent increase in the global demand for healthy young children and a decline in adoption opportunities have resulted in a rise in the 'price of young children' as well as an increase in the waiting time for their placement. International surrogacy and IVF are emerging as lucrative alternatives. In a more tongue-in-cheek comparison, Anoop Gupta, an Indian fertility doctor, has surmised that 'surrogacy is the new adoption' (quoted in Twine, 2011: 16). Whether this is so is debatable but the 'open' model of adoption can provide a guiding frame for future policies (Satz, 1992; Scherman et al., 2016).[10]

An open and transparent model of transnational surrogacy brings into focus another intricacy that has curiously escaped much of the discussion – the recognition that the *final 'product' of this market is a living child.* Unlike in the case of adoption, where many countries (including India) have ratified The Hague Adoption Convention (1993) and have devised comprehensive laws regarding the rights of the adopted child, the rights of children born out of surrogacy become a topic of discussion only during custody disputes.[11] More research is needed to gauge the impact of gestation on the lives of children. But for now we can reasonably assume that issues that have been relevant for intercountry adoption will arise in the future for transnational surrogacy. For instance, should the child born out of surrogacy be told about his/her womb mother? Should a child be allowed to contact his/her birth mother? These are just some of the questions that will need answering in a not so distant future.

Notes

1 This was reinforced in August 2016, when the Indian government approved the introduction of the Surrogacy (Regulation) Bill, 2016 in Parliament, to be discussed in the forthcoming winter session.

2 The origin of the term 'surrogacy' and its social and political implications have been widely discussed by feminists. Critics have argued that this terminology suggests that the womb mother is somehow less than the genetic or social mother. Although the phrase 'women who give birth for pay' or 'womb mothers' may be preferred over the term 'surrogates', in this article I use 'surrogacy' and 'surrogate' for purposes of brevity and clarity. The women refer to one another as 'surrogate mothers', and when I explained what the term 'surrogate' meant in English, most agreed that the description was fitting.

3 For the most recent ethnographic work on surrogacy in India see Pande (2014, 2015) and Rudrappa (2015).

4 See <http://lawcommissionofindia.nic.in/reports/report228.pdf>.

5 See <www.bionews.org.uk/page_576944.asp; http://indianexpress.com/article/india/india-news-india/supreme-court-asks-centre-to-bring-commercial-surrogacy-within-ambit-of-law>.

6 See <www.abc.net.au/news/2015-04-13/australian-couple-abandon-baby-boy-in-india-surrogacy-case/6387206>.

7 In Australia, it is illegal to pay a woman to carry a child for someone else, except in the Northern Territory where there are no laws concerning surrogacy. For more on recent debates in Australia, see <http://www.abc.net.au/news/2015-04-18/commercial-surrogacy-should-be-legalised-family-court-justice/6402924> and <www.couriermail.com.au/news/queensland/push-to-make-surrogacy-legal-in-australia/story-fnihsrf2-1227308579743>.

8 Humbyrd outlines, in some detail, what a formal international agreement governing intercountry surrogacy could look like. She advocates a model similar to The Hague Convention on Intercountry Adoption as well as more immediate regulations; for instance, clients must work with nationally accredited service providers. Within this regulatory framework, 'brokers and agencies involved in international surrogacy could be accredited based on their compliance with Fair Trade surrogacy standards, and the list of approved surrogacy service providers could be publicized on the State Department website as it is for adoption service providers'.

9 Shireen Ally, in her study of domestic work in South Africa, demonstrates that while state efforts to modernize and professionalize domestic work as a form of employment in post-apartheid South Africa have been remarkable, some domestic workers feel disempowered by these laws. Domestic workers value the intimate negotiations with their employers as much, if not more, than the rights-based benefits given by the state. When the state positions itself as the representative and protector of the interests of 'vulnerable' domestic workers, the workers themselves get demobilized, and their voices muted. Other scholars have reported similar findings. For instance, Latina day workers and part-time cleaners in the studies of Mary Romero (1992) and Leslie Salzinger (1991) are perceived to have 'upgraded' the occupation by establishing a business-like contractual relationship. However, Jennifer Mendez (1998) interviewed cleaners employed by a bureaucratic agency and found that many workers actually prefer private employment, in which they have the autonomy of selecting employers and can obtain personal favours. Similarly, Turkish maids and doorkeepers interviewed by Gul Ozyegin (2001) even embrace class hierarchies because they gain raises and extra benefits in a patron–client relationship.

10 Debra Satz has previously compared surrogacy and adoption and argued for an 'open' model: one that regulates the arrangement, that respects the surrogates' option to change her mind, and provides all relevant details about associated risks (Satz, 1992).

11 The Hague Convention on Protection of Children and Co-operation in Respect of Intercountry Adoption (1993) seeks to protect children and their families against the risks of illegal, irregular or ill-prepared adoptions abroad. In India (a signatory to this Convention) the Central Adoption Resource Authority (CARA) under the Ministry of Women & Child Development, functions as the nodal body for adoption of Indian children. CARA is mandated to monitor and regulate all in-country and inter-country adoptions. See <http://adoptionindia.nic.in/guideline-family/Post%20Adoption.html> for the specifics on 'Root Search', or the rights of the child to obtain information about his or her origins.

References

Ally S (2009) *From Servants to Workers: South African Domestic Workers and the Democratic State.* Ithaca, NY: Cornell University Press.

Anleu SR (1992) For love but not for money? *Gender & Society* 6(1): 30–48.

Chavkin W (2010) The globalization of motherhood. In: Chavkin C and Maher JM (eds) *The Globalization of Motherhood: Deconstructions and Reconstructions of Biology and Care.* New York: Routledge, pp. 180–202.

Davison N (2012) Chinese surrogate mothers see business boom in year of the dragon. *Guardian*, 8 February. <www.guardian.co.uk/world/2012/feb/08/china-surrogate-mothers-year-dragon>

Ehrlich RS (2011) Thai company accused of trafficking Vietnamese women to breed. *Washington Times*, 6 March. <http://www.washingtontimes.com/news/2011/mar/6/thai-company-accused-traffick-vietnam-women-breed>

Humbyrd C (2009) Fair trade international surrogacy. *Developing World Bioethics* 9(3): 111–18.

Liberto H (2013) Noxious markets versus noxious gift relationships. *Social Theory and Practice* 39(2): 265–87. <http://wp.hallie-liberto.

philosophy.uconn.edu/wp-content/uploads/sites/1026/2015/02/Noxious-Markets-versus-Noxious-Gift-Relationships-January-2013-re-submission.docx.pdf>

Mendez J (1998) Of mops and maids: contradictions and continuities in bureaucratised domestic work. *Social Problems* 45(1): 114–35.

Millbank J (2015) Gammygate II: surrogacy law must not be based on the latest tabloid story. *BioNews*, 27 April. <www.bionews.org.uk/page_519793.asp>

Ochert A (2015) Mexico bans surrogacy for gay couples and foreigners. *BioNews*, 21 December. <www.bionews.org.uk/page_599021.asp>

Ozyegin G (2001) *Untidy Gender: Domestic Work in Turkey*. Philadelphia, PA: Temple University Press.

Pande A (2014) *Wombs in Labor: Transnational Commercial Surrogacy in India*. New York: Columbia University Press.

Pande A (2015) The kin labor in kinship travel: intended mothers and surrogates in India. *Anthropologica: Canada's Anthropology Journal* 57(1): 53–62. Special Issue on Kinship Travel.

Pande A and Bjerge DM (2014) Made in India: sketches from a baby farm. *Global Dialogue* 4(3): 19–21.

Pennings G (2002) Reproductive tourism as moral pluralism in motion. *Journal of Medical Ethics* 28: 337–41.

Qadeer I (2010) *New Reproductive Technologies and Health Care in Neo-liberal India: Essays*. New Delhi: Centre for Women's Development Studies.

Raymond J (1990) Reproductive gifts and gift giving: the altruistic woman. *Hastings Center Report* 20(6): 7–11.

Romero M (1992) *Maid in the U.S.A.* London and New York: Routledge.

Rotabi KS and Bromfield NF (2012) The decline in intercountry adoptions and new practices of global surrogacy: global exploitation and human rights concerns. *Affilia* 27: 129.

Rothman BK (2000) *Recreating Motherhood: Ideology and Technology in a Patriarchal Society*. New Jersey: Rutgers University Press.

Rudrappa S (2015) *Discounted Life: The Price of Global Surrogacy in India*. New York: NYU Press.

Salzinger L (1991) A maid by any other name: the transformation of 'dirty work' by Central American immigrants. In: Burawoy M, Burton A, Ferguson AA and Fox KJ (eds) *Ethnography Unbound: Power and Resistance in the Modern Metropolis*. Berkeley, CA: University of California Press, pp. 139–60.

Sama Resource Group for Women and Health (2010) *Unravelling the Fertility Industry: Challenges and Strategies for Movement Building*. New Delhi: Sama.

Satz D (1992) Markets in women's reproductive labor. *Philosophy and Public Affairs* 21(2): 107–31.

Scherman R, Misca G, Rotabi K and Selman P (2016) Global commercial surrogacy and international adoption: parallels and differences. *Adoption & Fostering* 40(1): 20–35.

Sengupta A (2010) Technology, markets, and the commoditisation of life. In: *Unravelling the Fertility Industry: Challenges and Strategies for Movement Building*. Delhi: Sama.

Spar DL (2006) *The Baby Business: How Money, Science, and Politics Drive the Commerce of Conception*. Cambridge, MA: Harvard Business School Publishing Corporations.

Storrow RF (2010) The pluralism problem in cross-border reproductive care. *Human Reproduction* 25(12): 2939–43.

The Hindu (2008) Japanese baby gets birth certificate. *The Hindu*, 11 August. <www.thehindu.com/2008/08/11/stories/2008081160180300.htm>

Twine FW (2011) *Outsourcing the Womb: Race, Class, and Gestational Surrogacy in a Global Market*. New York and Abingdon: Routledge.

US Embassy (2015) Surrogacy in Nepal. US Citizen Services, 30 October. <http://nepal.usembassy.gov/service/surrogacy-in-nepal.html>

Vora K (2015) *Life Support: Biocapital and the New History of Outsourced Labor*. Minneapolis, MN: University of Minnesota Press.

20 | GOVERNING TRANSNATIONAL SURROGACY PRACTICES: WHAT ROLE CAN NATIONAL AND INTERNATIONAL REGULATION PLAY?

Sonia Allan

Introduction

The previous chapters of this book have examined the significant issues raised by surrogacy practices, particularly in the context of commercial transnational arrangements. This final chapter provides an overview of current laws, policies and practices around the world in order to present a global picture of the position countries currently take. It shows that the majority of nations prohibit commercial surrogacy – a significant number of such nations prohibit *all* surrogacy arrangements; and a significant number of other nations have specific legislation permitting 'altruistic' arrangements, while maintaining prohibitions on commercial surrogacy. Other nations do not have specific legislation regulating surrogacy, but have other laws that are relevant, which limit or stop surrogacy practices. The *minority* of nations have permissive regimes.

The presence of permissive regimes, or countries that have (or had) no laws at all, has seemingly enabled transnational arrangements in which commissioning person(s) have been encouraged (often by agents in their home countries or via concerted internet and media campaigns)[1] to travel to engage in commercial surrogacy. It is in this context that many issues related to commercial surrogacy have been brought to global attention. The discussion of international law and regulation has therefore also been growing, noting that transnational commercial surrogacy arrangements have raised both private international law and public international law issues.[2] The second section of this chapter considers the international issues raised by transnational commercial surrogacy.

The third section then looks forward, asking the question of what regulatory approach should be taken. It considers international regulation, in terms of suggestions for a multilateral, legally binding instrument such as a convention, and approaches that may be taken domestically. It is concluded that, given that most of the world prohibits commercial surrogacy, a facilitative or permissive convention would be unacceptable. One that takes a united stance against such practices would be preferred, but it is noted that such a treaty would be unlikely to be signed by those few nations that wish to continue commercial practices. Domestic laws therefore need to be strong and enforced. Those countries that choose to prohibit commercial surrogacy should not practise a double standard by turning a 'blind eye' to their people engaging in such practices offshore. Countries that permit commercial surrogacy should restrict such practices to those permanently domiciled in their own communities. Ultimately, however, I argue that surrogacy should not be seen as a form of 'trade'; we should not acquiesce to the 'market' terms or practices, or notions that this is an acceptable way to 'form families'. Empowerment will not come through using women's bodies to bear children for others; children should not be commodified. We have a global issue that needs careful united work to see their needs and human rights put first.

Laws, policies and practices of countries around the world

Jurisdictions that prohibit all surrogacy arrangements A significant number of nations worldwide prohibit all surrogacy arrangements via laws, policies and/or religious decree. This includes all those nations and jurisdictions set out in Table 20.1.

The ethos underpinning such bans generally includes statements that view surrogacy as 'a violation of the child's and "surrogate" mother's human dignity'. Such jurisdictions often adopt the view that commercial surrogacy involves the commodification of women and children, and/or a multitude of other unacceptable risks and practices including (but not limited to) those of exploitation, sale and trafficking.

If surrogacy were to occur in any of these jurisdictions, the birth mother would be considered the legal mother of any resulting child, and the surrogacy arrangement would be void and unenforceable. Criminal sanctions may apply to the parties involved in the arrangement or, more commonly, for any intermediaries and/or medical institutions facilitating it.

Jurisdictions that expressly permit and regulate 'altruistic' surrogacy, but prohibit commercial surrogacy A number of other jurisdictions permit only altruistic surrogacy arrangements and provide criminal sanctions

TABLE 20.1 Jurisdictions that prohibit surrogacy arrangements[3]

Afghanistan	Albania	Algeria	Austria	Bahrain
Bangladesh	China[4] (mainland)	Croatia	Egypt	El Salvador
Ethiopia	Finland	France	Germany	Iceland
Indonesia	Italy	Jordan	Kuwait	Malaysia
Maldives	Malta	Mauritius	Mexico (e.g. Queretaro)	
Moldova	Morocco	Norway	Oman	Portugal
Qatar	Saudi Arabia	Serbia	Singapore	Slovenia
Spain	Sweden	Switzerland	Syrian Arab Republic	Taiwan
Tajikistan	Tunisia	Turkey	Turkmenistan	United Arab Emirates
Some jurisdictions within the US (e.g. Arizona and the District of Columbia)			Vietnam	Yemen

regarding commercial surrogacy. Such countries include those listed in Table 20.2.

In addition to the jurisdictions listed in Table 20.2, Hong Kong prohibits commercial surrogacy and does not recognize other surrogacy arrangements.

A number of these jurisdictions allow reimbursement of 'reasonable expenses'. This is generally limited to costs actually incurred – noting that places like the UK of late have been criticized for 'blurring' the lines and granting much higher payments (equivalent or more, in some cases, to what is paid to women involved in commercial surrogacy arrangements in other nations).

Under this approach there is also a 'strong trend' to permit only surrogacy arrangements where at least one commissioning person is genetically related to the child, and in some jurisdictions only 'gestational' surrogacy is allowed.

In several of these jurisdictions, women and commissioning persons must meet certain criteria before being able to enter into a surrogacy agreement. For the woman, these may include such things as age requirements, satisfactory completion of medical and psychological screening, having already had a living child and/or having completed

TABLE 20.2 Jurisdictions that permit altruistic surrogacy but prohibit commercial surrogacy arrangements

Australia (all states and territories except the Northern Territory where surrogacy is not practised)	Belarus	Belgium	Brazil
Bulgaria	Canada	Denmark	Greece[5]	Hungary
Ireland	Latvia	Lithuania	Mexico (some states)	Netherlands
New Zealand	South Africa	South Korea	Thailand	United Kingdom
Uruguay	Peru			

her family, civil status and having received independent legal advice. For the commissioning person(s), criteria may include such things as infertility, a particular relationship status, criminal record and child protection checks, age, counselling, legal advice, residence requirements and more.

Jurisdictions that do not have specific laws governing surrogacy Under this approach, there may be no direct legislation pertaining to the practice of surrogacy, or explicit prohibition in law regarding commercial surrogacy.[6] This is the current situation in countries including (but not limited to) Argentina, Belgium, Brazil, the Czech Republic, Ireland, Japan, Mexico (Mexico City) and some jurisdictions in the US (e.g. Michigan) and Venezuela.

However, these are not necessarily 'destination' countries for international commercial surrogacy, as the transfer of legal parentage to customers may not be possible. In these countries a contractual obligation for a surrogate mother to surrender a child to commissioning person(s) would be void and unenforceable under general law. The birth mother is the legal mother of the child. Also while in some such jurisdictions there is no specific regulation of surrogacy, commercial surrogacy is banned in a number, either through express legal provision or general laws pertaining to, for example, child trafficking in Turkmenistan and Azerbaijan. Other jurisdictions have other laws, guidelines or practice that govern their position on surrogacy, or have indicated an intention to pass laws as follows:

- In **Argentina** the courts have recognized an altruistic surrogacy arrangement, using a couple's own eggs and a close friend who carried the child. Commercial surrogacy is prohibited, and specifically for foreigners.
- In **Belgium**, commercial surrogacy is prohibited on public policy grounds. Altruistic surrogacy is not regulated and is therefore possible. Contracts are not enforceable and adoption is required to transfer legal parenthood; a small number of such arrangements occur in the country each year. In 2010, a Belgium Court of Appeal recognized a commercial surrogacy agreement that had taken place in California, granting partial relief sought by the two men who had commissioned it.[7] The Court decided to recognize and give effect to the birth certificates issued in California in so far as they form the basis for the legal link between the female children and their biological father. The other male partner was not legally recognized as a 'parent'. There was some indication that he would have to adopt the children in order to be seen as such. In general, this reflects the position under Belgian law that filiation is a preliminary question to the determination of Belgian nationality and parentage.
- In **Brazil**, altruistic surrogacy is permitted pursuant to guidelines in limited circumstances. The surrogate must be related to the commissioning husband or wife, but exemptions may be allowed by regional medical councils. No payment is permitted. Commercial practices associated with gamete or embryo donation or surrogacy are prohibited (Part IV and Part VII of the Resolution CFM No 1957, 2010).
- In **Ireland**, consideration of laws to permit altruistic surrogacy, and prohibit commercial surrogacy, is ongoing. Under the present law, transfer of parentage would not be possible.
- In the **Czech Republic**, the law does not permit surrogacy 'as a business' (i.e. commercial surrogacy). In 'altruistic' arrangements the commissioning couple pay medical expenses and health costs, although there is some indication that other payments are 'unofficially' made. The birth mother is the legal mother. A biological commissioning father may be recognized as the legal father; a biological mother (i.e. a woman whose egg has been used) would have to adopt the child. If the birth mother does not wish to give up the child, she does not have to.
- In **Japan**, the Japanese Society of Obstetrics and Gynecology prohibits any form of surrogacy. The reasons given were as follows:

1. Priority should be given to the welfare of the child and surrogacy offends such welfare.
2. Surrogacy is associated with the burden of mental and physical risk.
3. Surrogacy makes family relationships complex.
4. Surrogacy contracts are not acceptable in terms of social ethics (Nozawa and Banno, 2004: 194).

In 2008, a committee of the Science Council of Japan made public a draft report that called for enacting a law to ban surrogate pregnancy and birth by law. The general view is that surrogate pregnancy arranged for profit should be punished, and that such punishment should be applied to the medical doctor who provided treatment, mediators and commissioning persons, but surrogate mothers should be excluded. The birth mother is considered the legal mother of a child born as the result of a surrogate pregnancy. In cases of altruistic surrogacy, or special cases in which Japanese people have engaged in surrogacy overseas, establishment of legal parenthood between a child born as a result of surrogate pregnancy and the commissioning married couple has been recognized by way of an adoption or a special adoption.[8]

A permissive approach to surrogacy, including commercial surrogacy
Countries that take a permissive approach are few. They include Armenia, Georgia, Israel,[9] Kazakhzstan, Russia, Uganda, Ukraine, Liechtenstein and some US states.[10] In these jurisdictions commercial surrogacy is permitted and practised. Following a surrogacy arrangement, there are usually procedures in the state which enable legal parentage to be granted to one or both of the commissioning person(s); there may or may not be a domicile or habitual residence requirement for them; and differences are found regarding who is permitted to enter into such agreements, and requirements such people must meet. That is, policy perspectives in the countries that permit commercial surrogacy vary, and do not mean that people can access such services in all of these nations from abroad.

- In **Armenia**, legislation allows foreign residents, couples (including same-sex and/or LGBT) and/or individuals to undergo surrogacy.[11] However, there have been proposals in Armenia for new laws to prohibit foreigners from hiring Armenian women to

- be 'surrogate' mothers for them, because many believe that 'the usage of Armenian women's wombs for giving birth to foreigners' children is unacceptable' (Abramyhan, 2013).
- In **Georgia**, 'extracorporeal fertilization' is permitted for heterosexual couples, in the case of infertility, to avoid transmission of genetic disease and/or if the woman has no uterus, using the couple's or donor gametes. In such circumstances a 'surrogate' mother has no legal rights over the child born. However, it has been reported that experts and officials have become increasingly concerned about a lack of oversight, and have also considered banning surrogacy for a fee.
- In **Russia**, the prospective parents must be a heterosexual couple or single woman, who meet certain medical criteria regarding inability to conceive, carry or deliver a child. Stipulations concerning who may act as a surrogate also exist (regarding age, requirement of previous healthy child, medical certification of good health and signed permission from husband if married).[12] The 'surrogate' mother must not be the egg donor. Surrogates are encouraged to see the arrangement as a financial one, and those who appear altruistically motivated may be rejected. Christina Weis (2015), a PhD candidate in Anthropology whose research draws on ethnographic fieldwork on commercial surrogacy in St Petersburg, describes the policies of surrogacy agencies as being based 'in the notion that money-oriented women make better workers, as they will do whatever is necessary to maximise their profit. Emotional involvement and a friendly relationship between the intended parents and the surrogacy workers are considered messy and as having the potential to spoil both process and outcome.' Russia has also seen proposals to prohibit surrogacy arrangements (Tétrault-Farber, 2014).
- The **Ukraine**, is currently promoted as a 'destination' country for transnational commercial surrogacy in that it allows heterosexual married couples to access surrogacy and register them on the child's birth certificate (see Demény, Chapter 7). The registered 'parents' would, however, still have to apply for citizenship and a passport for the child in their home country.

In the above countries, it is very clear that financial hardship is a driving factor for women agreeing to act as surrogates.

'Destination' countries move to prohibit international and commercial surrogacy

The absence of uniform legislation worldwide, combined with the ability of some people to travel to countries in which commercial surrogacy may occur, has led to an increase in 'fertility tourism' over the past few years and the potential for exploitation of women who are economically, socially or legally disadvantaged, many of whom live in developing nations (Leibowitz-Dori, 1997). In 2012 the Permanent Bureau of The Hague noted in this regard (Hague Conference on Private International Law, 2012: 7):

> [t]he unease expressed by some concerning the practice of engaging surrogates in States with emerging economies to bear children for more wealthy intending parents ... has dimensions similar to those discussed in the preparatory reports on inter-country adoption.

Destination countries such as Thailand, India, Nepal and Mexico have, however, increasingly responded to close such practices down.

In **Thailand**, the Protection of Children Born of Assisted Reproductive Technologies Act 2014 was passed in February 2015 to prohibit commercial surrogacy (section 23); brokering, acting as a middleman or arranging surrogacy agreements for reward; advertising and promotion of surrogacy arrangements; and the buying or selling of eggs, sperm or embryos. In-country surrogacy agreements were also limited to those between family members and must be altruistic. The laws passed 160 votes to 2, following several surrogacy scandals including the 'Baby Gammy' case, as well as another in which a Japanese man had fathered at least sixteen babies using numerous Thai 'surrogate' mothers. A member of Thailand's National Legislative Assembly told Reuters, 'This law aims to stop Thai women's wombs from becoming the world's womb' (Niyomyat, 2015).

In **India**, there was first a move to restrict access by foreigners to surrogacy; and then, in November 2015, a letter from the Indian Council of Medical Research (ICMR) officially ended surrogacy services for non-Indians – effective immediately. The letter was issued at the behest of the Health Ministry and requires fertility clinics 'not to entertain any foreigners for availing surrogacy services in India'. In addition, the Indian government banned the import of human embryos for IVF and surrogacy purposes. In a notification dated 26

October, the 'Import policy of the item "Human Embryo"' has been changed from requiring a 'No Objection Certificate' from the ICMR to 'Prohibited except for research purposes based on the guidelines of the Department of Health Research'. The government also advised the Supreme Court that foreigners 'cannot rent a womb in India'. Surrogacy services would only be available for Indian couples and there would be prohibitions on the import of human embryos for the purpose of commercial surrogacy for foreigners. From now on, the scope of surrogacy would be limited to 'needy Indian married couples only', with the ultimate aim of 'prohibiting and penalising commercial surrogacy services', while allowing altruistic surrogacy. The Bureau of Immigration, Ministry of Home Affairs, India, now provides on its website the following notice: 'Government of India guidelines dated 03.11.2015, the foreign nationals including OCI/PIO card holders are not allowed to commission surrogacy in India.' Again, such laws were enacted following numerous stories that had exposed the exploitation of women, abandonment of babies and selling of babies on the black market.[13]

In **Nepal**, in October 2015, three weeks after the country's Supreme Court issued an interim order to halt surrogacy in Nepal, a meeting of government ministers decided to ban surrogacy altogether. The Minister for Information and Communications, Minendra Rijal, announced a government ban on surrogacy services in Nepal, describing a situation the previous year in which several private hospitals had managed to secretly acquire a 'permission letter' through the Personnel Administration Division (PAD), which is not an authorized division of the Ministry of Health and Population (MoHP), and started surrogacy services. He noted that Indian women had been flown into Nepal via 'agents' to serve as 'surrogate' mothers, and that this was not acceptable. The Minister said: 'The Government has rescinded its earlier decision to allow surrogacy services for foreigners in Nepali hospitals. From now onward, the hospitals cannot provide surrogacy services.' The Department of Immigration has also stopped issuing visas to the babies born to 'surrogate' mothers.[14]

In **Mexico**, in December 2015, the congress of the Mexican State of Tabasco approved a reform to the Civil Code, with twenty-one votes in favour and nine against, banning surrogacy for foreigners and limiting in-country arrangements to heterosexual couples. The new law, which will come into effect in mid-2016, also prohibits agencies from offering services for surrogacy, including intermediaries acting between the 'surrogate' mothers and commissioning persons.

The law also restricts surrogacy in country to require that intended parents be Mexican citizens, in a heterosexual couple and must provide evidence via a medical certificate of an accredited institution that a woman is unable to carry a pregnancy herself. Among other requirements, birth certificates will contain notation of the method of conception and birth being assisted by a legal surrogacy agreement. The commissioning persons will pay the private insurance, and expenses for the pregnancy, birth and recovery. All will be overseen by the Ministry of Health.[15]

With options narrowing in terms of international surrogacy, agents, lawyers and the industry, as well as some people seeking children, have been lobbying for an opening up of local laws, to support their demands and/or interests. They also branch into other nations, in an attempt to access potential surrogates in the next 'destination' country. Only a few countries remain. For example, the Ukraine continues to be advertised as a 'favourable' destination for heterosexual commissioning person(s). In addition, due to an absence of laws, agents and clinics moved into Cambodia, promoting it as a destination for people seeking surrogacy arrangements. Agencies appeared to be working hard to convince that country's government to pass laws to facilitate such arrangements, rather than shut them down. However, in October 2016 an interim directive issued by the Cambodian Health Minister completely banned surrogacy due to concern about exploitation, human trafficking and human rights issues.

The question for the rest of this chapter is what human rights issues are raised, and how should countries respond?

International law engaged

In the realm of private international law, cross-border surrogacy came to the attention of The Hague Conference on Private International Law in early 2010 in relation to the issue of legal differences across nations leaving some children with 'unresolved legal parentage' and/or 'statelessness'. This was identified as possibly placing such children at risk of suffering legal disadvantages, having their rights impeded and being discriminated against due to the circumstances of their birth. In response, there has been some suggestion and discussion of developing some kind of multi-lateral treaty to resolve such issues.

However, transnational commercial surrogacy also raises matters relating to child welfare, exploitation of the vulnerable (particularly in the context of global economic disparities), health policy and regulation, and equality issues. Broader public international law considerations, including human rights, are therefore also raised.

Here it is important to note that while The Hague Conference has recognized the need to also include such considerations, international human rights should not just be seen as 'needs to be met'. Tobin (2014) has identified that such a view is problematic for a number of reasons. He states that first, international human rights instruments 'impose binding international legal obligations that states parties must comply with in good faith' (p. 320). Second, he notes that seeing them as such 'risks marginalising the role of public international law in resolving the issues associated with international surrogacy'. He stresses (p. 321):

> it may not be enough to acknowledge the relevance of international human rights to a private law multilateral instrument, because such an approach overlooks the threshold question of whether surrogacy arrangements are compatible with human rights law at all.

To this end, human rights should not merely be seen as 'ends to be protected' when developing a private international law response to international surrogacy, rather they may serve as a 'means by which to inform this response'. Finally, Tobin notes the moral significance of human rights as agreed upon by states that reflects an 'admittedly incompletely theorised, moral conception of the relationship between state and individual, and what it means to live a life of dignity and self-worth' (p. 321). He therefore emphasizes that human rights discourse can play an informative role in resolving the ethical dilemmas associated with international commercial surrogacy arrangements – and points to a substantive human rights analysis[16] of the competing human rights in order to do so.

International human rights and surrogacy

No international human rights instrument specifically addresses surrogacy, but a number may be relevant to the issues it raises. These include the International Covenant on Civil and Political Rights (ICCPR), International Covenant on Economic, Social and Cultural Rights (ICESCR), Convention on the Elimination of All Forms of Discrimination against Women (CEDAW)[17] and the Convention on the Rights of the Child (CRC).

It is useful, in the first instance, to identify which rights may be engaged in relation to the practice of surrogacy and/or issues raised by it, and to consider how they might apply (and their relevance) to surrogacy arrangements. One should, however, keep in mind that whether a state is a signatory to a treaty is relevant to whether it has undertaken to be bound by it,[18] that such articles should not be superficially applied, that international human rights law is complex, that rights may 'compete' and need to be balanced against one another, and that some rights are not 'absolute'.

Rights relevant to 'intending parents' The ICCPR states that 'No one shall be subjected to arbitrary or unlawful interference with his privacy, family, home or correspondence' (Article 17). It defines the family as 'the natural and fundamental group unit of society' (Article 23) and states that it is entitled to protection by society and the State (Article 24(1)). The ICESCR contains similar language about the family (Article 10). To this end, it may be (and has been) argued that the right to reproductive health and autonomy, the right to found a family, and the right to respect for privacy and family life are relevant in the context of surrogacy.[19]

However, the content of such rights arguably does not provide an entitlement to enter into surrogacy agreements. The right to reproductive health could not be held to go so far as creating an entitlement to enlist the reproductive capacity of another woman to enable a person to bear children. Rather, the right has been identified to apply in the context of access to sexual and reproductive health education, information about the healthy spacing of children and an entitlement to have a healthy sex life.

While the 'right to found a family' may be argued to include modern family formations, it again could not be said to create an obligation to provide women to those people who cannot bear children themselves.

The right to respect for privacy and family under Article 17 of the ICCPR has however been recognized as a broad concept that 'encompasses ... [among other things] the right to respect for the decisions both to have and not to have a child'. To this end, 'the right of a couple to conceive a child and to make use of medically assisted procreation for that purpose is also protected'. Arguably, medically assisted procreation may include surrogacy. However, even if the right to respect for privacy and family life encompasses a right to enter surrogacy arrangements, this right would not be absolute. It remains 'subject to a state's capacity (and potential obligation) to restrict this where it is reasonably necessary to (a) protect the rights of persons other than the intending parents and/or (b) protect public morality' (Tobin, 2014: 326). Thus states must consider competing rights and the broader theme of public morality in any response to transnational commercial surrogacy.

Rights relevant to children The preamble of the CRC, among other things, recognizes the family as the fundamental group of society and the natural environment for the growth and well-being of all its members, and particularly children, that it should be afforded the necessary protection and assistance so that it can fully assume its responsibilities within the community, and that the child, for the full and harmonious development of his or her personality, should grow up in a family environment, in an atmosphere of happiness, love and understanding.

Article 3(1) also provides: 'In all actions concerning children, whether undertaken by public or private social welfare institutions, courts of law, administrative authorities or legislative bodies, the best interests of the child shall be a primary consideration.'

The following Articles may be further engaged when considering surrogacy arrangements:

- Article 7(1) provides for birth registration and a right to know one's parents. This requires that the child be registered immediately after birth and shall have the right from birth to a name, the right to acquire a nationality and as far as possible, the right to know and be cared for by his or her parents. This accords with the ICCPR, which states that every child has the right to be 'registered immediately after birth' (Article 24(2)) and has 'the right to acquire a nationality' (Article 24(3)).
- Article 8(1) relates to the preservation of identity, again requiring that States Parties undertake to respect the right of the child to preserve his or her identity, including nationality, name and family relations as recognized by law without unlawful interference.
- Article 9.1 requires States Parties to ensure that a child shall not be separated from his or her parents against their will, except when competent authorities subject to judicial review determine that such separation is necessary for the best interests of the child. Such determination may be necessary in a particular case, such as one involving abuse or neglect of the child by the parents, or one where the parents are living separately and a decision must be made as to the child's place of residence.

Such Articles raise a number of issues in relation to surrogacy. Many such arrangements take place in countries that do not honour a child's rights to information about their conception; they do not provide information about the providers of gametes (i.e. their genetic 'parents'); nor about the woman who carried and gave birth to the child (whether or not she is genetically related to them). The child's right to be cared for by her or his parents 'as far as possible' leads to questions of who the 'parents' actually are.

Children's rights to preserve their identity, including nationality, name and family relations, are influenced by how identity, nationality, name and family relations are determined – for example, whether they are determined by their link to their birth mother, the donor(s), commissioning person(s) or all of them. Questions arise regarding the extent to which genetic connection matters and why it appears to be answered differently when a commissioning person(s) sperm/eggs have been used as opposed to a donor. We might also ask whether the child's birthplace matters, whether the birthplace of any gamete donor(s) and/or the surrogate mother matter, and whether the birth mother is always the legal mother in first instance.

None of the above issues necessarily preclude or compete with the 'rights' of intending parents to family and private life, nor determine whether or not to accept any or all types of surrogacy. They do, however, call for much better systems to address and honour such rights.

The CRC also raises issues about the sale of children. Article 35 requires States Parties to take 'all appropriate national, bilateral and multilateral measures to prevent the ... sale of or traffic in children for any purpose or in any form'. Article 2 of the Optional Protocol to the CRC on the Sale of Children, Child Prostitution and Child Pornography further defines the sale of children as 'any act or transaction whereby a child is transferred by any person or group of persons to another for remuneration or any other consideration'. Using the ordinary meaning[20] of 'transfer', 'remuneration' and 'consideration', it is clearly arguable that a commercial surrogacy will fall within the definition of the sale of a child as it is *an act* or *transaction* whereby a child *is transferred by any person* or group of persons (the surrogate, the clinics, the brokers) *to another* (the commissioning person(s)) *for remuneration or any other consideration*. This is so regardless of how payments are made (for example, in monthly instalments) or presented as not being for the child, as ultimately, the child is exactly what the 'contract' is about. That is, whether 'commercial surrogacy' is framed as the purchase of a child, the purchase of reproductive labour or the purchase of parental rights, they all involve the transfer, for a fee, of a child from the woman who carried it throughout pregnancy and gave birth to it, to the commissioning person(s). There is in all instances a failure to reasonably justify payment.

Denial, indifference and/or ignorance regarding the needs, interests and well-being of the child(ren) born as a result of commercial surrogacy also do not change some of their lived experiences of commodification, sale and/or trafficking. The question thus becomes, how can nations support a practice that denies or ignores the interests of the children that are the very reason that the practice is said to exist? When seen as something that meets the definition of sale of children, there is a strong case that commercial surrogacy is contrary to international law. In addition, moral objections to a practice seen to commodify children, or to compromise their human dignity or well-being, are sufficient to fall within a state's margin of appreciation to prohibit commercial surrogacy. This is so whether or not the surrogate is a wholly autonomous and willing party to the transaction, or whether she is herself commodified or exploited in terms of the arrangement. In the latter instance, she could not be held morally culpable, but the nature of the transaction remains the same.

Rights relevant to women who may be engaged as 'surrogate' mothers
International human rights issues are also raised in relation to women who are commissioned as 'surrogate' mothers. CEDAW requires 'the proper understanding of maternity as a social function' (Article 5b) and calls for special protection for women during pregnancy in work proved to be harmful to them (Article 11.2). It also requires the provision of health services, and specifically to ensure services to women during pregnancy and postnatal confinement (Article 12).

It is not clear whether CEDAW's focus on the health of pregnant women is relevant to surrogacy arrangements, but such a focus would not be inconsistent with the practice. The requirement here would be to ensure that women are treated well, and that they receive adequate health care pre- and postnatally.

In contrast, CEDAW's definition of maternity as a social function may preclude commercially contracted pregnancy. It would also preclude seeing (or regulating) the arrangement within some kind of 'fairtrade' or 'labour' related model (as suggested by Pande, Chapter 19). Non-commercial surrogacy arrangements, for example between relatives or friends, may nevertheless still be considered acceptable.

To the extent that CEDAW requires non-discrimination of women, one may argue either way. That is, some argue that it is discriminatory not to allow a woman to do what she wishes with her own body; others emphasize the social and economic disparities that exist, particularly in commercial surrogacy arrangements, and view the practice as entirely discriminatory and potentially coercive.

Financial disparities between women who serve as 'surrogate' mothers and those who commission them are also relevant. Prohibitions on commercial surrogacy may be seen as a way to prevent the exploitation of financially disadvantaged women and/or to prevent coercion due to a woman's poor financial status. Further, even if one argues that the woman has not been coerced, her relative financial disadvantage calls into question the justice of the arrangement. Here we might look to the 'lack' of available surrogates for altruistic surrogacy arrangements as an indication that most women do not wish to act as surrogates; nor do they wish to be exposed to the multitude of risks described in previous chapters, and only choose to do so in exceptional circumstances (for example, for a close friend or relative), or in circumstances in which money is offered.

What regulatory approach should be taken?

International regulation At a global level some have called for a multilateral, legally binding instrument that would establish a global, coherent and ethical practice of international surrogacy (e.g. Davis and Dalessio, 2000; Fiandaca, 1998; Lee, 2009; Leibowitz-Dori, 1997; Trimmings and Beaumont, 2012; *X & Y (Foreign Surrogacy)* [2008] EWHC 3030 (Fam), 29). However, a convention serves no purpose if states are not willing to ratify it.[21] Given that most countries prohibit the practice of commercial surrogacy, and that recent legislation in nations that have moved to regulate the practice has also taken this stance, the only convention that would gain signatories would appear to be one that prohibits *commercial* surrogacy (or in other terms financial transactions in the context of surrogacy arrangements which involve financial gain).

Prohibitions on commercial surrogacy would also be consistent with the other international instruments discussed above, which explicitly prohibit the sale of children and the transfer of children in the somewhat analogous situation of intercountry adoption for financial gain. In addition, a prohibition on commercial surrogacy would be consistent with the European Parliament's Resolution on the Trade of Human Egg Cells (the European Resolution).[22] This Resolution affirmed that payment for ova should be prohibited, recognizing that the harvesting of egg cells constitutes a high medical risk for the life and health of women (see also Beeson and Lippman, Chapter 5):

(a) the planned egg cell trade would exploit the economic situation of women who lived in impoverished regions; and
(b) despite the possibility of serious effects on women's life and health, the high price paid for egg cells incites and encourages donation, given the relative poverty of the donors.

As commercial surrogacy poses virtually the same risks, it may be decided to recommend that it be similarly banned.

Tobin (2014: 351) has also taken this view, stating:

> The idea that the mere regulation of international commercial surrogacy is a pragmatic and functional response to the dilemmas associated with this practice is misplaced. On the contrary, in a global environment where prohibition of this practice remains the norm rather than the exception, it could be incongruous for prohibitionist states to ratify a multilateral treaty, which obliges them to recognise commercial surrogacy arrangements entered into in permissive jurisdictions. Thus, far from being a pragmatic and functional response, multilateral regulation is unlikely to be a realistic option in the current global environment ... Indeed, if anything, a prohibitionist treaty is a far more realistic option and would be consistent with international human rights law, if it accepted that commercial surrogacy arrangements amount to the sale of a child. This conclusion may not provide comfort to those who have a legitimate and understandable desire to have children. Their desire, however, does not demand tolerance of a practice that arguably maintains gender inequality and potentially violates the rights of 'surrogate' mothers and the children to whom they give birth.

The difficulty, of course, is that an international convention is not an instrument that can achieve a global ban on commercial surrogacy unless all nations concur. The few states that continue to permit such arrangements may simply not become signatories. This may particularly be so in those countries that have encouraged commercial surrogacy based on the money it brings to them, and therefore would not protect women and/or children. Nevertheless, at best, a prohibitive convention would represent a strong and united stance taken by the international community that wishes to see an end to exploitative, risky and unacceptable practices.

I note that the argument that such a position might simply drive commercial surrogacy underground (Keyes and Chisholm, 2013) is not in itself reason to establish a permissive regime. That is, while some argue that a ban would create a black market, others argue that laws that regulate surrogacy end up promoting it and that even if surrogacy was 'outlawed', thereby driving it underground, 'the number of surrogate arrangements would be miniscule compared to the explosive growth that would result from permissive regulation' (Smerdon, 2009: 83). In fact, what we have recently seen is that countries that were once 'destinations' have closed their doors, refusing to let their women be used as 'wombs' for the world and prohibiting or restricting surrogacy practices on their own shores. This surely will lead to a decline in transnational arrangements and lower the number of children who will be moved across borders, as the border authorities are on notice not to permit such things.

The alternative – a convention that is permissive or facilitative in its approach – is likely to be rejected by the majority of nations that prohibit commercial surrogacy, which is the majority of nations worldwide. It could also be seen as extremely worrisome (if not completely unacceptable) for a nation to sign a convention that permits the use of commercial surrogacy abroad but continues to ban such practices in its home country.

Whether or not an international convention is ultimately seen as necessary or able to put an end to commercial surrogacy, or address the issues transnational surrogacy raises, these will not be resolved without also having strong domestic laws. It is to consideration of what these might be that the discussion now turns.

Domestic regulation International convention or not, strong domestic regulation is absolutely necessary in order to properly address issues raised by surrogacy practices. Such regulation speaks loudest to the stance a nation wishes to take. Domestic laws may also determine what a particular nation will do when surrogacy has occurred in another country and the commissioning persons wish to bring the resulting child back to their country of residence.

The question then becomes what legal position should jurisdictions take towards commercial surrogacy practices, both domestically and in relation to transnational practices?

Some people have argued that the solution would be to permit commercial surrogacy domestically, rather than continue to prohibit it, in order to stop people from travelling abroad (see e.g. Skene, 2012). In Australia, Millbank (2013) further suggests 'cautious' commercial surrogacy or a flat rate compensatory fee, as the way to resolve such issues. She proposes a set fee for profit – which is not too low, but not too high – to prevent exploitation. Allegedly, the minimum (small) payment will serve to avoid 'unfair inducements', while being fair compensation for the surrogate mother's risk and burden. However, arguably this would not address the ethical issues that are raised by commercial surrogacy. In fact, I argue that such a suggestion is simply cause for further concern as it is contradictory to argue that, in order to reduce exploitation, surrogates should receive a *minimum* fee. Who would act as a surrogate in such circumstances? One can only suppose that perhaps it will be the most vulnerable or financially needy, the low-income single mother, immigrant, unemployed woman, or mother unable to work and care for the children at the same time, enticed (or induced) by the minimum payment, which to her may not be that small. The 'solution' would only bring the global inequities seen in commercial surrogacy to yet another nation; it would not resolve the issues at all. Perhaps what will follow, however, will be arguments that accepting low payments for commercial surrogacy reflects that such surrogate mothers are not really doing it for the money after all – which of course is yet another unacceptable position to take.

It is the position of this author that it would also be unacceptable to change laws because of arguments that focus upon the 'plight' of commissioning persons and claims that people who desire children may face 'serious harms' due to being 'excluded from their preferred or only available, family formation avenue' (Millbank, 2011: 191).[23] In the context of such family formation, issues pertaining to legal parentage of the resulting children have taken primary place in terms of discussion of what is in the child's best interests. However again, while best interest determinations regarding the legal parentage of a resulting child may be relevant in such context, analysis of the broader ethical and legal issues for children raised by such practice should not be lost, and in fact should take precedence when considering regulatory options.

I also reject again the market language and views that some people adopt. The interpretation of the surrogacy 'contract' as something that is simply 'fairtrade', a 'service' or even a 'job' dismisses arguments that commercial surrogacy is 'baby selling' by changing the nature of how one views the 'contract' between the commissioning person(s) and the 'surrogate' mother. However, even if one sees the transaction in these terms, it does not make it acceptable to 'engage' a woman to provide 'services' to bear children for other people with the 'clause' that she will be 'compensated' (paid) to do so during and upon the 'success' of the arrangement (i.e. the birth of the child). I submit that neoliberal[24] and market views that permeate discussions, practice and some people's acceptance of 'commercial' (aka 'compensated') surrogacy are only reason for concern. The language of contract law, payment for 'services', 'success clauses' and 'markets' has a profound impact on how surrogacy is viewed. When those in favour of 'commercial' surrogacy speak in such terms, they move people away from other issues and the human face of surrogacy, reducing the process to a market transaction, upon which everyone simply agrees to the terms (of course absent of any possible agreement by the child to be born as a result).

Rather than accept such views as justifications for commercial surrogacy, we should be questioning them, pointing to the fact that, even if we use such terms, surrogacy is an example of neoliberal ideology at its worst, exploiting people financially, using unstable outsourced 'employment' and requiring people to 'work' under oppressive conditions defined by the terms of 'contracts' or 'service' arrangements. Let's also not forget that the 'terms of contract', which are said to simply convey the 'intentions' of the parties, include both the sale of the procreative 'service' provided by 'surrogate' mother(s) and possibly 'donor(s)' *but also* the agreement to transfer 'custodial rights' to a child (whether such 'transfer' takes place prior to or after the child's birth) as well as the 'physical possession' thereof.

Permitting commercial surrogacy in jurisdictions that currently ban it may thus further risk broadening a practice (or 'market') that reflects the financial, social and cultural disparities between commissioning person(s) and surrogates, and does not address issues surrounding the nature of the transaction, for example, regarding the sale or commodification of women and children, nor risks related to trafficking. Note that commissioning person(s) may also be vulnerable. They may be 'sold' the idea that commercial surrogacy is simply a business transaction that can be performed with ease. They are told they will achieve emotional fulfilment and a family of their own using commercial surrogates who are really giving, altruistic women, who want to help (for a fee/compensation). Interestingly, in an environment in which only altruistic surrogacy is available, the ready availability of such giving, altruistic women is rather limited, and perhaps is evidence in itself that it is the commercial nature of transactions elsewhere that increases participation.

Nevertheless, there is scope for domestic laws to be improved worldwide. For instance, there is a need to create consistency in countries that permit reimbursement of reasonable expenses to ensure that such 'reasonable expenses' are not a guise for commercial arrangements (see Davaki, Chapter 8). It is also necessary to ensure that laws apply equally to all, regardless, for example, of sexuality, and to determine how legal parentage issues should be resolved.

When a request is made regarding an arrangement that has taken place abroad it is clear that special consideration and close scrutiny of any such arrangement needs to occur. If we reflect on the chapters in this book, a very extensive list of considerations is indicated before any transfer or recognition of legal parentage might occur. Box 20.1 sets out the information and evidence that a court or some other authority may need to consider in any given case.

Box 20.1 Considerations to be had in relation to surrogacy arrangements

a. A presumption against granting 'parental responsibility' and/ or 'legal parentage' to commissioning person(s) in the case of commercial surrogacy arrangements in any jurisdiction in which such transactions are illegal.

b. An expectation of live testimony being given by all parties involved including the 'surrogate' mother, which will enable evidence gathering, and assessment of the agreement, and what would be in the 'best interests' of the child (i.e. a signature or thumb print from the 'surrogate' mother is not enough).

c. The application being made no less than six weeks and no more than six months after the child's birth (giving time for the birth mother to change her mind, allowing early bonding with caregivers).

d. Evidence regarding:

   i. the jurisdiction in which the surrogacy arrangement took place;
   ii. the names, addresses, date of birth, nationality of any 'surrogate' mother(s), egg donor(s), sperm donor(s), and/or embryo donor(s) used;

iii. how the 'surrogate' mother, and/or donor(s), were recruited.

e. Details of any clinic(s), hospital(s) or other facility at which the respective people (surrogate mother, donors, commissioning persons) underwent medical procedures and/or were treated, including details of:

  i. practice standards and compliance with any regulatory requirements or guidelines of any such place;
  ii. any fees paid to the fertility service providers, and/or people, agents; companies associated therewith, noting details of such fees and receipts.

f. Details of independent legal advice provided to the 'surrogate' mother; the person(s) making the application; and any partners of such people, including details of:

  i. the names, qualifications, and registration status of the respective providers;
  ii. evidence of any relationship the providers of such legal advice had/have with the fertility treatment providers, agents or intermediaries;
  iii. the type of advice provided, including e.g. whether the parties were informed of all legal rights and not just provided information regarding the surrogacy 'contract' (e.g. rights to claim compensation for negligent treatment, etc.); and
  iv. any fees paid to the providers of legal advice, including signed costs agreements, and details of who paid such fees (noting in the case of the legal advice provided to a potential 'surrogate' mother and/or donor of reproductive materials, in which commissioning person(s), agents, intermediaries, clinics, or otherwise paid such fees, a sworn undertaking that such advice was not affected by a conflict of interest).

g. Details of independent counselling provided to all parties, (including 'surrogate' mother, egg, sperm and/or embryo donors, the person(s) making the application and any partners of the previous listed people), detailing:

i. the names, qualifications, and registration status of the respective providers;
ii. evidence that the providers of such advice do not have a relationship with the fertility treatment providers, agents, intermediaries and/or legal advisers;
iii. evidence of the type of counselling, its frequency, and purposes of counselling;
iv. evidence that such counselling included discussion of a child's right to identity, knowledge about the circumstances of its birth, and its genetic and biological heritage; and
v. any fees paid to such counsellors (noting in the case of counselling provided to a potential 'surrogate' mother, in which commissioning person(s), agents, intermediaries, clinics or otherwise paid such fees, a sworn undertaking that such advice was not affected by a conflict of interest).

h. Details of any agent or intermediary or other person(s) or organization used to arrange or facilitate the surrogacy agreement (and the legality of such arrangements), including:

i. the names, qualifications, and registration status of any such person(s) or organizations;
ii. any relationship with the fertility treatment providers that any such person(s) or organizations had or have;
iii. the role such agents, intermediaries or other person(s) or organizations played. For example:

a. international agents/agencies that liaise with foreign couples and clinics;
b. agent-facilitators overseeing surrogacy/'surrogate' mother;
c. neighbourhood/local recruiter); and

iv. any fees paid to agents/intermediaries/facilitators/other person(s) or organizations.

i. The surrogacy agreement – including details of who drafted the agreement, any negotiations that took place among the parties to the agreement, any changes to the agreement that were made, whether the agreement was translated into any other languages, how the agreement was communicated to all parties involved, and any other matter the Court/Authority requires. This should include information regarding the legality of any such agreement entered into, and/or the payment of money to any of the parties involved (including agents, etc.). (In cases in which an illegal transaction has occurred the appropriate authorities should be notified.)

j. The number, name and address of any other children the 'surrogate' mother has.
k. The 'surrogate' mother's full and prior informed consent, and how such consent was obtained.
l. Whether the 'surrogate' mother has undergone prior surrogacy arrangements, and if so, the number of children that have resulted (and whether there is ongoing contact with such children).
m. Any payment made to the 'surrogate' mother, including reimbursement of expenses associated with the pregnancy, birth and/or postnatal care, and evidence of receipts for such expenses; or evidence of any other payments that she received either directly or indirectly.
n. Any pre-existing relationship between the 'surrogate' mother and the commissioning person(s).
o. Information regarding whether the arrangement was a 'traditional' or 'gestational' arrangement, and in both cases evidence of who else provided gametes.
p. Information regarding the number of embryos implanted in the woman.
q. Information regarding the number of fetuses that resulted.
r. Any reduction of pregnancy that occurred and, in such circumstances, evidence of the woman's counselling by an independent counsellor and her consent to such reduction.
s. Information about the prenatal and postnatal care that the 'surrogate' mother received and whether such care is ongoing.
t. Information about the mode of delivery at birth, and if a caesarean, evidence that this was necessary for the well-being of the woman and/or child.
u. Details of any complications with the pregnancy or birth, and how they were addressed.

> v. Details of the number of attempts at surrogacy made prior to the arrangement before the court, including:
>
>   a. any other treatment of women in the attempt to cause a pregnancy;
>   b. any pregnancies that resulted in miscarriage, abortion or stillbirth;
>   c. details of the names and addresses of all of the women used;
>   d. details of the care provided to any such woman who experienced treatment, miscarriage, abortion or stillbirth.
>
> w. Details of whether a family study has been conducted on the commissioning person(s) (applicants for 'legal parentage'), and if so the results thereof.
> x. Evidence of criminal record and child protection checks on the commissioning person(s).
> y. Details of how the child will have access to information concerning the child's genetic, gestational and cultural origins. This should include details of any contact arrangements or plans for contact that have been made for contact between the child with the 'surrogate' mother, donors of genetic materials, and/or siblings or other children (this includes other related or unrelated children associated with the 'surrogate' mother, including any child that lives with her and may have witnessed the pregnancy), and how such contact will be maintained.
> z. Details of any support services available for, and follow-up with, all parties including the children of respective families involved.

The matters listed may in turn influence behaviours due to knowledge that practices will be extensively scrutinized. It would enable countries to uphold their preferred position on prohibiting commercial surrogacy by maintaining a presumption against treatment. It would also mean that courts or the relevant authority would not grant Parenting Orders in circumstances that do not satisfy them that all parties have been suitably treated and protected or in which laws have been breached.[25] Such scrutiny may also ultimately serve to curb the practice of people engaging in arrangements abroad, given legal parentage may not be granted in their home country.

The presumption against granting legal parentage orders in cases of commercial surrogacy arrangements may of course be rebutted. For example, it may be argued not to apply in Europe in cases that meet the *Mennesson* requirements, i.e. in which one of the intended parents *has a biological connection to the child, and recognition of parental status has been legally established in another foreign state*, as pursuant to the European Court of Human Rights (ECtHR), legal parentage should be recognized in such instances.[26] However, the case would need to be made about why the presumption should be rebutted, and would still be subject to significant scrutiny in relation to all aspects of the agreement.

The requirement for scrutiny would be consistent with *D and Others v. Belgium*, a case that also went before the ECtHR in 2014, in which the Court issued a unanimous ruling that Belgian authorities had been in their rightful authority to insist on 'carrying out checks before allowing a child who had been born in the Ukraine to a surrogate mother to enter Belgium', and rejected the applicants' claim that Belgian authorities had interfered with 'their right to respect for their family life'. The ECtHR held that 'Belgium had acted within its broad discretion (a wide margin of appreciation)' and denied any further application for a claim in this case.

It should here be noted also that the decision in *Mennesson* referred to above *does not* require countries to change their laws prohibiting all, or particular kinds of, surrogacy arrangements. That is, the ECtHR did not call into question France's ban on surrogacy in that case, but rather addressed the interests of the children subject of the application, in having certainty regarding legal parentage status, in the circumstances of the cases before the Court. French Family Minister, Laurence Rossignol, reminded parliament following the decision that 'several penal provisions allow for the prosecution of those who resort to surrogacy abroad'. That is, people who engage in acts prohibited by law may still be subject to prosecution.

It is of utmost importance, therefore, to remember that, beyond determining legal parentage or deciding on final nationality of a child born as a result of such arrangement, which are end-point problems resulting from transnational surrogacy practices, there remains the need to address the wider ethical, social and policy issues raised by such practices altogether. While in Europe parties to the European Human Rights Convention appear to need to include some scope to evaluate nationality and legal parentage, they, like the rest of the world, must also continue to work to protect the rights and welfare of children, women and other parties involved with such arrangements, in line with established global human rights standards. Such work may in fact be focused upon better enforcement of prohibitions on commercial surrogacy, and a reduction in, or end to, such practices.

To such an end, focus should also be upon how to address the actions of lawyers, brokers and other agencies who make a business (and handsome profit) out of giving 'advice' to people about commercial surrogacy arrangements abroad, and who may encourage or facilitate people to engage in commercial surrogacy that is in fact against the laws of their state. The practices of clinics and 'fertility services' must also be scrutinized.

Further, for those countries that continue to prohibit commercial surrogacy within their borders, there is the option to introduce prohibitions that apply extraterritorially. That is, residents of those states would be committing a crime if they travelled elsewhere to engage in practices that are prohibited in their own territory. This is the position taken in three Australian states (New South Wales, the Australian Capital Territory and Queensland),[27] Malaysia and Turkey (Storrow, 2011). Arguably, such extraterritorial prohibition may lead to a reduction in online forum shopping and limit the number of people willing to engage in such practices abroad.

However, the counter-argument is that extraterritorial laws are extremely difficult to enforce, and there are clearly dilemmas still facing children when such laws are breached (Storrow, 2011). Perhaps, yet another alternative or simultaneous option is to encourage the view that, if a country chooses to allow commercial surrogacy,[28] *they should restrict access to people permanently domiciled in their own jurisdiction.* That is, such countries should not offer their own citizens for commercial surrogacy arrangements with people from countries where the practice is banned.

It is also important to recognize that in those few countries that may continue to allow commercial surrogacy, protective domestic regulation must go beyond prohibiting foreigners onto their shores. Regardless of a country's position, legal regulation that reflects the above listed criteria, giving children access to information, safeguarding women's health, ensuring pre-screening of commissioning person(s), legal advice, counselling, and more, is needed to govern any surrogacy arrangement. Of course, this will also require capacity and will to establish and effectively enforce any such laws (Tobin, 2014: 347).

Conclusion

Advances in assisted reproductive technology, increases in its use and positive social progress in recognizing and accepting different family formations and ways of achieving parenthood have all contributed to an upsurge in surrogacy arrangements. At the same time, commercial surrogacy practices have raised many ethical and legal issues and been the subject of heated debate related to the actual, or potential, commodification and exploitation of women and children. Concurrent arguments exist that women should be free to exploit their reproductive capabilities and to act as they wish. Surely, there are not only stories of exploitation and inequities but also stories of joy. Finding suitable solutions to the ethical, social and legal problems posed is difficult. Women should be free to contract, bargain, work and to make informed choices about what they do with their bodies. Opportunities for women to rise out of poverty, provide for their families and build better lives should also exist. However, given the negatives that can and do occur, it is apparent that the world of commercial surrogacy is not a place where this takes place.

We have seen throughout the chapters in this anthology that the world of domestic and/or transnational commercial surrogacy can be full of inequality and unequal bargaining power, lack of freedom and less than informed decision-making. In worst-case scenarios, it is a world that is exploitative and dangerous. Children may in many (or even most) circumstances be dearly wanted and loved by the commissioning person(s) who desire to form a family, but at the same time they may be commodified. Surrogacy practices can also lead to significant risks of some children being sold, trafficked or exploited or abused. While the arguments on both sides regarding how to address such issues are complex, most jurisdictions have decided that commercial surrogacy creates unacceptable risks for women and children, and therefore prohibit its practice.

Domestic laws should not be changed to permit commercial surrogacy in those jurisdictions that currently prohibit the practice solely based upon dilemmas created by people who have engaged in global surrogacy arrangements (sometimes against the law of their own jurisdiction). As stated earlier, such cases should be dealt with by the courts on a case-by-case basis and/or the legislature should speak as to what should occur. Any such cases must be extensively scrutinized both for the purposes of singular examination, but also to expose the practices of an industry that is clearly driven by profit and perhaps as a way to drive change.

More broadly, the issue remains as to what must be done given the international nature of commercial surrogacy and the problems it raises. This chapter has examined regulatory actions that may serve to address discrimination, exploitation, inequities, trafficking and/or the commodification of women and children, while still permitting certain forms of surrogacy. I believe that commercial practices should continue to be prohibited in those jurisdictions that choose to do so, and restricted to within the borders of those that choose not to prohibit them – with minimal regulatory standards in all such jurisdictions.

In closing, it is noted that if the concern is that women should have a way to prosper and move out of poverty, the focus needs to be on other opportunities for them to do so. Similarly, while we should accept and encourage different family formations, commercial surrogacy should not be 'sold' as the preferred option to women and men seeking to form a family. While clearly many people simply long to love and care for a child – and it is not the intent to discourage such people from seeking to form a family (complete with children) – the issues discussed in this book arise and exist beyond individual families, surrogates and circumstances. Decisions about addressing these issues must take precedence over any singular desire to have a family, and must include consideration of all factors that shape the situation of people seeking children, women who may consider bearing children for others and the children that may be born as a result.

Notes

1 See e.g. Riggs and Due (Chapter 2) regarding the marketing to gay couples of commercial surrogacy that tells them they will 'realise their dreams', become 'whole' or 'complete' their family.

2 *Private international law* is defined as a body of law developed to resolve private, non-state disputes involving more than one jurisdiction or a foreign law element. It focuses on such things as marriage, birth rights, divorce, property settlements or commercial disputes that take place across borders. *Public international law* is the body of international law that governs the activities (and rights and duties) of governments in relation to other governments, as well as increasingly individuals, corporations and international organizations. Note – they are not mutually exclusive, with some private international law instruments (e.g. the 1993 Hague Intercountry Adoption Convention and the 1996 Hague Child Protection Convention) being said to provide a framework that enables States Parties to better implement international human rights obligations in a cross-border context; and public and private international law often being considered together.

3 For further information please see Center for Genetics and Society, BioPolicy Wiki, at <http://biopolicywiki.org/index.php?title=Countries>. The information provided was researched by the author in 2015 while engaged as a consultant to the US Center for Genetics and Society pursuant to a John D. and Catherine T. MacArthur Foundation grant awarded for their collaborative work on cross-border surrogacy and commercial egg retrieval. The grant was to build on efforts to bring a human rights and social justice perspective to the assisted reproduction industry.

4 Note that the law in China simply bans trade in fertilized eggs and embryos

and forbids hospitals from performing surrogacy procedures. It is reported that such regulations are not always adhered to (e.g. Xinhua, 2012).

5 Note that in Greece, due to youth unemployment hitting over 50 per cent, women are reported to have been attracted into surrogacy agreements by the offer of significant sums of money for arrangements that are represented as 'altruistic'. Also see Davaki (Chapter 8).

6 The Hague referred to these countries as 'largely unregulated', but in fact some (e.g. Argentina) have guidelines; in some of these jurisdictions the Court has offered a view; and in others there exist laws that would prevent commercial surrogacy.

7 Court of Appeal of Liège, 1st Chamber, ruling of 6 September 2010, docket No 2010/RQ/20.

8 E.g. see *Baby Manji Yamada v. Union of India & Anr*, 29 September 2008.

9 Israel authorizes monthly 'compensation payments' to the surrogate for pain and suffering which are seen by many as thus placing it in the category of permissive states.

10 There is affirmative case law or legislation allowing commercial surrogacy in California, Maryland, Massachusetts, Ohio, Pennsylvania, South Carolina (case law); and Alabama, Arkansas, Connecticut, Illinois, Iowa, Nevada, North Dakota, Oregon, Tennessee, Texas, Utah, West Virginia (statutes).

11 Law of the Republic of Armenia 'On reproductive health and reproductive rights of a human'. No. 474 of 26 December 2002, Articles 11–19.

12 The use of ART is regulated by order No. 107H of the Ministry of Healthcare of Russia dated 30 August 2012, 'On the Procedure for the Use of Assisted Reproductive Technologies, Contraindications and Restrictions to their Application.' See <http://www.garant.ru/products/ipo/prime/doc/70218364>.

13 For discussion of the inequities, practices, and issues raised by surrogacy in India see e.g. Nadimpally and Majumdar (Chapter 4).

14 For details of practices that were taking place in Nepal in the wake of the 2015 earthquake, see Shalev, Eyal and Samama (Chapter 3).

15 See Fulda and Tamés (Chapter 14).

16 As opposed to other approaches that may be described as 'invisible', 'incidental', 'selective', 'superficial' or 'rhetorical'.

17 Opened for signature 18 December 1979, 1249 UNTS 13 (entered into force 3 September 1981).

18 Thus being bound by such a treaty.

19 One may also raise the right to non-discrimination under the ICCPR, Articles 2 and 26, in relation to LGBTIQ access to reproductive services equivalent to those that are accessible by heterosexual couples.

20 Pursuant to the interpretation method for treaties set out in the Vienna Convention on the Law of Treaties, Article 31.

21 Note, initial consideration was given by The Hague Permanent Bureau on Private International Law as to whether HIAC was applicable to commercial surrogacy, but it was determined that it was not due to the significant differences between adoption and surrogacy. It is also noted that the success of HIAC was made possible because the starting point was general international consensus that adoption is an acceptable practice in certain circumstances. Clearly this differs regarding commercial surrogacy, in that there is no such consensus.

22 European Parliament resolution on the trade in human egg cells, P6_TA(2005)0074, adopted 10 March 2005.

23 Note here Millbank refers to the work of Campbell, *Sister Wives, Surrogates and Sex Workers: Outlaws by Choice* (Aldershot: Ashgate, 2013).

24 In which the only legitimate purpose of the state is to safeguard individual, especially commercial, liberty.

25 Orders could of course be made to place a child in other suitable care.

26 Following *Mennesson v. France* (application no. 65192/11) and *Labassee v. France* (no. 65940/11), States Parties to the European Convention on Human Rights would be expected to grant legal recognition of the parent–child relationship between a child born as a result of surrogacy treatment and the intended parent(s) in circumstances in which *one of the intended parents has a biological connection to the child; and where recognition of parental status has been legally established in a foreign state.*

27 Surrogacy Act 2010 (NSW), section 11; Parentage Act 2004 (ACT), section 45; Surrogacy Act 2010 (Qld), section 54.

28 On the assumption that total prohibition globally might not become a reality.

References

Abramyhan G (2013) Birth rights and concerns: issue of surrogate birthing raises debate. *Society*, 11 February. <http://www.armenianow.com/society/36243/armenia_surrogate_mothers_legislation>

Baker H (2013) A possible future instrument on international surrogacy arrangements: are there lessons to be learnt from the 1993 Hague Inter-country Adoption Convention? In: Trimmings K and Beaumont P (eds) *International Surrogacy Arrangements*. Oxford and Portland, OR: Hart Publishing, pp. 417–18.

Bureau of Immigration (2015) *Surrogacy*. Ministry of Home Affairs, Government of India, 3 November. <http://boi.gov.in/content/surrogacy>

Davis W and Dalessio J (2000) Reproductive surrogacy at the Millennium: proposed model legislation regulating 'non-traditional' gestational surrogacy contracts. *McGeorge Law Review* 31: 673.

Ellena M (2014) Georgia considers ending fee-based surrogacy. *Eurasianet*, 25 March. <www.eurasianet.org/node/68188>

Fiandaca S (1998) In vitro fertilization and embryos: the need for international guidelines. *Albany Law Journal of Science and Technology* 8: 337.

Hague Conference on Private International Law (2012) *A Preliminary Report on the Issues Arising from International Surrogacy Arrangements*. Preliminary Document No. 10. The Hague: Permanent Bureau. <www.hcch.net/upload/wop/gap2012pd10en.pdf>

Keyes M and Chisholm R (2013) Commercial surrogacy – some troubling family law issues. *Australian Journal of Family Law Issues* 105: 132. <https://www.ag.gov.au/FamiliesAndMarriage/FamilyLawCouncil/Documents/flc-submission-professor-mary-keyes-griffith-university-16july2013.pdf>

Krim T (1996) Beyond Baby M: international perspectives on gestational surrogacy and the demise of the unitary biological mother. *Annals of Health Law* 5: 193.

Lee RL (2009) New trends in global outsourcing of commercial surrogacy: a call for regulation. *Hastings Women's Law Journal* 20: 275.

Leibowitz-Dori I (1997) Womb for rent: the future of international trade in surrogacy. *Minnesota Journal of Global Trade* 6: 329.

Millbank J (2011) The new surrogacy parentage laws in Australia: cautious regulation or '25 brick walls'? *Melbourne University Law Review* 35(1): 165–207.

Millbank J (2013) Paying for birth: the case for (cautious) commercial surrogacy. *Guardian*, 22 September. <www.theguardian.com/

commentisfree/2013/sep/02/australia-commercial-surrogacy>
Nozawa S and Banno K (2004) Surrogacy. *Japan Medical Association Journal* 47(4): 192–203.
Niyomyat A (2015) Thailand bans surrogacy for foreigners in bid to end 'rent-a-womb' tourism. *Reuters*, 19 February. <www.reuters.com/article/us-thailand-surrogacy-idUSKBN0LO07820150220>
Skene L (2012) Why legalising commercial surrogacy is a good idea. *The Conversation*, 10 December. <http://theconversation.com/why-legalising-commercial-surrogacy-is-a-good-idea-11251>
Smerdon UR (2009) Crossing bodies, crossing borders: international surrogacy agreements between the United States and India. *Cumberland Law Review* 60: 81–3.
Storrow R (2011) Assisted reproduction on treacherous terrain: the legal hazards of cross-border reproductive travel. *Reproductive BioMedicine Online* 23(5): 538–45.
Tétrault-Farber G (2014) Russian lawmaker proposes ban on commercial surrogate motherhood. *Moscow Times*, 24 April. <http://www.themoscowtimes.com/news/article/russian-lawmaker-proposes-ban-on-commercial-surrogate-motherhood/498901.html>
Tobin J (2014) To prohibit or permit: what is the (human) rights response to the practice of international commercial surrogacy? *International and Comparative Law Quarterly* 63(2): 317–52.
Trimmings K and Beaumont P (2012) International surrogacy arrangements: an urgent need for legal regulation at the international level. *Journal of International Private Law* 7(3): 627–47.
Weis C (2015) Workers or mothers? The business of surrogacy in Russia. *Open Democracy*, 15 December. <https://www.opendemocracy.net/beyondslavery/christina-weis/workers-or-mothers-business-of-surrogacy-in-russia>
Xinhua (2012) China's female lawmakers call for surrogacy ban. *ChinaDaily.com*, 3 August. <www.chinadaily.com.cn/china/2012-03/08/content_14782835.htm>

ABOUT THE AUTHORS

Sonia Allan is associate professor of health law at Macquarie University, Sydney, and an independent consultant to government. She has published in leading national and international journals, authored books and contributed to several government inquiries regarding the regulation of ART, surrogacy, legal parentage and adoption. She was a 2011 Churchill Fellow which supported her international research on the release of information about donors to donor-conceived people. Her work has been influential in the development of government policy.

Diane Beeson, professor emerita of sociology, California State University, has published numerous articles in medical and sociological journals on the social consequences of developments in genetics and reproductive technologies. Her research over the last three plus decades has fuelled her activism and inspired her to co-found the Alliance for Humane Biotechnology, of which she is currently associate director.

Eric Blyth is emeritus professor of social work at the University of Huddersfield, UK, co-chair of the British Association of Social Workers' Project Group on Assisted Reproduction and international editorial adviser at the *China Journal of Social Work*. He is co-editor of *Faith and Fertility: Attitudes towards Reproductive Practices in Different Religions from Ancient to Modern Times* (Jessica Kingsley Publishers, 2009) and *Third Party Assisted Conception across Cultures: Social, Legal and Ethical Perspectives* (Jessica Kingsley Publishers, 2003).

Ayesha Chatterjee is a programme manager for the Our Bodies Ourselves Global Initiative, where her leadership has resulted in the development of resources based on Our Bodies Ourselves in 12 languages and counting. Ayesha is also part of a collaborative project with the Center for Genetics and Society and global partners in South Asia to advance public awareness on international commercial surrogacy. She is a DONA-certified postpartum doula, associate editor for DONA International's quarterly print magazine, *International Doula*, and an active member of her local childbirth community.

ABOUT THE AUTHORS

Wendy Chavkin MD, MPH is professor of public health and obstetrics and gynecology at the Columbia University Mailman School of Public Health in New York City. She was a founding member and former board chair of Physicians for Reproductive Health, and co-founded Global Doctors for Choice in 2007 and is a member of its board of managers. She has received numerous honours for advocacy for reproductive health and rights. She has written extensively about women's health and rights, including on globalized motherhood and assisted reproductive technologies.

Marilyn Crawshaw is honorary fellow (formerly senior lecturer) at the University of York and chair of the British Association of Social Workers' multi-agency PROGAR group. She has researched surrogacy, donor conception, cancer related fertility, adoption and birth registration, and has been an adviser to the UK Human Fertilisation and Embryology Authority (HFEA) and UK DonorLink.

Marsha Tyson Darling is professor of history and interdisciplinary studies and director of the Center for African, Black and Caribbean Studies, Adelphi University, New York City. She has written extensively on race and gender as well as on the interests of children in relation to new reproductive technologies. Recent published work includes: 'The welfare principle in children of surrogacy' (DasGupta and Dasgupta, *Globalization and Transnational Surrogacy in India*, 2014); 'Considering the Hague's Best Interest of the Child in Gestational Surrogacy Agreements' (under review at an academic journal); and 'Commercial surrogacy and the cost of reproductive freedom' (*Genewatch*, June/July 2011).

Konstantina Davaki is a research fellow in social policy at the London School of Economics in the UK. Her background in law, sociology and social policy is reflected in her main research interests: gender, comparative social policy, bioethics, care, work/life balance, violence against women, mental health policies and welfare ideologies in a globalized world. Since 2010 she has been advising the Committee on Women's Rights and Gender Equality (FEMM) of the European Parliament, for which she has produced and presented studies on gender equality, maternity leave, work/life balance and intersectional discrimination of women with disabilities. Her publications include the first study on the regime of surrogacy in the EU (Brunet *et al.*, *A Comparative Study of the Regime of Surrogacy in EU Member States*, 2013), funded by the European Parliament, to which she contributed the section on policy.

ABOUT THE AUTHORS

Enikő Demény is associate research fellow at the Central European University (CEU) Center for Ethics and Law in Biomedicine (CELAB). Her research interests include the impact of new reproductive technologies on identity and the family; ethical, legal, social and policy aspects of new converging technologies; social sciences and bioethics; gender and science; feminist epistemology; and the anthropology of international bioethics governance. She has contributed chapters to numerous publications, most recently 'From eugenics and "race protection" to preventive medicine and family planning in Hungary' (in Moskalewicz M and Przybylski W (eds) *Understanding Central Europe*, Routledge, 2017) and 'Medically assisted reproduction: challenges for regulation in Romania' (Sándor, CELAB, 2013).

Deborah Dempsey is associate professor of sociology at Swinburne University in the Australian city of Melbourne. She has a longstanding fascination with how assisted reproductive technologies and clinical practices (ART) influence family formation and meanings of family and is best known for her work on family formation in LGBTI communities and the socio-legal aspects of same-sex relationships. Recent publications include: *Qualitative Social Research: Contemporary Methods for the Digital Age* (Sage, 2016, with Vivienne Waller and Karen Farquharson); *Families, Relationships and Intimate Life*, 2nd edition (Oxford University Press, 2014, with Jo Lindsay); and *Same-Sex Parented Families in Australia* (Australian Institute of Family Studies, 2013).

Clemence Due is a lecturer in the School of Psychology at the University of Adelaide, South Australia. Her research interests focus on the well-being of marginalized children and families, including gender diverse children, refugee children and children with autism spectrum disorder.

Kajsa Ekis Ekman is a Swedish journalist, writer and activist. She is the author of several works about the financial crisis, women's rights and capitalism critique, most recently *Being and Being Bought: Prostitution, Surrogacy and the Split Self* (Spinifex Press, 2013) and *Silent Spring* (Kerdos, 2014), about the economic crisis in Greece.

Andy Elvin is chief executive of TACT (The Adolescent and Children's Trust), the UK's largest fostering and adoption charity providing families for vulnerable children.

Hedva Eyal is a doctoral student at the Hebrew University of Jerusalem where her research focuses on the regulation of medical experiments on humans in Israel. She recently took part in policy design related to reproductive technologies in the country and served for five years as the head of the Haifa-based feminist organization Isha L'Isha (Woman to Woman), where she was founding director of the Women and Medical Technologies project. The project deals with feminist ethics and policy change concerning medical technologies, such as ova donations, surrogacy and abortions.

Patricia Fronek is senior lecturer in social work at Griffith University, Australia, and president of the Australian and New Zealand Social Work and Welfare Education and Research.

Isabel Fulda joined GIRE in 2012, where she developed as a researcher with a particular interest in surrogacy and assisted reproductive technologies in Mexico. She recently completed a master's degree in legal and political theory at University College London.

Generations Ahead was the first organization in the United States to work with a diverse spectrum of social justice stakeholders – including reproductive health, rights and justice, racial justice, LGBTQ, and disability and human rights organizations – on the social and ethical implications of genetic technologies. After its closure in 2012, executive director Sujatha Jesudason moved on to create a new project, the CoreAlign Initiative, dedicated to supporting people to fight for resources, rights and respect for their sexual and reproductive lives. Meanwhile Generations Ahead reports and resources continue to be available at www.generations-ahead.org/resources.

Linn Hellerström holds a bachelor's degree in political science and economics from Lund University and has wide experience of working with women's rights issues in various organizations in Sweden and the US. **The Swedish Women's Lobby**, for whom she worked in 2015, is a politically and religiously independent umbrella body representing a wide range of women's organizations in Sweden. Its work is feminist with foundations in the UN Convention of the Elimination of All forms of Discrimination Against Women (CEDAW) and the Beijing Platform for Action.

Fiona Kelly is an associate professor in the Law School at La Trobe University, Melbourne, Australia. The primary focus of her research is the law's response to non-normative families. Her publications address issues such as the judicial and legislative treatment of families created by lesbians and single mothers by choice, the legal regulation of parentage in the context of assisted reproduction and the ethics of sperm donor anonymity.

Ari Laurel grew up in Oakland, California, and has lived near the ocean for most of her life. She is a blog editor for *Hyphen* magazine and is currently living in the city of Missoula while pursuing an MFA in fiction writing at the University of Montana.

Abby Lippman is a longtime feminist activist and researcher with special interests in women's health and women's health policies. Now a professor emerita, she has one foot still based in academia (specifically at McGill and Concordia Universities) and the other, the foot she favours, remains firmly planted in social justice and reproductive justice activism with diverse community groups in Montréal and beyond its borders.

Anindita Majumdar is an assistant professor in the School of Liberal Arts, Indian Institute of Technology-Hyderabad.

Emma Maniere is a graduate of the University of Michigan, where she earned her BA in women's studies and political science. During her time there, she was involved in reproductive rights activism and research. Emma wrote her chapter for this book as a communications and program associate for the Center for Genetics and Society, Berkeley, California. She now works at Gynuity Health Projects in New York.

Sarojini Nadimpally is a founder member of Sama Resource Group for Women and Health and has coordinated national and international level research studies on reproductive and medical technologies including commercial surrogacy, clinical trials and ethics and access to medicines. She has contributed several articles/papers to national and international journals and has been a visiting scholar at the University of Massachusetts. Currently, she is a part of the Mission Steering Group of the National Health Mission (NHM) of the Government of India and a member of the Central Ethics Committee on Research of the Indian Council of Medical Research (ICMR).

Amrita Pande is a social scientist and academic, who conducted extensive ethnographic research of surrogacy practices in India between 2006 and 2014. Her findings are published in *Wombs in Labor: Commercial Surrogacy in India* (Columbia University Press, 2014). Her work on surrogacy has appeared in many journals, including *Signs:*

Journal of Women in Culture and Society, Gender & Society, Qualitative Sociology, Feminist Studies, Indian Journal of Gender Studies, Reproductive BioMedicine and in several edited volumes. Amrita is also an educator-performer and is currently involved in a multi-media theatre production, *Made in India: Notes from a baby farm* (Global Stories Production, Denmark) based on her surrogacy work.

Damien W Riggs is associate professor in social work at Flinders University, Adelaide and an Australian Research Council Future Fellow. He is the author of over 200 publications in the fields of gender/sexuality studies, family studies and marginalization, including (with Elizabeth Peel) *Critical Kinship Studies: An Introduction to the Field* (Palgrave Macmillan, 2016) and (with Clemence Due) *Surrogacy, Psychology and Health: A Critical Perspective* (Routledge, 2017).

Etti Samama is director of the Division of Medical Technology Policy at the Ministry of Health, Israel. She lectures in the field of medical policy at Haifa and Tel Aviv Universities. She holds a BA in nursing, an MA in social work from the Hebrew University of Jerusalem and a PhD in health systems management from Ben-Gurion University of the Negev. Her master's thesis and doctoral dissertation researched surrogate motherhood in Israel over the years. She lectures in the field of surrogacy and has published articles on the topic including a co-authored report on the state of surrogacy in Israel, published by the Isha L'Isha (Woman to Woman) feminist organization in 2011.

Carmel Shalev is a human rights lawyer and ethicist and the founding head of the Department for Reproduction and Society at the International Center for Health, Law and Ethics, Haifa University, Israel. Her publications include *Birth Power: The Case for Surrogacy* (Yale University Press, 1989) and *Health and Human Rights in Israeli Law* (Ramot, 2003) [Hebrew].

Laurel Swerdlow recently earned her master's in public health from the Columbia University Mailman School of Public Health in New York City, where she obtained a certificate in sexuality, sexual and reproductive health. She has managed projects focusing on a range of sexual and reproductive health issues, including family planning insurance coverage, abortion regulation, conscientious objection and transnational surrogacy. She currently serves as advocacy director for planned parenthood advocates in Oregon.

ABOUT THE AUTHORS

Regina Tamés, JD from Universidad Iberoamericana in Mexico City and a master's degree in international law from Washington College of Law, American University, became GIRE's executive director in April 2011. She has previously held positions with the United Nations Mexican Office of the High Commissioner for Human Rights and Planned Parenthood Federation of America, as well as other human rights organizations.

The Centre for Social Research (CSR) is a leader in the Indian women's movement as a facilitator of grassroots programmes and training, a research institute, and a lobbyist, advocate and adviser to government institutions. Key areas of work include: violence against women, prenatal sex selection, engendered governance, women and economy, and gender sensitization for and mainstreaming within all sectors of society.

France Winddance Twine is a documentary filmmaker and professor of sociology and black studies at the University of California at Santa Barbara. As an ethnographer and critical race feminist, she teaches courses on race/class/gender, critical race theory, sociology of the body, qualitative research methods and black Europe. Twine is the author and editor of 10 books. She is the series editor for Routledge's 'Framing twenty-first century social issues' collection. Her recent publications include *Outsourcing the Womb: Race, Class and Gestational Surrogacy in a Global Market* (2015, revised edition), *Geographies of Privilege* (Routledge, 2013) and *A White Side of Black Britain: Interracial Intimacy and Racial Literacy* (Duke University Press, 2010). She is currently completing a book titled *Geek Girls: Race, Gender and Sexuality in the tech industry* (forthcoming, Cambridge University Press).

Sally Whelan, a co-founder of Our Bodies Ourselves (OBOS), directs the organization's Global Initiative where her leadership has resulted in the development of 19 cultural adaptations of Our Bodies Ourselves used in health literacy and advocacy projects for women and girls around the world. Currently, Sally is part of a collaborative project with the Center for Genetics and Society and global partners in South Asia to advance public awareness on international commercial surrogacy and paid egg retrieval, as well as to step up the call for best practices in assisted reproduction.

INDEX

23 and Me website, 211

60 Minutes news programme, 232

abandonment of babies by intending parents, 56, 171, 187, 224, 329, 331
ableist systems, critique of, 284
abnormalities in babies *see* birth defects
abolitionist perspective, in feminism, 314, 322–5
abortion, 6, 27, 61, 119, 125, 150, 152, 199, 223, 237, 254, 278, 288, 290, 368; forced, 113, 269; illegal, deaths from, 125; initiated by surrogate mother, 257, 269; legalization of, 144 (in Romania, 125); results in reduced fee for surrogate mother, 255; spontaneous, 73 *see also* fetuses, reduction of *and* sex selection
Abourezk, James, 107
Abram, in Book of Genesis, 3
accountability, 234, 337
adoption, 20, 23, 27, 28, 37, 39, 128, 153, 164, 166, 169, 211, 247, 265, 301, 313, 348, 349; difficulties of, 38, 112; identity development in, 11; intercountry, 174, 175–6, 336, 339, 340 (conventions for, 172); legislation regarding, 339; of Romanian children, 125; regulatory model of, 52; triangle of, 7
Adoption and Children Act (2002) (UK), 173
African American women, and breast cancer, 286
age, of surrogate mother, 88, 91, 127, 149, 252
agencies, 234–8, 352; advertising copy of, xv; in Israel, 55–6; use language of altruism, 295
agency: and autonomy of women, 31; meaning of, 314, 316–19; of surrogate mothers, 267; constrained, 119
agents, facilitators and middlemen, 7, 65–81, 133–4, 249, 252, 321, 351, 370; elimination of, 259; registration of, 366
Akanksha clinic (Gujarat, India), 29, 229
Al Jazeera, 232
alienated labour, 322, 324–5 *see also* reproductive labour
Allan, Sonia, 321–2
Almeling, Rene, 215; *Sex Cells*, 214
altruism, 132–3, 149, 151, 155, 351; rhetoric of, 154, 156, 228, 230, 239, 295, 363–4; reason for rejection of surrogate mothers, 350
altruistic surrogacy, 68, 79, 80, 112, 126, 127, 188, 195, 298, 304, 307, 320, 328, 330, 335, 338, 344, 348, 349, 363–4; global permissive regimes, 345–50; lack of candidates for, 359; non-existent, 306–7; permitted in Greece, 143; socially constructed, 338
American Civil Liberties Union (ACLU), 289
American Indian Movement (AIM), 107
American Society of Reproductive Medicine (ASRM), 94
anaesthesia, risks of, 84
AnaLize journal, 123–4
ancestry testing, 287
Anleu, Sharyn, 338
anonymity, 58, 208, 214, 215, 216, 259; banning of, 207; difficulty of maintaining, 205–6; of donors and surrogates, mandatory or permitted, 204; of donors, in Greece, 149; of surrogate mothers, 174–5
Anonymous v. Ministry of Welfare and Social Services (Israel), 60
Appleton Foundation, 225
Arely, a surrogate mother, 270–1
Argentina, altruistic surrogacy in, 348
Armenia, 60; surrogacy practices in, 349–50; permissive approach to surrogacy, 349
arrests, arising out of operations of fraudulent clinics, 130, 131

'ART Banks', 67
ART (Regulation) Bill (2010) (India), 246, 248–52, 257
Artavia Murillo et al. (In vitro fertilization) v. Costa Rica, 262
artificial insemination, 22, 249
Asian women: egg donations by, 292; pressured to use genetic technologies, 281
asking for additional money, 10, 59–60, 62, 114–15, 150
assisted reproductive technologies (ARTs), 1, 110; additional services provided by clinics, 235; contradictions and inconsistencies of, 26–9; demand for, 21, 129; development and commercialization of, 4; fast-growing sector, 221; global aspect of, 23; global value of market in, 105; growth of, 8, 22, 190; health risks of, 82–104; in different communities, 279–85; numbers of babies born from, 105; numbers of players in, 79; predominantly in private sector, 224; pressure to use, 227; principles of, 29–31; promotion of, 66; public education regarding, 99; variety of, 20
Association for Fertility Support (Greece), 151
Association of Romanian Women, 136
asthma, among c-section children, 96
attachment to child, of surrogate mother, 134
Audi, Tamari, 112
Australia, 163; altruistic surrogacy in, 307; commercial surrogacy banned in, 206; surrogacy practices in, 207, 362, 335–6
Australian Capital Territory, extraterritorial prohibition in, 370
autism, risk of, 25
autonomy, 314, 317; of decision-making, 359; of women, 152; reproductive, 285, 289
Azerbaijan, 347

Baby Cotton, 4–5, 164
Baby Gammy, 56, 171, 199, 232, 233, 331, 351
Baby Joy, 8, 41
Baby L, 195
Baby M, 4–5, 229, 231, 233, 322, 330
Baby Manji, 233, 250–1
Baby Samuel, 194
'bad mothers', 107
Baillieu, Ted, 209
Banerjee, Amrita, 119
banning of surrogacy *see* surrogacy, prohibitions of
Basset, Angela, 299
BBC, *Hard Talk* programme, 230–1
Beck, Ulrich, 216; with Elisabeth Beck-Gernsheim, *Distant Love*, 204–5
Beck-Gernsheim, Elisabeth, 216
Belgium: altruistic surrogacy in, 348; citizenship issue in, 193–5; surrogacy practices in, 369
'best friends', acting as surrogates, 149
Beta hcG testing, 73
Bible, references to surrogacy in, 163
Bihar, recruitment of women in, 55, 56
Bilhah, in Book of Genesis, 4
bio-capitalism, in transnational commercial surrogacy, 3, 105–22
bio-colonialism, 279, 281, 287
bio-crossings, 68
bio-markets, 339
bio-piracy, 49, 50, 61–3, 279
bio-politics, 111–18
bio-prospecting, 279
biology: disaggregated from care, 19–32; variable primacy of, 26
BioTexCom company, 130, 132
birth, presence of commissioning parents at, 39
birth certificates, 27, 128, 130, 132, 251, 257, 266, 271–2, 348, 350, 353; issuing time of, 272; social and medical meanings of, 28
birth defects, 28, 93, 94, 97, 254–5, 258, 260, 269, 283; risk of, 24
birth mother, identification of, 19
birth weight, low, 24, 92, 93
birthrates, decline of, 21–2 (in Romania, 125)
'bits and pieces' use of women's bodies, 61
black market for commercial surrogacy, 361 *see also* underground existence of commercial surrogacy
Black women regulating fertility of, 108 *see also* women of colour

Black Women's Health Imperative (USA), 289
bleeding, intra-abdominal, 87
blood tests, of surrogate mothers, 75
blood transfusions, to be avoided by surrogate mothers, 248
bodily integrity of women: compromised, 113–14; right to, 112
'bodily labour', 10
body: of Black women, exploitation of, 282; woman's control of, 27, 359; woman's relationship with, 303
bonding with the child, 156, 168, 174, 257, 364
bonuses for surrogate mothers, in HIV cases, 231
Boone, Sarah, 323
border controls: training of staff, 179; visa process for surrogate children, 170
Brazil, altruistic surrogacy in, 348
breastfeeding, 96, 257; prevention of, 86
British Association of Social Workers (BASW), 173
Bromfield, Nicole Footen, 339
Brown, Lesley, 83
Brown, Louise, 4–5, 83, 164
Building Futures agency, 74, 75
Bulgaria, pro-natalism in, 227

c-section delivery, 10, 26, 49, 56, 57, 63, 86, 115, 223, 236, 238, 257, 299; an outcome of market and social pressures, 95; as exploitation, 239; for convenience of commissioning parents, 231; proof of necessity of, 367; rising rates of, 85 (in Greece, 155); risks of, 95–6, 270; viewed as problematic, 58
California, 163, 169, 190, 192; eugenics programmes in prisons, 107; health and safety advertising requirements, 90; passing of eugenics law in, 106; sterilizations in (forced, banned, 109; in prisons, 109); surrogacy laws in, 39; surrogacy practices in, 3, 10, 206, 307, 348
Cambodia, market for gay people, 353
Canada: citizenship issue in, 195; surrogacy practices in, 228
cancer, 89, 90, 209; breast cancer, affecting African American women, 286; environmental, 286; of prostate, 90; relation to IVF, 86; vaginal, 98
Cancun (Mexico), 238, 266, 270, 271
Carmen, a surrogate mother, 268
Caucasian babies, preference for, 57
Caucasian surrogate mothers, preference for, 235
Ceaușescu, Nikolae, 125
Center for Bioethics and Culture (CBC) (USA), 137
Center for Genetics and Society (CGS) (USA), 2, 225, 226, 227, 240
Center for Reproductive Rights (USA), 289
Centre for Social Research (CSR) (India), 1, 114, 228, 233, 245–6; national conference of, 257
Centro Medico Nacional 20 de Noviembre (Mexico), 264
Change, Arlene, 112
changing of minds, by either party, 265
chaperoned contact between intending parents and surrogate mothers, 236, 237
Chavkin, Wendy, 336
Cheney, Kristen, xv, 2
child, as marker of family, 41–2, 43
child abuse, 224; by commissioning parents, 232, 329
Child and Family Court Advisory and Support Service (UK), 177
Child Citizenship Act (2000) (USA), 197
child protection checks, on commissioning persons, 368
child selling, 171–2
childless couples, stigmatization of, 150
Childlessness Overcome Through Surrogacy (COTS), 166
children: bear consequences of adult agency, 186, 189; best interests of, 11, 133, 138, 146, 163–84, 185–203, 191, 196, 200, 209, 224, 273, 325, 349, 356, 358, 362, 364 (paramount, 192, 193, 195; responsibility for, 187, 190); born 'out of wedlock', 197, 198; born through surrogacy, in Mexico, 271–4; identity needs of, 178; marginalization of, 2; of surrogate mothers, 179, 367, 368 (impact of surrogacy on, 167; support for, 62); protecting privacy of, 266; rights of, 142, 232, 340, 353–4, 356–8 (to citizenship, 187, 189, 200)

China: one-child rule, 334; surrogacy driven underground, 334; surrogacy practices in, 333-4
choice: meaning of, 314, 316-19, 324; of donors, 207; rhetoric of, 38, 317
churches: Catholic, 136, 163; in Romania, attitude to surrogacy, 135-8; Orthodox, 136, 150; position on surrogacy, 12
Circle Surrogacy, 8, 40
citizenship, 210, 224, 257, 335; case of Baby Manji, 250-1; denied to children, 187, 191; humanitarian grounds for, 195 *see also* children, right to citizenship
clandestine markets, 265
'clans', of donor siblings, 213
class, issues of, 133
clinics: in India, survey of, 256-7; regulating operations of, 249, 370 *see also* agencies
Colen, Shellee, 105-6
Collectif pour le Respect de la Personne (CoRP) (France), 137
colonialism, 319
commercialized contract motherhood (CCM), 323
commissioning parents, 7-11, 49, 131-2, 185, 187, 344; assessment of, 175; celebrity parents, 230; 'exchanging' of, 268; in Mexico, 271-4; interests of, 164, 165; judgements in favour of, 188; motivations of, 146; prioritizing interests of, 221; relations with egg donors, 296; screening of, 198-9; seen as evil, 329; survey of, 255-6 *see also* intending parents, *and* rights, relevant to intending parents
commissions: charged for arranging surrogacy, 70-1; given to surrogate mothers for recruiting others, 78
commodification, 152, 322-3, 329, 338, 345, 363; of biological labour, 113; of children, 251, 358, 371; of intimate relationships, 65; of life, 172; of motherhood, 332; of reproduction, 24; of surrogacy, 154, 155, 259; of surrogate mothers, 43, 44, 304, 323; of women, 227, 285, 314
communities of connection and support, 205, 206

community-based research, need for, 187-8
compensation, 363; right to claim, 365
concierge-style services, 234, 235
confidentiality, 249
consent, informed, 62, 63, 89, 92, 98, 130, 153, 154, 170, 223, 267, 269, 314, 331, 367; compromised, 152; impossibility of, 222; record-keeping of, 251; video recording of, 258; of surrogate mother, for parental orders, 196; problematics of, 119; to fetal reduction, 367
constraints on reproduction, 22; growth of, 19
consumer voices, power of, 240
contact between surrogates and commissioning parents *see* relations between surrogate mothers and commissioning parents
contact information of intending parents, 62
contraception, 6, 7, 108, 119; made illegal in Romania, 125
contract labourers, female, 115-18
contracts, 62, 70, 86, 114, 132, 143, 145, 150, 168, 193, 221, 222, 237, 238, 256, 267, 270-1, 273, 331, 366-7; administration of, 337; codification of, 321; contain prohibitions, 61; copies not given to surrogate mothers, 253-4; enforceability of, 194, 322; ensuring understanding of, 120; in context of liberalism, 325; language of, 75; loopholes in, 250; non-enforceability of, 128, 137, 191, 348; signing of, 253, 268-9; terms of, 363; to be made in local languages, 259; unreadability of, 223, 237
convention on surrogacy, proposed, 344-5
Convention on the Elimination of All Forms of Discrimination against Women (CEDAW), 354, 358-9
Corea, Gena, xv, 323
corruption, 175
cosmetics, not to be used by surrogate mothers, 61
Costa Rica: prohibition of IVF in, 263; surrogacy issues in, 262-3

costs: of surrogacy, 66, 79, 130, 145, 152, 229, 365 (discounting of, 236, 238; in selected countries, 155); of treatment of children born through surrogacy, 93 *see also* fair price in regional context
Cotton, Kim, 4, 164
Council of Europe, 191
counselling, provision of, 259; to all parties, 321, 365–6; to surrogate mothers, 367
criminal checks for surrogacy partners, 235
cross-departmental collaboration, 176; establishment of working groups, 173
cryopreservation, safety and efficacy of, 25
culture mediums, commercial secrecy of, 95
cytoplasmic transfer, 26
Czech Republic, altruistic surrogacy in, 348

D and Others v. Belgium, 193
Daaar, Judith, 314–16
Damian, Cornel, 136
Daniel, a surrogacy agent, 55–8
Das Dasgupta, Shamita, 318–19
DasGupta, Sayantani, 318–19
data: ethnic, disaggregation of, 282; for birth defects, lack of, 97; informed consent as basis for, 98; lack of, 86, 89–91, 124, 148, 171; legislation to provide protection of, 260; limited size of research base, 97; need for collection of, 170; recording of, not obligatory for clinics, 114
death: of commissioning parents, 259; of donors, 170; of fetus, 271; of surrogate mothers, 25, 84, 88, 170 (pregnancy-related, 25)
decision-making: by commissioning parents, 27; medical, 26 *see also* surrogate mothers, decision-making powers of
Decree No. 770 (Romania), 125
delayed childbearing, 6, 19, 21, 22, 23, 30
Delhi, surrogacy practices in, 252–60
demographic transition, second, 21
Dempsey, Deborah, 215

Denmark, amends nationality law, 192
'designer babies', 277, 278
desire to have children, 360, 362, 372
detective work, by donor-conceived people, 210, 214
diabetes, gestational, 59
diet, of surrogate mothers, 70, 71, 269, 270; control of, 73
diethylstilbestrol (DES), risks of, 98
Dietrich, Heather, 324
dignity, 306, 358; of labour, 336–40, 339; of parenting, 290
disability rights, 289
disabilities: children rejected because of, 199 *see also* women with disabilities
disclosure to children of birth origins *see* informing child of circumstances of conception
discussion forums and blogs, 124, 128, 151, 155
disparities: between surrogate mothers and commissioning parents, 315, 359, 363; of power relations, in surrogacy, 324
Diva Donors, 23
divorce, 21
DNA: collection of, 285 (from Indigenous peoples, for research, 286); creation of databases of, 287; dragnets, for solving crimes, 285; preventing transfer of defects in, 190; testing of, 54, 168, 189, 209 (for forensics, 287; for parentage, 187, 194, 195, 196, 198, 214 (compulsory in India, 247; marketing of, 205); in relation to disability, 283; prenatal, 285; via internet, 210)
doctors: accountability and criminal responsibility of, 260; investment in surrogacy industry, 149; opinions about surrogacy, 256
documentation, safe storage of, 258
domestic workers, as surrogate mothers, 10, 154, 252
donor conception, changing attitudes to, 205
donor linking, 208
Donor Sibling Registry (DSR), 212–13
donor siblings: creation of registers of, 205; relationships between, 212–13

double implantation *see* two gestational mothers impregnated
Down's syndrome, 199, 331; reason for abandoning baby, 56; screening for, 285
Draft ART (Regulation) (2008 and 2010) (India), 329, 330
Draft ART Regulation Bill (2014) (India), 79, 197
Draft Law on Medically Assisted Human Reproduction (Romania), 127
Dworkin, Andrea, 302

education: children's ineligibility for, 186, 193; community-based, 287; of children of surrogate mothers, 253; of surrogate mothers, 252; of the public, 241
Edwards, Robert G., 83–4
'egg catalogue', xiii, xiv
egg providers, narratives of, 239
eggs: donation of *see* eggs, provision of; donors of (definition of, 27–8; rendered invisible, 40); ethnic discrimination of, 40; freezing of *see* freezing, of eggs; harvesting of, 5, 25, 28, 87, 263, 296, 360 (health risks of, 29, 82–104, 223; in excess, 294; preference for 'white' eggs, 29); market in, 26, 55, 57, 79, 351 (in China, banned, 334; in USA, 89); ownership of, 145; provision of, 44, 52, 53, 57, 66, 69, 78, 112, 129, 196, 206, 207, 221, 227, 234, 292–7 (by Asian donors, 281; by Roma women, 130; by Romanian donors/sellers, 128; by university students, 130; by women from South Africa, 49); commercial (illegal, 130, 133); from Eastern Europe, 224; in USA, 88; motivations of donors, 295, 296; payment for, 295; risks to providers, 87–9, 90; commercialization of, 79; unauthorized splitting of, 231 *see also* freezing of eggs
Ekman, Kajsa Ekis, 12, 323, 324, 325; *Being and Being Bought*, 298
embassies and consulates, enhancing staffing in, 179
embryos: protocols for handling of, 95; sensitivity of, 94–5

empathy, 151
empowerment, 172, 345
endometriosis, 90, 153
epigenetic alterations, 28, 94, 95, 100
epigenetic inheritance, 28–9
equality, fiction of, 114
Ergas, Yasmine, 27
errors committed by fertility clinics, 195, 198, 199
Esteban, a commissioning parent, 272–3
ethical questions of surrogacy, xiv, 1, 12, 61, 65, 68, 119, 123, 136, 142, 150, 152, 156, 227, 232, 245–61, 277, 285, 299, 313, 316, 319, 325, 354, 362, 371; clinical, 62–3
eugenics, 224, 239, 278, 282, 283, 292; movement for, 106; negative, 110
European Charter of Human Rights, 193
European Court of Human Rights, 188, 190, 191, 192, 193, 273, 369
European Court of Justice, 188, 192; decision on legal parenthood, 138
European courts, role of, 191–4
European Human Rights Commission, 369
European Parliament: resolution on trading of eggs, 359–60; resolution on Human Rights (2015), 305–6
European Society for Human Reproduction and Embryology, 178
European Women's Lobby, 137
exploitation, 142, 172, 259, 351, 354, 308; of egg donors, 296; of surrogate mothers, 119, 172, 239, 251, 303, 313, 319, 329, 352, 359; of women, 305, 325; of women of colour, 282, 287
extraterritorial laws, difficulty of enforcement, 370

face recognition software, use of, 214
Facebook, use of, 51; as means of donor sibling contact, 213–14
failure of pregnancy, 91, 177
'fair price in regional context', 336–7
fair-skinned women, chosen as surrogate mothers, 257
'fairtrade surrogacy', 328, 336–40, 358, 362
false or misleading information, provision of, 175
falsifying of medical records, 197

familial identities, medicalization of, 210
family: can only be achieved through children, 43; concept of, 41; creation of, 42; definition of, 355–6; 'extended', 214; formation of, 362; Greek traditional ideas of, 144, 151; importance of, 285; new forms of, 1, 163, 205, 301, 315, 372 (acceptance of, 29); right to found, 355
family studies, of commissioning person(s), 368
Family Tree DNA.com, 210–11
father, biological connection of, not questioned, 301
fatherhood, desire for, 42
fees and payments for surrogacy, xv, 56, 69–71, 115, 118, 129, 130, 150, 154, 177, 228, 229, 236, 239, 249, 254, 257, 265, 266, 270, 313, 317, 319, 320, 339, 346, 348, 365, 366, 367; disparities in, 117–18, 313; documentation of, 248; flat fee proposed, 362; forbidden, in UK, 195, 196; impossible to verify, 236; in Africa, 227; inequality in, 286; non-payment of, 247, 271; of staff at surrogacy centres, 72; paid in instalments, 236, 247, 337; paid to counsellors, 366; paid to providers of legal advice, 365; proposed uniformity of, 321; repayment of, 237; request for additional payment *see* asking for additional money; standardized base of, 259; uncertainty about, 254 *see also* reasonable expenses *and* costs
feminism, 12, 52, 118, 136, 137, 144, 150, 151, 153–4, 298–309; critique of surrogacy, 152–4, 304–8 (diversity of positions, 314); in Romania, 123–4; views of commercial surrogacy, 313–27
Feminist No to Surrogacy network (Sweden), 305
Feminists for the Abolition of Surrogacy, 137
feminization of survival, 77
fertility: declining rates of, 21–2; regulation of (in India, 109–11; in USA, 106–8); time limits of, 19, 22
fertility continuum, 105–22
Fertility Institutes, The, 37, 235, 236, 237, 238

fetuses, reduction of, 86, 92–3; consent to, 367
Food and Drugs Administration (USA), 90
Foreign and Commonwealth Office, statement regarding legal advice, 176
France: denial of citizenship in, 192; prohibition of commercial surrogacy in, 163, 192–3, 369
Franks, Trent, 288
fraud by fertility clinics, 223, 232, 247, 258
Freeman, T., 212–13
freezing of eggs, 1, 5, 57
frozen embryos, 238–9; black-marketing of, 259

gamete donors, identity registration of, 206, 207, 208
gametes: donation of, 22; primacy ascribed to, 28; third-party, health risks of, 24
Gammy *see* Baby Gammy
gay communities, targeted outreach to, 238
gay couples, 1, 6; access to surrogacy (in Israel, 51–2; niche market, 206); disclosure of origins to children, 208; excluded from surrogacy, 227, 238; surrogacy needs of, 36 *see also* India, prohibition of surrogacy, for gay couples
gay men: drawn to commercial surrogacy, 34; inclusivity of, 333, 348; reproductive desires of, 33–45; seeking parenthood, 5, 8
gender, 322; hierarchies, reinscription of, 323–4; norms, challenging of, 315
gender inequality, 119
gender selection *see* sex selection
gender wage gap, inequity of, 30
General Health Law (Mexico), 263
Generations Ahead (USA), 1, 3, 276–91 *passim*
genetic characteristics, desired, seeking of, 223
genetic determinism, 286
genetic relatedness, 165, 347; desire for, 34, 36, 39–41, 43, 57, 152, 153, 301; required for citizenship, 60
genetic research, privatization of, 286

390 | INDEX

geneticization of social and environmental problems, 278
genetics: dominant paradigm in society, 287; foregrounding of, 44
Genographic Project, 285; boycott recommended, 286
Genovese v. Malta, 192
Georgia, surrogacy practices in, 350; permissive approach to, 349
gestation, misconstrued as care, 20
gestational mothers *see* surrogate mothers
Ghilain, Laurent, 194–5
globalization, 22, 336; counter-geographies of, 77; of motherhood, 23
Goncharik, Alesia, 301
grassroots knowledge about surrogacy, 226–9
grassroots movements, need for, 98
Grech, Narelle, 209–10
Greece, 206; anonymity permitted in, 207; austerity measures in, 143; becomes market for ARTs, 147, 149, 154; Civil Code, 143, 146; IVF centres in, 130; Law 3089/2002, 144, 146, 147; Law 3305/2005, 143, 145, 146; Law 4272/2014, 147
opposition to surrogacy in, 12; residency requirement in, 9; role of family in, 143; surrogacy practices in, 9–10, 142–60
Green Cards, obtained by surrogate mothers, 284
Growing Generations, 36
Grunberg, Laura, 137
Grupo de Información en Reproducción Elegida (GIRE) (Mexico), 1, 9, 262–75 *passim*
guaranteed incomes for surrogate mothers, 119
Guardian Wards Act (1890) (India), 330
Guatemala, 339; surrogacy practices in, 334
Gupta, Anoop, 316, 339
Gupta, Jyotsna Agnihotri, 317, 321

Hagar, in Book of Genesis, 3
Hague Conference on Private International Law, 2, 136, 172, 351, 353, 354; Permanent Bureau, 224

Hague Convention on Protection of Children and Co-operation in Respect of Intercountry Adoption, xv, 187, 188, 336
Hague Forum, 9, 12
handover of baby *see* relinquishment, of baby
happy families, portrayal of, 299–300, 303
health, reproductive, right to, 355
health risks, 6; for children, 171; for surrogate mothers *see* surrogate mothers, health risks of; in fragmentation of motherhood, 30
healthcare: children ineligible for, 186, 193; free provision of, 173; of surrogate mothers, benchmarks for, 322 *see also* public health ramifications of ARTs *and* surrogate mothers, healthcare of
Hedley J., Justice, 195
Hellerstrøm, Linn, 298–309
Helsinki Foundation for Human Rights, 189
Hertz, Rosanna, 212, 213
Hindu Marriage Act (1955) (India), 259
HIV: risk of, 9; sperm from donors with, 231; status of commissioning parents, 268
Home Box Office (HBO) *Vice* series, 231–2
Home Office (UK), statement warning parents, 176
homonormativity, in desire to have a child, 42
homophobia, 151
Hong Kong, prohibition of commercial surrogacy, 346
hormone replacement therapy (HRT), 98
hormone treatments, 57, 84, 223, 296; risks of, 25, 87, 156; unknown effects of, 89
hospitals: corporate, in India, 67; links with agencies, 68
human capital, theory of, 111, 115
Human Fertilisation and Embryology (HFE) Act (1990), 164, 165, 166
Human Fertilisation and Embryology (HFE) Act (2008) (UK), 165, 169
Human Fertilisation and Embryology Authority (HFEA) (UK), 173, 195, 196, 316

human rights, 12, 79, 172, 186, 222, 257, 262–3, 273, 285, 305, 354, 369–70; international framework of, 354–9 *see also* children, rights of
Humbyrd, Casey, 336–7
husbands, 73, 265; concerns of, 75, 117, 134 (pivotal, 77); consent of, 145; pressure on wives to enter surrogacy, 253; promote wives as surrogates, 69, 76; visit sex workers, 257
hypertension, 25, 86

Iceland, prohibition of surrogacy in, 335
in vitro fertilization (IVF), 1, 4, 7, 22, 83, 94, 95, 99, 110, 131, 189; clinics, 67 (number of, in India, 222); health risks of, 24, 82; principles of, 164; regulation of, 126
India, 60, 163, 169, 216; as surrogacy destination for Israelis, 53; first surrogate birth in, 246; jurisdiction in, 246, 247–52; landscape of surrogacy in, 246–7; medical tourism in, 222; Ministry of Women and Child Development, 245; non-support for donors and surrogates, 215; prohibition of surrogacy in, 53, 55, 320–1, 328, 332–6, 351–2 (for non-Indian nationals, 6; for single persons, 79; for gay couples, 56, 62, 79); regulation of fertility in, 109–11; residency requirement in, 222; restricted access to surrogacy, 206, 226, 231, 233, 238; surrogacy market in, 169–70, 221–2 (growth market, 246, 307, 313, 332 (limiting of, 196–7)); surrogacy practices in, 6, 10, 27, 38, 52, 65–81, 105–22, 196, 199, 207, 225, 233, 234, 238, 240, 317; transnational commercial surrogacy in, 328–43; use of English in, 7
'India Bundle', 237
Indian Council of Medical Research (ICMR) *Guidelines*, 67, 75, 80, 247, 329–30; statement on surrogacy, 351
Indian Health Services (IHS) (USA), sterilization policies in, 107
Indian Society for Assisted Reproduction, 222
Indigenous communities: exploitation of, 172; medical practices and ceremonies of, 281; researchers' role in, 280; treated as historic artefacts, 286
Indigenous women, 12; and new genetic technologies, 276–91; effects of genetic technologies on, 279–81; targeted for sterilization, 107
inequality, xv, 152, 325, 333, 361, 362, 371; in surrogacy relationship, 142, 322; structural, confronting women, 277 *see also* disparities, between intending parents and surrogate mothers
infertility, 91, 94, 129, 131, 145, 151, 207, 276, 313; among women of colour, 277, 283; increase in, 5, 6
information: about biographical and genetic heritage, access to, 166, 171, 173, 176, 186, 205, 206, 207, 215, 216, 232, 237, 249, 340, 356, 357, 366, 368 (as human right, 208; gathering of, 97, 178; importance of, 174–5, 209; pursuit of, 204–17; right to, 168); as source of power and exploitation, 176–7; for commissioning parents, 225; for surrogate mothers, 86; industry-biased, 241; not recorded in birth data, 41; reliability of, 234; standardized, provision of, 178
informing child of circumstances of conception, 166, 208
injection, of self, 296
Institute of Medicine (IOM) (USA), report on IVF, 89
insurance cover for surrogate mothers, 120, 223, 258, 353
intending mothers: profiles of, 153; required qualifications of, 145–6
intending parents *see* commissioning parents
Inter-American Court of Human Rights, ruling on ARTs, 262
International Association of Schools of Social Work (IASSW), 172
International Convention of Surrogacy, proposed, 179
International Covenant on Civil and Political Rights, (ICCPR), 355–6
International Covenant on Economic, Social and Cultural Rights (ICESCR), 355

International Federation of Fertility
Societies (IFFS), 178
International Federation of Social
Workers (IFSW), 172, 173, 178
International Forum on Intercountry
Adoption and Global Surrogacy, xv, 1,
82, 173-4
International Institute of Social Studies
(ISS) (The Hague), xv, 2, 173, 178
International Union for the Abolition of
Surrogacy, 136
Internet, 133, 247; data bases on, 234;
harnessing power of, 210-14;
promotion of commercial surrogacy
on, 33-45, 124; survey of surrogacy,
233-8; survey of US fertility clinic
websites, 34; treatment of surrogacy,
225-6; use of, 11, 66, 128, 224 (as
resource for 'origins' information,
204-17; as source of recruitment,
129)
intersectional analysis, 278, 285, 287, 288,
289, 332
intra-cytoplasmic sperm injection (ICSI),
22, 24-5, 94; mainstreaming of, 25;
reducing use of, 99
invisibility: of risks to surrogate mothers,
92; of surrogate mothers, 66, 70, 299,
319
involuntary childlessness, 175
IQ testing, for egg donors, 292
Ireland, altruistic surrogacy in, 348
Islam, 163
Israel, 163; surrogacy practices in, 318
(permissive approach to, 349); pro-
natalism in, 227; reaction to Nepal
earthquake emergency, 49-64, 231,
233; regulation of surrogacy in, 50,
51-3; use of photo profiles in, 211
Israeli doctors arrested in Romania, 130
Italy, prohibition of surrogacy in, 163

Jackson, Michael, 299
Jacob, in Book of Genesis, 4
Jadva, V., 213
Jagland, Thorbjorn, 191
Japan: altruistic surrogacy in, 348-9;
citizenship issues in, 250-1;
prohibition of surrogacy in, 348-9
Japanese man, fathers sixteen babies, 351

Japanese Society of Obstetrics and
Gynecology, 348-9
jealousy, used as means of control of
women, 72
Jesudason, Sujatha, 276
John, Elton, 299
Johnson, Corey G., 109
Jönsson, Kutte, 299, 301
jus sanguinis, 189, 191, 197, 198
jus soli, 189, 197
Juvas, Sören, 301

Kazakhstan, permissive approach to
surrogacy in, 349
Kenya, growing markets for surrogacy,
227
Khan, Aasia, 114-15, 117-18
Kidman, Nicole, 299
kidney donors, women as, 338
kinship: conflated with genetics, 44;
privileging of certain forms of, 43
knowledge of birth circumstances, 11, 28
Kramer, Ryan, 212
Kramer, Wendy, 212
Krølokke, C. H., 113
Kumar, Deepal, 69-73, 76, 77

La Maruta TV show, 134
Labbassee v. France, 193, 273
labour markets, gendered, 24
lactation, risks of skipping of, 96
languages: doctors act as go-betweens,
255; English, 55, 75 (spoken by doctors,
7, 247); Hindi, used in contracts, 75;
of commercial surrogacy, 362-3; of
contracts, 259 (to be understandable,
267); shared, not available, 62
Latina women in the USA relation to
genetic technology, 284
law and legislation, 232, 322, 259:
capacity of keeping up with
developments, 190-1; citizen
litigation, 188; creation of, 191;
domestic (bypassing of, 188; changes
in, 371-2); global laws, 345-50, 353-4
(limits of, 187-90); in India, 329-31; in
Mexico, 264-6; in Romania, 126, 135;
in UK, 195-6; inadequacy of, 245; lack
of, 347; need for, 258; legal action
against clinics, 256

Law Commission of India, *228th Report...*, 329-30
legal advice, provision of: to all parties, 321, 365; to surrogate mothers, 228, 237, 346-7
legal representation of surrogate mothers, 223, 267; lack of, 2
Lemke, Thomas, 111
lesbian couples, 6; choice of sperm donors, 40; disclosure of birth origins to children, 208; interest in donor identities, 213; surrogacy needs of, 36
LGBTQI community, 288; and new genetic technologies, 276; rights of, 289
libertarian approach, in feminism, 314-16
Liechtenstein, permissive approach to surrogacy in, 349
life: new forms of, 112; stewardship of and respect for, 281
life processes, transformability of, 111
light skins, preference for, 36
live testimony, required of all parties, 364
Luke, a parent, xiii
Lundgren, Bo, 299
Lupron (leuprolide acetate), 90-1; classified as hazardous drug, 91

MacArthur Foundation, 225
Made in India film, 114-15, 117
Madge, Varada, 318
Malaysia: extraterritorial prohibition in, 370; prohibition of cross-border surrogacy in, 335
Malm, H. M., 302-3
Mark, Karl, 324
Market Data Enterprises, 105
market for surrogacy, 345, 362-3; shifts across borders, 320
marketing of surrogacy, aggressive, 223
marriage, stipulation of, 197
Martin, Ricky, 299
Marwah, Vrinda, 316, 317
maternity, definition of, 358
Mattes, Jane, 212, 213
media: coverage of transnational surrogacy by, 225-6, 229-33; sensationalist reporting in, 329
medical tourism, 6, 22, 67-8, 105, 110, 120, 163, 222, 246, 307, 331; deregistration of fraudulent clinics, 258

Mehta, Pritiben, 250
Mendiola, Alejandra, 9
Mennesson, Dominique, 192-3
Mennesson, Sylvie, 192-3
Mennesson v. France, 192-3, 273, 369
menopause, onset of, 89
menstrual cycle abiding by, 83
mental retardation, risk of, 25
Meurrens, Peter, 194-5
Mexico, 169, 206, 216; anonymity in, 207; growth market for ARTs, 274; preferred destination for transnational surrogacy, 63; residency restrictions in, 265; surrogacy practices in, 2, 9, 228, 234, 238, 240, 262-75, 352-3 (legal for gay couples, 35)
Mexico Surrogacy, 42
middlemen, culture of, in India, 67 *see also* agents, facilitators and middlemen
migration for work, 134
milder stimulation protocols, requirement for, 99
military wives, as surrogate mothers, 3
minimally invasive approaches, requirement for, 99
Ministry of Health and Family Welfare (MoHFW) (India), 329
Miroiu, Mihaela, 137
miscarriage, 75, 368; forfeiture of part of fee, 247
Mitochondrial Replacement Therapy (MRT), 190
mitochondrial transfer, 26
modes of delivery, decisions regarding, 26
Modi, Narendra, 6
money, as source of power and exploitation, 176-7
monitoring of pregnancy, 78
Mor-Yosef Commission (Israel), 51
moral pluralism, 335
moral relativism, 325
'moral safety valve', 315
morality, questions of, 10, 61, 68, 135
mortality, maternal, 99
motherhood, 357; biological, 29 (non-primacy of, 20); definition of, 19, 323; disaggregation of, 21; dissolving concept of, 301; fragmentation of, 19-32 (value ascription in, 26-7); globalization of, 23; liberatory

motherhood (cont.):
construction of, 31; proletarianization of, 323; understanding of, 358 *see also* commercialized contract motherhood; military wives, as surrogate mothers; *and* surrogate mothers
mothering, social ascription of, 20
multiple births, extra children resulting from, 172 *see also* twins and multiples
multiple embryo implantation, 25, 118, 171; risks of, 85, 91–2, 231
multiple embryos, selective reduction of, 25–6
Mumbai, surrogacy practices in, 252–60
Mutcherson, Kimberley, 314–16
My Body, My Rights radio show, 227

nannies: migrants as, 20, 23; use of, 19
National Asian Pacific American Women's Forum (NAPAWF), 288, 289
National Commission for Women (NCW) (India), 245, 259
National Independent Authority for Medically Assisted Reproduction (Greece), 145
National Latina Institute for Reproductive Health (USA), 289
National Perinatal Association (NPA) (USA), 99
National Socialist Party (Germany), 107
nationality, 322, 369; of surrogate children, 185–203; right to acquire, 356
Nayak, Preeti, 316, 317
neoliberalism, 36, 43, 106, 108, 111–18, 314, 318, 363; logics of consumption, 38; treatment of women under, 98
Nepal, 206; earthquake in, 2, 49, 231, 233, 334; prohibition of commercial surrogacy in, 328, 352; surrogacy market in, 221–2; surrogacy practices in, 56, 225, 228, 233, 238, 240, 334 (legal for gay couples, 35)
Nepal Supreme Court, moratorium on transnational surrogacy, 63
Netherlands: altruistic surrogacy in, 307; eligibility for citizenship in, 189
networks of reproduction, 123–41
New Life clinic, 155

New South Wales, extraterritorial prohibition in, 370
New York Times, 231, 233
Northwest Surrogacy Center, 37, 39, 41
Norway, prohibition of surrogacy in, 335
not-for-profit surrogacy, 165, 166, 177, 262
notaries, interests of, 268
Novas, Carlos, 210
Nuffield Council of BioEthics, 176
nutrition and exercise, of surrogate mothers, to be controlled, 61

Ohlsson, Birgitta, 298
Oliari and Others v. Italy, 190
Oliver, Kelly, 114, 323, 324
ombudsman for surrogacy, recommended, 259
Omnitrace.com, 211
orphanages: children left in, 187, 193, 194, 200, 258; in Romania, 125
Our Bodies Ourselves (OBOS) (USA), 1, 99, 225, 226, 227, 228, 232, 240; *Our Bodies Ourselves*, 226, 228
outcomes, 37, 66, 99, 144, 148, 176, 186, 247, 256; lack of research into, 166 (for commissioning parents, 174; for surrogate children, 174); need for large-scale study of, 94; of IVF, 83 *see also* failures
outsourcing of reproduction, 1, 22
ovarian hyperstimulation syndrome (OHSS), 85, 87–8, 99, 171, 223, 227; mitigating the symptoms of, 295; risks of, 292–3
ovarian stimulation, 5, 22, 57, 83, 84, 259; affects uterus lining, 88; risks of, 58, 293–4
ovulation, natural cycle of, 84

Pakistan, prohibition of surrogacy in, 163
Pande, Amrita, 10, 11, 78, 119, 316, 317, 318, 320–1; *Wombs in Labor*, 10, 109–10, 116
Pant, S., 113
parallel pregnancies, 57
parentage, 137, 148, 206, 224, 236, 257, 264, 265, 272, 322, 349, 350, 351, 353, 362, 369; definition of, 357; in Greece, 144, 145, 146; legal, determination of, 179, 189; recognition of, 39, 127, 130, 138, 150, 186, 193, 250, 271–2, 273

(standards for, 136); transfer of, 165, 348, 353, 363, 364
parental and visitation rights, 5
Parental Orders, 165–6, 173, 177, 195, 196; choosing not to apply for, 178; costs and complexity of, 168, 170; deadlines for, 167; disincentives of, 179; rising number of, 169; timescale of, 178 (delays in, 168)
Parental Orders (Human Fertilisation and Embryology) Regulations (2010) (UK), 165
parenthood: concept of, challenged, 301; contested, in Romania, 123; right to, 51; social, 301
parenting: desire for, universality of, 41–2; preparation for, 175–6 *see also* commissioning parents
Parker, Sarah Jessica, 299
Paromita, a supervisor of surrogate mothers, 73–5
Pasok party (Greece), 144
passports, 271–2, 299, 350; application for, 168; denied to children of male couples, 272, 273; of surrogate mothers, confiscated, 334 *see also* travel documents *and* visas
Patel, Nayna, 229, 230–1, 236, 250
paternity, desire for, 34
people with disabilities, and new genetic technologies, 276
permissive approach to surrogacy, 349–50, 361
Phillips, Anne, *Our Bodies, Whose Property?*, 112
photographs, used as means of identifying donors, 211
pituitary gland, 90; operation of, 87
placenta, decreased efficiency of, 86
placenta previa, 85–6, 95
Planet Hospital (Mexico), 112, 114, 232, 233, 235, 237, 238; bankruptcy of, 231
Planned Parenthood (USA), 289
Poland, citizenship restrictions in, 189–90
police checks, on surrogate mothers, 176
Policy Dialogue on Issues Surrounding Surrogacy in India conference, 245
policy solutions, proposed, 320–2
poor women, as surrogate mothers *see* surrogate mothers, poor women as

Portugal, prohibition of surrogacy in, 163
post-colonialism, in transnational commercial surrogacy, 105–22
postpartum care of surrogate mothers, 223, 258, 331, 367; lack of, 85, 86
poverty, 324; role of, 228 *see also* surrogate mothers, poor women as
pragmatic attitudes to surrogacy, 135
Pre-Conception and Pre-Natal Diagnostic Techniques, 258
precautionary principle, 30, 90, 98, 100
preeclampsia, 25, 86
pregnancy: desire to experience, 152, 306; protection during, 358
premature birth, 58, 86, 92, 93, 115, 227; resulting from Nepalese earthquake, 56
presumption against treatment, 364, 368
prisons, sterilization abuses in, 109
privacy, 216, 314; varying views of, 215
profiling of donors, xiii
prohibition, of commercial surrogacy *see* surrogacy, prohibitions of
prohibitionism: at world level, 345; in India, 332–6; viewed as detrimental, 320
Project Group on Assisted Reproduction (PROGAR), 173, 176, 178; roundtable, 176, 177–9
prostitution, 60, 302–3
public attitudes to surrogacy: in Greece, 150–1; in Romania, 135–8
public health ramifications of ARTs, 24–6
public knowledge of transnational surrogacy, gaps in, 221–44
punishment of commercial surrogacy, 349, 369
Purdy, Laura, 319–20

Qadeer, Imrana, 337
Queensland, extraterritorial prohibition in, 370
queer community, oppression of, 283

race, issues of, 133, 315, 322
race hierarchies, reinscription of, 323–4
race selection, 290
Rachel, in Book of Genesis, 4
racism, 3; confronting women, 277; in transnational commercial surrogacy, 105–22; scientific, 278

Raymond, Janice, 323, 324, 338
'reasonable expenses', 145, 149, 165, 168, 177, 195, 346, 364
reception staff, at surrogacy centres, 72
recording systems for surrogacy data, 11, 63; bypassing of, 169; ensuring maintenance of, 215; inadequacy of, 82, 168, 174; lack of, 212
recruitment: discourse of, 78; of donors, 365; of surrogate mothers, 65–81, 129, 222, 232, 234, 248, 365 (tactics of, 223; agencies for, 233; by surrogate mothers, 68; chain system of, 70, 71, 72; tiered structure of, 76)
reduction of fetuses, 85, 236, 237, 238; forced, 223
reformist perspective, in feminism, 314, 316–22
registers: of donor siblings, 205; of surrogate mothers, proposed, 127; web-based, for donor-conceived people, 210
registration, 207, 266; for information about genetic origin, 208; of all providers, 366; of babies at birth, 356; of identity, of surrogacy parties, 215; of surrogacy arrangements, 258; of surrogate mothers, 251, 259
registries: lack of, 82; of donor siblings, 212–13; of donors, 214; requirement of, 89, 97
regulation: of ARTs, 263, 264; of contracts, 10; of egg donation, lack of, 296; of surrogacy, xiv, 7, 23, 84, 120, 124, 138, 142, 144, 148, 178, 188, 190, 207, 222, 248, 252, 316, 321, 372; at international level, 359–61; domestic, 362–70; in Romania, 126; in USA, 315; lack of, 6, 7, 69, 87, 137, 164, 174, 177, 191, 238, 245, 246, 271, 274, 339 (in Sweden, 304; *see also* legislation, lack of); problems of, 165; of transnational surrogacy, 119, 344–75; state's role in, beneficial, 320
rejection: of babies, 171, 199, 255, 258; of babies with disabilities, 232; of surrogate mothers, 74 (by doctors, 77)
relations between surrogate mothers and commissioning parents, 167, 215–16, 236, 237, 253, 255, 338, 350, 367

relationships of surrogacy: obfuscation of, 30; transparency of, 339–40
relinquishment: of baby, 86, 128, 156, 236, 238, 255, 256, 306, 347; of parental rights, 249
remittances, of nannies, 23
'remote control' of pregnancy, 58
reporting, of medical problems, lack of, 87
reproductive exiles, use of term, 33
reproductive justice, 106, 108, 118–20, 276–91, 333
reproductive labour of women, 8, 10, 41, 42, 105–6, 118–19, 149, 152, 239, 302, 332, 337, 338, 363
reproductive liberalism, concept of, 324
reproductive rights, 3, 115, 131, 263, 314, 316, 332; of Indigenous women, 277; of women of colour, 277
reproductive tourism, 6, 9, 22–3, 33, 78, 110, 116, 125, 128, 138, 142, 144, 147, 206, 282, 285–6, 330, 335, 351; in India, 246–7
repropreneurs, 37–8, 43, 115–18, 119; use of term, 33, 113, 116
research, evidence-based, need for, 99
residency requirements for surrogacy applicants, 145, 147, 349, 370
Riggs, Damien, 215
right not to have children, 290
right of blood *see jus sanguinis*
right to bodily integrity, 307
right to choose, 152
right to found a family, 355
right to have a child, 12, 118, 180, 290, 329, 355
right to knowledge, 185
right to raise children with dignity, 118
right to reproductive health, 355
rights: of children, 245, 259, 307, 356–8; of intending parents, 245, 355–6; of surrogate mothers, 245, 307–8, 358–9; of women, 2; reproductive *see* reproductive rights
Rijal, Minendra, 352
risks: of drugs used in surrogacy, 249; of surrogacy, 9; need for follow-up research, 97; psychological, 82; shared by pregnant women and infants, 95–6; to embryos, fetuses and infants, 91–5;

to Indigenous peoples, 280 see also surrogate mothers, health risks for
Roberts, Dorothy, 108
Roma women, as surrogate mothers, 133
Romania: Law No. 287/2009; opposition to surrogacy in, 12; surrogacy practices in, 2, 123–41
Romanian Women's Lobby (ROWL), 137
Rose, Nikolas, 116, 210
Ross, Loretta, 118
Rossingnol, Laurence, 369
Rotabi, Karen Smith, 339
Rothman, Barbara Katz, 322–3
Rudrappa, Sharmila, 27; *Discounted Life*, 332–3
Rupak, Rudy, 113
Russia, surrogacy practices in, 350; permissive approach to, 349;

sacredness: of bond between mother and child, 332; of the body, 280
safety of gestational surrogacy, 82–104
Sama Resource Group for Women and Health (India), 1, 65, 114, 222–3, 226, 233; *Birthing a Market*, 65; *Can We See the Baby Bump Please?*, 228
same-sex couples, xiv, 25, 194; civil unions of, 143 (recognized in Greece, 151); difficulties faced by, 272; discrimination against, 189–90; inclusivity of, 190, 260, 350 (in USA, 315); suitability for parenting, 29; surrogacy for, 143, 165 (not available to, 146, 147–8, 151, 169, 266) see also gay couples *and* lesbian couples
Sarai, in Book of Genesis, 3
scandals: regarding surrogacy, 329–31, 351; regarding sums of money involved, 156
Scholz, Sally J., 301
science, non-questioning of, 282
screening: of commissioning parents, 198–9; of surrogate mothers, 346–7
self-determination, 172
self-ownership, 112
selling of children, 329, 352, 357, 359, 362–3, 371 *see also* trafficking, of children
Senegal, surrogacy practices in, 227
separation, risks and realities of, 194–5
Seventh Generation, concept of, 281

sex of child, 258; choice of, 256 *see also* sex selection
sex offenders, commissioning babies, 199
Sex Purchase Act (1999) (Sweden), 304
sex selection, 236, 238, 254, 278, 290; banning of, 288–9 (in India, 258); selecting traits of intelligence, 282
sexuality: disclosure of, 295; question of, 226
shame of using fertility treatment, 281
Shanley, Mary Lyndon, 317, 320
Sinaloa (Mexico), surrogacy practices in, 264, 265–6
single embryo transfers (SET): becomes standard, 92, 93; preference for, 99
single embryos, risks to, 93–5
single men, surrogacy not available to, 146, 148, 151
single mothers, 9; as surrogate mothers, 267; interest in donor identities, 211, 213
single parents, 1, 21, 29
single people: access to surrogacy, in Israel, 51–2; difficulties faced by, 272; discrimination against, 167; excluded from surrogacy, 227, 238, 266; inclusivity of, 260, 350; restrictions on, 169; surrogacy rights of, 165 *see also* India, prohibition of surrogacy in, for single persons
Sistare, C. T., 302
SisterSong Collective, 118, 288, 289
slavery, 282
slaves, used as surrogates, 163
Slovenia, citizenship in, 190
Smith, Andrea, 108; *Conquest: Sexual Violence and American Indian Genocide*, 107
social media, 53; as source of birth information, 205, 214
social work perspectives on surrogacy, 163–84
social work response to challenge of transnational surrogacy, 172–6
son preference, 289
South Africa: egg providers from, 49; growing market for surrogacy, 227; surrogate mothers from, 53, 56–7, 62
Spain, anonymity permitted in, 207
Spar, Debora, 325, *The Baby Business*, 321

sperm, donation of, alternating between male partners, 34, 40
sperm banks, 212
sperm donors, anonymous, tracking of, 210–11
state, role of, in regulation, 320, 321
stateless babies and children, 3, 11, 185–7, 331, 353; dangers of, 185–203
Steiner, Leslie Morgan, *The Baby Chase*, 313
Steptoe, Patrick, 83
sterilization, 7, 119; coerced, 107, 283; in USA, 106–8
Stern, Elizabeth, 5
Stern, William, 5
stigmatization of surrogate mothers, 222, 285, 319, 333
stillbirth, 92, 368
Stoicea-Deram, Ana-Luana, 137
Stop Surrogacy Now campaign, 325
stratified reproduction, 105–6
subverting of established clinical policies, 210
success rates *see* outcomes
surprise monitoring visits to surrogate mothers, 72, 74
surrogacy, 5–7, 5, 82–104, 347; arguments for and against, 8; as career, 117; as equal trade, 318; as human rights issue, 262–3; as labour, 302; as lesser of two evils, 319; as revolutionary act, 300–2; as the new adoption, 339; banning of *see* surrogacy, prohibition of; calls for banning of, 126; commercial (amounts to sale of a child, 357; definition of, 177; feminist views on, 308, 313–27; promotion of, 33–45; punishment of, 349); commercialization in, 178; definition of, 8, 248; engages numerous actors, 66; in Greece, 142–60; in India, 105–22; in Mexico, 262–75; likened to prostitution, 298, 304; motivations of, 131–5; not necessarily exploitative, 320; opposition to, xv, 136–7, 150, 151, 298–309; prohibitions of, 11, 12, 166, 188, 314, 344, 348, 359–60, 361, 372 (global, 345–50); portrayed as fast and simple, 37; viewed as vocation, 151 *see also* complexity; fairtrade surrogacy; prostitution *and* transnational commercial surrogacy

Surrogacy360 clearing house, 225–6, 240–1
Surrogacy Abroad, 235, 236, 238
Surrogacy Alternatives, 37–8, 39–40
Surrogacy Arrangements Act (1985) (UK), 4, 164
Surrogacy Beyond Borders, 9, 235, 236, 237, 238
Surrogacy Cancun, 8, 40–1
Surrogacy Center Nepal, 42
surrogacy homes, 256, 257, 268, 269, 270; women's movements restricted, 223
Surrogacy Mexico, 36–7
Surrogacy (Regulation) Bill (2016) (India), 79
Surrogacy UK, 166
Surrogate Mother Agreements Law (1996) (Israel), 51
Surrogate Motherhood: Ethical or commercial? report, 245
surrogate mothers, 8–11, 25–6, 53, 55–6, 185, 323, 328; advocacy for, 225; agency of, 270 (as workers, 116); arrests of, 131; asymmetrical conditions of power, 266 (*see also* disparities); change and replacement of, 155; changing of minds, 258; cheaper when recruited overseas, 169; commodification of, 43–5; controlled by fertility industry, 62; criteria for selection of, 132, 145, 248, 346–7, 350; daily realities of, 319–20; decision-making powers of, 269, 338–9 (lack of, 228, 237, 256); erased from documents, 28; extended perspective on, 230; health care of, 74, 265, 266, 270 (right to, 119); health risks for, 25, 82–104, 156, 171, 222–3, 238, 286 (downplaying of, 239; information regarding, 251); identity registration of, 206, 207; in Nepal, affected by earthquake *see* Nepal, earthquake in; inappropriate selection of, 231; lack of respect for, 156; loss of control of bodies, 86; maintaining contact with, 215–16; matching to commissioning parents, 269; measuring contribution of, 65; motivations of, 132–5, 146, 155, 253, 317, 319, 359; narratives of, 239; needs of, 221; not a uniform category, 142–3; oversupply of, 115, 119; poor women as, 4, 6, 8, 106, 114, 115, 132, 224, 236, 253, 254, 285, 319, 359, 360;

INDEX | 399

pressures on, 317; protection of, 252, 358; registering details of, 365; relation with intending parents *see* relations between surrogate mothers and commissioning parents, 44; rights of, 52, 233, 331, 333 (to privacy, 270); selection procedure for, 75; sought online, 233; study of, in India, 252–5; turnover of, 57; vetting and monitoring of, 237, 238; welfare needs of, 331; wishing to keep child, 128 *see also* domestic workers, as surrogate mothers; rejection, of surrogate mothers; relations between surrogate mothers and commissioning parents; *and* rights, relevant to surrogate mothers
Sweden: amends nationality law, 192; prohibition of surrogacy in, 335; surrogacy practices in, 304–8
Swedish Federation for Lesbian, Gay, Bisexual and Transgender Rights (RSFL), 298, 301
Swedish National Council on Medical Ethics, *Extended Opportunities for the Treatment of Involuntary Infertility*, 305
Swedish Women No to Surrogacy campaign, 298–309
Swedish Women's Lobby, xv, 1, 12, 298–309
Switzer, Brian, 114–15
Switzer, Lisa, 114–15
Syriza, 143
Szpigler, Daniel, 300, 303

Tabasco (Mexico), 266–74 *passim*; as gay surrogacy destination, 40–1; exclusion of foreign couples and gay men, 328; surrogacy practices in, 228, 238, 264, 265, 352–3
Taiwan, prohibition of surrogacy in, 334
Tamade, Yuki, 250
Tännsjö, Torbjörn, 301
Teman, Elly, 316, 320–1; *Birthing a Mother*, 318
termination of pregnancy, 223 *see also* abortion
Thailand, 216; anonymity in, 207; prohibition of commercial surrogacy in, 351; prohibition of transnational surrogacy in, 328, 331, 334; surrogacy practices in, 52, 56, 199, 232, 334 (restricted, 206, 238)
Tobin, J., 354, 360
Toboni, Gianna, 232
tourism *see* medical tourism *and* reproductive tourism
trafficking, 345, 363; of children, 54, 60, 171, 179, 272, 347, 357, 371; of women, 9, 50, 55, 60–1, 147, 334; reproductive, 49, 60–1
transfer at birth, 168
transnational commercial surrogacy, xiii–xiv, 1, 4, 7, 11, 20, 49–64, 132, 175–6, 313; debate in Israel, 61; governance of, 344–75; growing market, 3, 78–9, 169–71, 271; in India, 328–43; in media and online, 225–6; meeting challenges of, 187; recommendations for, 285–6; social inequities of, 24; terms used to define, 27
transnational co-operation, required, 321
transnational resilience and determination of agents, 239
transparency, 11, 142, 154, 174, 222, 228, 260, 329, 337; in egg donation process, 297; medical, 338–9; of fees and payments, 321, 337–8; of relationships, 339–40
travel documents, of children, 330, 335
Turkey, 348; extraterritorial prohibition in, 370; prohibition of cross-border surrogacy in, 335
twins and multiples, 57, 75, 92, 114, 115, 118, 127, 148, 192, 195, 196, 199, 224, 227, 236, 270, 331; compensation for, 259; fees related to, 255; payment for, 199; probability of, 24; rejection of, 187; risks of, 223; unwanted, 171
two gestational mothers impregnated, 92, 237, 245

Uganda, permissive approach to surrogacy in, 349
Ukraine, 169, 194, 196, 299; citizenship issue in, 193–4; growth market for commercial surrogacy, 350, 353; IVF centres in, 132; surrogacy practices in, 193, 369 (permissive approach to, 349; legal, 129, 130)

ultrasound monitoring, 73, 75
unasked questions about surrogacy, 221–44
underground existence of commercial surrogacy, 333, 361; in China, 334
unemployment, among young women, 149
United Kingdom (UK), 163; altruistic surrogacy in, 307; issue of 'reasonable expenses' in, 346; social work perspectives on surrogacy in, 163–84; surrogacy legislation in, 195–6; surrogacy practices in, 164–7 (criticism of, 167–9)
United Nations Convention on the Rights of the Child (CRC), 163, 174, 187, 188, 189, 273, 354, 356–8
United States of America (USA): as market for surrogate services, 206; altruistic surrogacy in, 307; child's right to citizenship in, 189; citizenship issues in, 195, 197; fertility services market in, 105; legal position of surrogacy in, 197–8; regulation in, 315; study of egg and sperm donation in, 214; surrogacy practices in, 3, 6, 52, 234, 235, 238 (legal for gay couples, 35; permissive approach to, 349); use of photo profiles in, 211
university-based clinics, 234
unused gametes or eggs, disposal of, 263
US National ART Surveillance System, 88
uterus: sale of, 302; viewed as room, 29, 113

vaginal delivery, 26
vanishing twin (VT) syndrome, 93
Vaughan-Brakman Sarah, 301
Victoria (Australia), access to sperm donor records in, 209
Victorian Assisted Reproductive Treatment Authority (VARTA), 208
Vietnam, surrogacy practices in, 228
violence: against women, 226; domestic, 289
visas, medical, 246, 258
Viva Family, 38, 41
voluntary organizations, non-commercial surrogacy, 148
Vora, K., 29, 113
vulnerability, 265; of commissioning parents, 224, 231; of surrogate mothers, 60, 66, 119, 156, 267, 333; of women, 306

Warnock, Mary, 164
We Are Egg Donors advocacy forum, 292, 296
wedlock *see* children born 'out of wedlock'
Wennerholm, Christer G., 299
Westerlund, Ulrika, 301
White Anglo-Saxon Protestants, eugenics of, 106
Whitehead Mary Beth, 5
whiteness of babies, on fertility clinic websites, 36
Wiles family, 313
'win-win for everyone' rhetoric, 229, 256
Winfrey, Oprah, 229, 230
Winter, Renate, 185
womb: as container, 298; purchasing of, 285; 'renting' of, 27, 352; safeguarding of, 251; viewed as spare room, 29
wombs 'sans frontières', 329
women: as 'first environment', 280; bodies of, as source of profiteering, 98, 149; discrimination against, 21; poor, as surrogate mothers *see* surrogate mother, poor women as *see also* Black women; reproductive labour, of women; women of African descent; *and* women of colour
'women helping women' topos, 230, 233, 239
Women Human Rights Defenders, 226
women of African descent, and genetic technologies, 282
women of colour, 12; and new genetic technologies, 276–91
women with disabilities, and genetic technologies, 283–4
women's movement, 144
Women's Rehabilitation Centre (Nepal), 226
Woodward, Julia, 214
word of mouth operation of networks, 66, 68, 75, 78
'world babies', 112
World Health Organization (WHO), 270; recommendations of, 96

Yamada, Ikufumi, 250
Yamada, Yuki, 250